Essentials of Psychiatry in Primary Care
Behavioral Health in the Medical Setting

Notice

Medicine is an ever-changing science. As new research and clinical experience broaden our knowledge, changes in treatment and drug therapy are required. The authors and publisher of this work have checked with sources believed to be reliable in their efforts to provide information that is complete and generally in accord with the standards accepted at the time of publication. However, in view of the possibility of human error or changes in medical sciences, neither the authors nor the publisher nor any other party who has been involved in the preparation or publication of this work warrants that the information contained herein is in every respect accurate or complete, and they disclaim all responsibility for any errors or omissions or for the results obtained from use of the information contained in this work. Readers are encouraged to confirm the information contained herein with other sources. For example and in particular, readers are advised to check the product information sheet included in the package of each drug they plan to administer to be certain that the information contained in this work is accurate and that changes have not been made in the recommended dose or in the contraindications for administration. This recommendation is of particular importance in connection with new or infrequently used drugs.

Essentials of Psychiatry in Primary Care
Behavioral Health in the Medical Setting

Robert C. Smith, MD, MS, MACP
University Distinguished Professor
Professor of Medicine and Psychiatry
Michigan State University, College of Human
  Medicine
Department of Medicine, Clinical Center
East Lansing, Michigan

Gerald G. Osborn, DO, MPhil, dFACN, dLFAPA
Professor Emeritus of Psychiatry
Department of Psychiatry
Michigan State University, College of Human
  Medicine
East Lansing, Michigan

Francesca C. Dwamena, MD, MS, FACP
Professor and Chair
Department of Medicine
Michigan State University, College of Human
  Medicine
East Lansing, Michigan

Dale D'Mello, MD, Member APA
Associate Emeritus Professor of Psychiatry
Department of Psychiatry
Michigan State University, College of Human
  Medicine
East Lansing, Michigan

Laura Freilich, MD, FACP
Assistant Professor of Medicine
Department of Medicine
Michigan State University, College of Human
  Medicine
East Lansing, Michigan

Heather S. Laird-Fick, MD, MPH, FACP
Associate Professor of Medicine
Department of Medicine
Michigan State University College of Human
  Medicine
Director, Office of Assessment
East Lansing, Michigan

McGraw Hill

New York   Chicago   San Francisco   Athens   London   Madrid   Mexico City
Milan   New Delhi   Singapore   Sydney   Toronto

Essentials of Psychiatry in Primary Care: Behavioral Health in the Medical Setting

1 2 3 4 5 6 7 8 9   LCR   24 23 22 21 20 19

ISBN 978-1-260-11677-9
MHID 1-260-11677-8

This book was set in Minion Pro by Cenveo® Publisher Services.
The editors were Amanda Fielding and Kim J. Davis.
The production supervisor was Richard Ruzycka.
Project management was provided by Madhulika Jain of Cenveo Publisher Services.
The cover designer was W2 Design.

Library of Congress Cataloging-in-Publication Data

Names: Smith, Robert C. (Robert Charles), 1937- author.
Title: Essentials of psychiatry in primary care : behavioral health in the
  medical setting / Robert C. Smith [and 5 others].
Description: New York : McGraw-Hill Education, [2019] | Includes
  bibliographical references and index.
Identifiers: LCCN 2018048630 (print) | LCCN 2018049923 (ebook) | ISBN
  9781260116786 (ebook) | ISBN 1260116786 (ebook) | ISBN 9781260116779 (pbk.: alk. paper) |
  ISBN 1260116778 (pbk. : alk. paper)
Subjects: | MESH: Mental Disorders—diagnosis | Primary Health Care | Mental
  Disorders—therapy
Classification: LCC RC473.D54 (ebook) | LCC RC473.D54 (print) | NLM WM 140 |
  DDC 616.89/075—dc23
LC record available at LC record available at https://lccn.loc.gov/2018048630

The authors dedicate this book to the intrepid primary care clinicians who now provide most mental health care against great odds—and to the present students and residents and their teachers, upon whom will fall the responsibility for future mental health care in the United States—and to the patients with mental disorders who deserve so much more than they now receive.

Contents

Foreword *from Medicine*

Physical and Behavioral Health: Two Peas, One Pod

"The mind may undoubtedly affect the body; but the body also affects the mind. There is a re-action between them; and by lessening it on either side, you diminish the pain on both."

These words of Leigh Hunt (a contemporary of the 19th century romantic poet John Keats) capture precisely the inextricable connection between physical and mental disorders and consequently the need for every medical provider to have some fundamental skills in behavioral health. Depression and anxiety are the second and fifth leading cause of years lived with disability in the United States and are as prevalent in primary care as common medical disorders such as hypertension, diabetes and arthritis.[1] In addition, more patients with these common mental disorders are treated in primary care than in mental health settings.[2] Substance use disorders and somatization (medically unexplained physical symptoms that are often an expression of psychological distress) are two other prevalent conditions which along with depression and anxiety constitute the *DASS tetrad*, which should be a core behavioral health curriculum.

Smith and colleagues embrace this concept of a core curriculum and their efforts have produced an efficient manual for evaluating and managing the behavioral health conditions of greatest relevance to primary care as well as other nonmental health providers. Unusual for a textbook, however, this primer is also highly readable with many memorable messages and teaching points. It can be read cover-to-cover (for those desiring an overview) or referenced at point of care when treating a specific disorder. The style is neither turgid nor encyclopedic but rather crisp and succinct. For example, the authors suggest a useful therapeutic message to patients suffering from

anxiety: "Confronting what makes you anxious makes it better, avoiding what makes you anxious makes it worse." This is a patient-centered way of expressing one of the core tenets of exposure therapy for anxiety disorders. As another example, the authors offer a pearl for recognizing borderline personality disorder by "the phenomenon of 'splitting' where the patient pits some staff against another. Clinicians will often discover that clinic staff has wide-ranging opinions about these patients for this reason. For example, if you find that certain office staff can't stand the patient while others quite like them, look for a borderline personality."

I found this book to be organized into 3 major compartments. First, there are the disorders that often will be treated in primary care either exclusively or in collaboration with mental health. These are the DASS tetrad conditions, covered in Chapters 2, 4, 5, and 6. Useful screening tools are provided (which in some cases can also be used for monitoring treatment) that are essential to the measurement-based component underlying evidence-based mental health care. After all, we would not diagnose or treat hypertension and diabetes without blood pressure readings or glucose monitoring. The brief validated measures that exist for depression, anxiety, somatization, and other mental disorders are invaluable instruments for busy clinicians. The authors also provide concise tables on disorder-specific medications and other treatments.

A second compartment of the book covers those disorders which may best be treated by psychiatrists, psychologists, or other specialists but require recognition in primary care as well as comanagement of medical problems. These include the psychotic disorders (schizophrenia and bipolar disorder), personality disorders, and other mental disorders such as attention deficit-hyperactivity disorder, eating disorders, cognitive impairment, and end-of-life palliative care issues. Chapters 8, 9, and 10 will assist the clinician in recognizing these disorders as well as sorting out what to manage in primary care versus when to refer.

A third and particularly unique compartment of this book are those chapters articulating the models and processes for behavioral health care. These include three axioms of mental health care (Chapter 1), the mental health care model (Chapter 3), and the diagnostic interview (Chapter 7). Whereas the first 2 compartments focus on the knowledge needed to care for common behavioral conditions, this third compartment focuses on the requisite skills. The authors have done seminal studies over several decades on interviewing and communicating with patients, and their findings are encapsulated in these chapters. Building on George Engel's foundational work on the biopsychosocial model of clinical care, Smith and colleagues have done more evidence-based work in this area (including randomized trials) than any other educators while at the same time distilling their science into what is actually workable in clinical practice. Three examples are illustrative. Chapter 3 uses the ECGN acronym to capture the 4 principles of behavioral treatment: **E**ducating the patient, obtaining a **C**ommitment to treatment, establishing **G**oals for treatment, and **N**egotiating a specific treatment plan. The same chapter operationalizes a way to be empathic. To cite the authors:

> While teachers often told you to "be empathic," they seldom indicated exactly how to do that. Yet many clinicians feel helpless or confused when their patients become emotional, wondering with discomfort, "What do I do? He's crying." Consequently, we have devised an effective way to deal with this. In our model, we identify four empathic skills, sometimes descriptively called emotion-handling skills …, *that help you respond to a patient's emotions: Name the emotion. Understand the emotion. Respect the emotion. Support the emotion. They are recalled by the mnemonic* **NURS**. *For example, the clinician might say:* "You were pretty angry (naming). I can understand that (understanding) after all you have been through (respecting). Thanks for sharing that (respecting). This helps me to better meet your needs (supporting)."

Chapter 5 provides an A-B-C model for patients distressed by the physical symptoms accompanying an anxiety disorder. For example, a person experiencing a panic attack is *alarmed* by the cardiopulmonary symptoms, *believes* a heart attack is eminent, and *copes* by calling 911 or going to the emergency room. After a successful intervention, the A-B-C is converted to: **A**LARM: "Here we go again, the emergency room doctor and my primary care doctor said this might happen again before my medication started to work fully." **B**ELIEF: "I'm having another panic attack. This will be unpleasant but not dangerous to me." **C**OPING: "I will sit down, start my mindfulness and breathing control exercises and manage this."

This is not just another psychiatry book but instead a reconceptualization of mental health care and its education. It integrates rather than partitions the management of physical and psychological symptoms. It enables the nonmental health provider to manage the common problems seen on a daily basis and to recognize who and when to refer. It operationalizes Engel's biopsychosocial model in a way that it can be actually implemented rather than given mere lip service. It also tackles in some detail topics that are particularly timely, such as the opioid crisis and how to manage tapering or discontinuation. Whereas the target audience is primary care, the messages in this book are also salient to all medical and surgical specialists. The DASS tetrad and the essential communication skills to identify and deal with symptoms related to mental health (if only to recognize, acknowledge, and refer) are relevant to all health care disciplines. This book can serve as a core text for behavioral health curricula that are used in the training of medical students, residents, and other health care professionals as well as a companion guide to practicing clinicians.

The famous Roman orator, Cicero, once said: "In proportion as the strength of the mind is greater than that of the body, so those ills are more severe that are contracted in the mind than those contracted in the body." Smith and colleagues' goal is to prepare clinicians caring for the "body" to give proportionate attention to illnesses traditionally associated with the "mind." In modern parlance, we might preferentially use terms such as "body-brain," "physical-psychological," or "medical-mental." Whatever the terminology, this Cartesian dualism is not only dated but in some cases counterproductive for patient-centered care. Medical and behavioral symptoms are 2 peas coexisting in 1 pod.[3] Treating one category while ignoring the other is detrimental to the outcomes of both.

Kurt Kroenke, MD
Chancellor's Professor of Medicine, Indiana
University School of Medicine
Research Scientist, Regenstrief Institute
Indianapolis, Indiana

REFERENCES

1. Kroenke K, Unutzer J. Closing the false divide: sustainable approaches to Integrating mental health services into primary care. *J Gen Intern Med*. 2017;32(4):404-410.

2. Olfson M, Kroenke K, Wang S, Blanco C. Trends in office-based mental health care provided by psychiatrists and primary care physicians. *J Clin Psychiatry*. 2014;75(3):247-253.

3. Kroenke K. A practical and evidence-based approach to common symptoms: a narrative review. *Ann Intern Med*. 2014;161(8):579-586.

Foreword *from Psychiatry*

I am pleased to write this Foreword to Bob Smith's textbook on psychiatry in primary care. We were both friends and colleagues of Dr. Wayne Katon who was a pioneer in the diagnosis and treatment of psychiatric disorders in primary care settings. Dr. Katon was also a mentor to me here at the University of Washington where I worked with him for 30 years before his untimely death in 2015. It was Wayne's genius to recognize that depression and other common psychiatric disorders more often present themselves in the form of physical symptoms to primary care providers than in the form of psychological symptoms to mental health providers. Primary care is indeed our "de facto mental health care system."

In this book, Dr. Smith builds on the research of the past 30 years by presenting an accessible and comprehensive approach to diagnosing and treating common psychiatric disorders in primary care. He begins by addressing the dualism that still infects much of medical care. This dualism can be found in the belief that clinicians should consider mental disorders only after physical disorders have been "ruled out" as a cause for presenting symptoms. This dualism is a serious mistake because "mental and medical disorders often coexist," which is Axiom 1 in Smith's model. Indeed, the likelihood of mental disorders *increases* in the presence of chronic or severe medical disorders.

These mental disorders often present with physical symptoms (Smith's Axiom 2). For example, a small minority of patients presenting to the emergency department with chest pain have myocardial ischemia. An even smaller minority are having a myocardial infarction. Yet this is where all our clinical attention is directed. Perhaps this is necessary in the emergency department, but it is clearly inadequate in primary care practice, where comprehensive and longitudinal care of patients is provided. Some patients presenting with chest pain may have panic disorder and no myocardial ischemia. Other patients presenting with chest pain may have panic disorder and myocardial ischemia. This is an example of Smith's Axiom 3, that "there are two types of chronic physical symptom presentations of a mental disorder—medical disease and medically unexplained symptoms." Appropriate care of the patient with both panic disorder and myocardial ischemia must address both of these disorders. It is not adequate to address the ischemia and hope that the panic disorder will go away. Many of these patients will continue to return to the emergency department until they have received effective treatment of their panic disorder.

I currently provide psychiatric consultation in the University of Washington Medical Center Regional Heart Center and in our Center for Pain Relief. All the patients I see in the Regional Heart Center have both heart disorders and psychiatric disorders. This pattern of comorbidity can lead to worse quality of life, increased symptom burden, impaired function, poor adherence to medications and exercise, persistent unhealthy behaviors like smoking and drinking, and difficult relationships with medical providers. I started consulting in this cardiology clinic after a decade of research into the effects of depression on cardiac outcomes. Initially, many of the cardiologists in the clinic wondered what I was doing in their clinic. But now they send me many of their most difficult patients and my schedule is always full.

My role may be yet more essential in our Center for Pain Relief. This clinic specializes in the treatment of patients with chronic noncancer pain. We see patients with chronic painful conditions of various kinds: low back pain, fibromyalgia, neck pain, headache, and neuropathic pain. Psychiatric comorbidity is even more common and important here than in the cardiology clinic. Depression is very common, but we are recently coming to appreciate the importance of post-traumatic stress disorder (PTSD) as well. We encourage all new patients coming to the clinic to complete a battery of outcome and risk stratification measures called PainTracker.[1] In a recent study, we were able to show that the number of PTSD symptom domains endorsed by new patients was significantly associated with ALL the outcome and risk measures that we assessed with PainTracker.[2] This included not only the severity of anxiety (GAD-7) and depressive (PHQ-9) symptoms and sleep disturbance, but pain severity, pain activity interference and physical function. Substance abuse risk (including both alcohol and opioids) were also significantly related to PTSD symptoms.

The strong association of chronic pain with depression has been recognized for some time. Chronic pain increases the risk of depression, and depression increases the risk of chronic pain. They also interfere with treatment of the other condition. Antidepressants and psychotherapy don't work as well to treat depression in patients who also have chronic pain. Similarly, opioid and nonopioid treatments of chronic pain don't work as well in the presence of depression. It is difficult to activate patients with chronic pain who are also depressed.[3]

The rise of opioid therapy for chronic pain presents another important reason to integrate psychiatric expertise into primary care.[4] Although early 20th century psychiatric textbooks often recommended opioids for treatment of both mania and melancholia (depression), there is no controlled evidence of lasting benefit. Patients may obtain some relief of anxiety and insomnia at the cost of opioid dependence and its many side effects. In fact, there are multiple observational studies that suggest that long-term opioid therapy may increase the risk of incident, recurrent and treatment-resistant forms of major depression.[5,6] There is also evidence that depression increases the risk that patients prescribed long-term opioid therapy will progress to nonmedical use of opioids and possibly opioid use disorder. Attention to depression is a necessary component of responsible administration of long-term opioid therapy.[7]

Perhaps the most important reason of all for developing psychiatric expertise in the primary care work force is that comorbid psychiatric disorders make the management of chronic illness—that is the bread and butter of primary care—much more difficult. Not only are the symptoms, functional status and quality of life of patients with chronic illnesses like diabetes much worse, their participation in their own health care is also impaired. Depressed patients often do not adhere to recommendations concerning medications, diet, and exercise. They are not effective agents in their own health care. Indeed, depressed patients are not effective agents in their lives generally. Restoring this agency is a core responsibility of health care.[8]

In summary, Dr. Smith has produced an eminently practical and readable guide to the diagnosis and treatment of psychiatric disorders in primary care. I urge you to read it and take it to heart. Your patients will thank you for it.

Mark D. Sullivan, MD, PhD
University of Washington
Seattle, Washington

REFERENCES

1. Langford DJ, Tauben DJ, Sturgeon JA, Godfrey DS, Sullivan MD, Doorenbos AZ. Treat the patient, not the pain: using a multidimensional assessment tool to facilitate patient-centered chronic pain care. *J Gen Intern Med*. 2018;33(8):1235-1238.
2. Langford DJ, Theodore BR, Balsiger D, et al. Number and type of post-traumatic stress disorder symptom domains are associated with patient-reported outcomes in patients with chronic pain. *J Pain*. 2018;19(5):506-514.
3. Sullivan MD, Vowles KE. Patient action: as means and end for chronic pain care. *Pain*. 2017;158(8):1405-1407.
4. Howe CQ, Sullivan MD. The missing 'P' in pain management: how the current opioid epidemic highlights the need for psychiatric services in chronic pain care. *Gen Hosp Psychiatry*. 2014;36(1):99-104.
5. Scherrer JF, Salas J, Sullivan MD, et al. The influence of prescription opioid use duration and dose on development of treatment resistant depression. *Prev Med*. 2016;91:110-116.
6. Mazereeuw G, Sullivan MD, Juurlink DN. Depression in chronic pain: might opioids be responsible? *Pain*. 2018;159(11):2142-2145.
7. Sullivan MD. Depression effects on long-term prescription opioid use, abuse, and addiction. *Clin J Pain*. 2018;34(9):878-884.
8. Sullivan MD. *Patient As Agent of Health and Health Care*. New York, NY: Oxford University Press; 2017:448.

Preface

INTRODUCTION

We wrote this book for physicians, nurse practitioners, physician assistants, and nurses—and for students in each discipline, particularly for their family medicine, medicine, and psychiatry clerkships. Our aim is to provide help for clinicians in providing mental health care and to guide educators in their training of students, residents, and practitioners in these areas.

There is a compelling reason for all health care professionals to become skilled in caring for patients with mental disorders, which we define as mental and substance use disorders.[1] Mental health care is severely deficient in the United States. Only 25% of patients receive any care whatsoever, compared to 60% to 80% of those with cardiac and other medical diseases who receive expert care.[2,3] Psychiatrists now provide care for only 15% of all patients[4] reflecting a chronic, severe national shortage.[5,6] As a result, medical practitioners provide sole mental health care for 85% of mental health care patients.[7-10] However, untrained for mental health care,[11-21] they sometimes have difficulty with diagnosis and management.[2,3,22] And it's not just mental health care that suffers when mental health problems aren't treated. With the frequent co-occurrence of a medical disease and a mental disorder,[23] we know that medical care suffers until the mental disorder also is recognized and treated effectively.[24-26]

Greatly compounding this problem, mental disorders are the most common health problem in the United States, more common than heart disease and cancer combined.[27] One-half of the entire US population will have a mental disorder at some point during their lives,[28,29] one-fourth in any given year.[30] In the average clinic, approximately one-half of patients will have some mental disorder.[28]

From the societal perspective, careful actuarial analysis tells us that integrating mental and medical care would produce a savings of $26 to 48 billion per year,[31] over three-fourths of the savings from improved medical care.[24] Thus, we can improve medical care itself and save money for society when we diagnose and treat co-occurring mental disorders.

There have been many yeoman efforts to correct the problem, for example, collaborative care, the patient-centered medical home, alleviating clinicians' competing demands, and improved billing for mental health care. Despite these effective efforts, however, Healthy People 2020 tells us the mental health problem is becoming worse.[32,33] Why? Because the "root cause" has never been addressed—training the clinicians who provide the care.[19] This failure leads not only to suffering in our patients but also to our own frustration and burnout as clinicians.[34,35] It's hard to give care you're not trained to provide. That's why we've written this book—to offer you some help.

The authors are psychiatrists and general internists, and we have trained medical students, faculty, and internal medicine and family medicine residents since 1986. Our clinical trials and other research[36-46] and that of others from multidisciplinary pain clinics,[47] consultation liaison psychiatry,[48] and primary care[49,50] demonstrate that the training we outline is effective and associated with improved mental and physical health outcomes.

We do not propose to make psychiatrists out of you but, rather, to prepare you to manage the common mental disorders you are likely to encounter in practice. Psychiatrists and other mental health professionals will still be needed for consultation.

Specifically, this book:

1. Describes how to diagnose and treat a common core of mental disorders for which clinicians need significant mastery—depression and anxiety disorders and substance use problems.

2. Describes how to identify less common and more severe mental disorders that require early recognition and early referral—for example, schizophrenia, severe substance abuse, personality disorders.

3. Does not address counseling, psychotherapy, or specialty techniques (eg, electroconvulsive treatment or drug detoxification clinics). Some behaviorally skilled clinicians, however, may later want to expand their scope and obtain the required formal training now available in some of these areas.

HOW THIS BOOK DIFFERS FROM STANDARD PSYCHIATRY TEXTBOOKS

Essentials of Psychiatry in Primary Care seeks to integrate medicine and psychiatry—as the systems-based biopsychosocial model proposes. The book identifies physical symptoms as a common mode of presentation of mental health problems and describes how to integrate them with psychological symptoms to make diagnoses of mental disorders. The book also proposes an overarching model for treatment, the Mental Health Care Model (MHCM), one that integrates medical and psychiatric care. The MHCM uniquely inserts the clinician-patient relationship as the centerpiece of mental health care, going still further to integrate motivational interviewing principles as vehicles to best ensure adherence to medications as other aspects of mental health care. Importantly, the MHCM has an extensive evidence base in clinical trials. It is a behaviorally defined, evidence-based mental health care model for medical settings.[36-46]

OVERVIEW OF THE BOOK

In Chapters 1, "Three Axioms of Mental Health Care for Medical Settings" and 2 "Evaluating Physical Symptoms," we introduce a new approach to diagnosing mental disorders. In contrast to some psychiatry textbooks' focus on psychological symptoms, we address how many patients with mental disorders present in medical settings with predominant physical symptoms, often of severe, disabling proportions. The physical symptoms, thus, often are "red flags" suggesting an associated mental disorder that we must actively inquire about to make a correct mental health diagnosis and provide effective treatment.

In Chapter 3, "Mental Health Care Model," we introduce the Mental Health Care Model (MHCM). This model provides the overarching structure for the mental health treatment we present in the book. Next, we begin to describe the psychological symptom profiles of the most common mental disorders. We advise that all clinicians need expertise with three major categories of mental disorders: "Major Depression and Related Disorders" (Chapter 4), "Generalized Anxiety and Related Disorders" (Chapter 5), and "Misuse of Prescription Substances and Other Substances" (Chapter 6). In these chapters, we address diagnostic criteria and integrate pharmacologic and other treatments into the overarching MHCM.

In Chapter 7, "The Diagnostic Interview," we present the diagnostic interview for mental disorders. This topic comes after discussing the core disorders so that you get a better idea of what you'll be looking for in the interview. Chapter 8, "Other Disorders and Issues in Primary Care," provides the details of some other important mental disorders in medical settings and guidance in managing them, especially when to seek consultation from mental health professionals. Chapter 9, "Psychotic Disorders," summarizes these severe disorders with an emphasis on early diagnosis to facilitate early referral to psychiatry and on the medical needs of these patients. Chapter 10, "Personality Disorders," describes the features of many personality disorders with emphasis on borderline personality disorder. Chapter 11, "Enhancing Your Own Care," focuses on 2 key issues for working with others: team care and referral. It then addresses important personal awareness issues that may arise in working with mental health patients with an emphasis on avoiding burnout.

We recognize that you face a difficult task in providing effective care for a wide range of patients. After completing this book, however, we believe that you will feel more confident and competent in addressing the basic mental health needs of your patients.

REFERENCES

1. Peek C. *A Consensus Lexicon or Operational Definition: Integrated Behavioral Health and Primary Care.* In: (AHRQ) AfHRaQ, ed. Washington, DC: AHRQ; 2012.
2. Department of Health and Human Services. *Healthy People 2010: Understanding and Improving Health.* In: Services USDoHaH, ed. 2nd ed. Washington, DC: U.S. Government Printing Office; 2000:76.

3. Croghan TW, Schoenbaum M, Sherborne CD, Koegel P. A framework to improve the quality of treatment for depression in primary care. *Psychiatri Serv.* 2006;57:623-630.

4. Wang PS, Lane M, Olfson M, Pincus HA, Wells KB, Kessler RC. Twelve-month use of mental health services in the United States—results from the National Comorbidity Survey Replication. *Arch Gen Psychiatry.* 2005;62:629-640.

5. Association of American Medical Colleges. *2012 Physician Specialty Data Book.* In: Studies CfW, ed. Washington, DC: Association of American Medical Colleges; 2012.

6. Department of Health and Human Services. *The Physician Workforce: Projections and Research into Current Issues Affecting Supply and Demand.* Health Resources and Services Administration: Department of Health and Human Services. Bethesda, MD: 2008.

7. Wang P, Demler O, Olfson M, Pincus HA, Wells KB, Kessler R. Changing profiles of service sectors used for mental health care in the United States. *Am J Psychiatry.* 2006;163:1187-1198.

8. Unutzer J, Schoenbaum M, Druss BG, Katon WJ. Transforming mental health care at the interface with general medicine: report for the presidents commission. *Psychiatr Serv.* 2006;57(1):37-47.

9. Butler M, Kane R, McAlpine D, et al. Integration of Mental Health/Substance Abuse and Primary Care No. 173 (Prepared by the Minnesota Evidence-Based Practice Center). Rockville, MD: AHRQ; 2008:190.

10. Melek S, Norris D. *Chronic Conditions and Comorbid Psychological Disorders. Millman Research Report.* Seattle, WA: Millman; 2008:19.

11. Association of American Medical Colleges. *Basic Science, Foundational Knowledge, and Pre-Clerkship Content—Average Number of Hours for Instruction/Assessment of Curriculum Subjects.* Association of American Medical Colleges. Washington, DC: 2012.

12. Chin HP, Guillermo G, Prakken S, Eisendrath S. Psychiatric training in primary care medicine residency programs. A national survey. *Psychosomatics.* 2000;41(5):412-417.

13. Eiff MP, Waller E, Fogarty CT, et al. Faculty development needs in residency redesign for practice in patient-centered medical homes: a P4 report. *Fam Med.* 2012;44(6):387-395.

14. Green LA, Jones SM, Fetter G Jr, Pugno PA. Preparing the personal physician for practice: changing family medicine residency training to enable new model practice. *Acad Med.* 2007;82(12):1220-1227.

15. Leigh H, Stewart D, Mallios R. Mental health and psychiatry training in primary care residency programs. Part I. Who teaches, where, when and how satisfied? *Gen Hosp Psychiatry.* 2006;28(3):189-194.

16. Loeb DF, Bayliss EA, Binswanger IA, Candrian C, deGruy FV. Primary care physician perceptions on caring for complex patients with medical and mental illness. *J Gen Intern Med.* 2012;27(8):945-952.

17. O'Connor PG, Nyquist JG, McLellan AT. Integrating addiction medicine into graduate medical education in primary care: the time has come. *Ann Intern Med.* 2011;154(1):56-59.

18. Petterson SM, Phillips RL Jr, Bazemore AW, Dodoo MS, Zhang X, Green LA. Why there must be room for mental health in the medical home. *Am Fam Physician.* 2008;77(6):757.

19. Smith RC. Educating trainees about common mental health problems in primary care: a (not so) modest proposal. *Acad Med.* 2011;86:e16.

20. Smith R, Fortin AH VI, Dwamena F, Frankel R. An evidence-based patient-centered method makes the biopsychosocial model scientific. *Patient Educ Couns.* 2013;90:265-270.

21. Norquist G, Hyman SE. Advances in understanding and treating mental illness: implications for policy. *Health Affairs.* 1999;18:32-47.

22. Kilbourne AM, Welsh D, McCarthy JF, Post EP, Blow FC. Quality of care for cardiovascular disease-related conditions in patients with and without mental disorders. *J Gen Intern Med.* 2008;23(10):1628-1633.

23. Druss B, Reisinger-Walker E. *Mental Disorders and Medical Comorbidity.* In: Foundation RWJ, ed. Synthesis Project: National Library of Medicine. Washington, DC: 2011.

24. Thorpe K, Jain S, Joski P. Prevalence and spending associated with patients who have a behavioral health disorder and other conditions. *Health Aff (Millwood).* 2017;36(1):124-132.

25. Gallo JJ, Hwang S, Joo JH, et al. Multimorbidity, depression, and mortality in primary care: randomized clinical trial of an evidence-based depression care management program on mortality risk. *J Gen Intern Med.* 2016;31(4):380-386.

26. Katon WJ, Lin EH, Von Korff M, et al. Collaborative care for patients with depression and chronic illnesses. *N Engl J Med.* 2010;363(27):2611-2620.

27. National Alliance on Mental Illness. *Prevalences of Illnesses. Support, Advocacy, Education, Research.* Gainesville, FL: National Alliance on Mental Illness; 2014.

28. Norquist GS, Regier DA. The epidemiology of psychiatric disorders and the de facto mental health care system. *Annu Rev Med.* 1996;47:473-479.

29. Kessler RC, Berglund P, Demler O, Jin R, Merikangas KR, Walters EE. Lifetime prevalence and age-of-onset distributions of DSM-IV disorders in the National Comorbidity Survey Replication. *Arch Gen Psychiatry.* 2005;62:593-602.

30. Kessler RC, Chiu WT, Demler O, Walters EE. Prevalence, severity, and comorbidity of 12-month DSM-IV

disorders in the National Comorbidity Survey Replication. *Arch Gen Psychiatry*. 2005;62:617-627.

31. Melek S, Norris D, Paulus J. *Economic Impact of Integrated Medical-Behavioral Healthcare—Implications for Psychiatry*. In: American Psychiatric Association, ed. Denver, CO: Milliman; 2014.

32. Koh HK, Blakey CR, Roper AY. Healthy People 2020: a report card on the health of the nation. *JAMA*. 2014;311(24):2475-2476.

33. Department of Health and Human Services. Mental Health and Mental Disorders—Healthy People 2020. Washington, DC: US Department of Health and Human Services (HHS); 2014. http://www.healthypeople .gov/2020/topicsobjectives/nationalsnapshot. aspx?topicId=28.

34. Brigham T, Barden C, Dopp A, et al. A Journey to Construct an All-Encompassing Conceptual Model of Factors Affecting Clinician Well-Being and Resilience. National Academy of Medicine; 2018.

35. Dyrbye LN, Massie FS Jr, Eacker A, et al. Relationship between burnout and professional conduct and attitudes among US medical students. *JAMA*. 2010;304(11):1173-1180.

36. Smith R, Gardiner J, Luo Z, Schooley S, Lamerato L. Primary care physicians treat somatization. *J Gen Int Med*. 2009;24:829-832.

37. Smith RC, Lyles JS, Gardiner JC, et al. Primary care clinicians treat patients with medically unexplained symptoms—a randomized controlled trial. *J Gen Intern Med*. 2006;21:671-677.

38. Lyles JS, Hodges A, Collins C, et al. Using nurse practitioners to implement an intervention in primary care for high utilizing patients with medically unexplained symptoms. *Gen Hosp Psychiatry*. 2003;25:63-73.

39. Smith RC, Lyles JS, Mettler J, et al. The effectiveness of intensive training for residents in interviewing. A randomized, controlled study. *Ann Intern Med*. 1998;128:118-126.

40. Smith R, Laird-Fick H, D'Mello D, et al. Addressing mental health issues in primary care: an initial curriculum for medical residents. *Patient Educ Couns*. 2014;94:33-42.

41. Smith RC, Dwamena FC, Fortin AH VI. Teaching personal awareness. *J Gen Intern Med*. 2005;20:201-207.

42. Smith RC, Marshall-Dorsey AA, Osborn GG, et al. Evidence-based guidelines for teaching patient-centered interviewing. *Patient Educ Couns*. 2000;39(1):27-36.

43. Smith RC, Dorsey AM, Lyles JS, Frankel RM. Teaching self-awareness enhances learning about patient-centered interviewing. *Acad Med*. 1999;74:1242-1248.

44. Smith RC. Unrecognized responses and feelings of residents and fellows during interviews of patients. *J Med Educ*. 1986;61:982-984.

45. Smith RC. Teaching interviewing skills to medical students: the issue of "countertransference." *J Med Educ*. 1984;59:582-588.

46. Smith R, Laird-Fick H, Dwamena F, et al. Teaching residents mental health care. *Patient Educ Couns*. 2018;101:2145-2155.

47. Kashner TM, Rost K, Cohen B, Anderson MA, Smith GR Jr. Enhancing the health of somatization disorder patients: effectiveness of short term group therapy. *Psychosomatics*. 1995;36:462-470.

48. Lin EH, Katon WJ, Simon GE, et al. Achieving guidelines for the treatment of depression in primary care: is physician education enough? *Med Care*. 1997;35(8):831-842.

49. Bower P, Gilbody S. Managing common mental health disorders in primary care: conceptual models and evidence base. *BMJ*. 2005;330(7495):839-842.

50. Kroenke K, Taylor-Vaisey A, Dietrich AJ, Oxman TE. Interventions to improve provider diagnosis and treatment in mental disorders in primary care—a critical review of the literature. *Psychosomatics*. 2000;41:39-52.

Acknowledgments

This new textbook stems most proximately from George Engel and his remarkable group of biopsychosocial scholars at the University of Rochester where Dr. Smith was fortunate to do fellowship work, later remaining of faculty. We also owe a debt of gratitude to Michigan State University, one of Engel's initial advocates and the home base for the authors, for the propitious atmosphere they have established encouraging new and different approaches. Paraphrasing Robert Kennedy, Michigan State challenged us not to focus on why mental health is so problematic in the United States, but rather to dream how we could improve it.

The research involved in developing the evidence-based content of this book would not have been possible without the generous support of the Fetzer Institute (Kalamazoo, MI), the National Institute of Mental Health, and the Health Resources and Services Administration. It simply is not possible to develop rigorous educational interventions without such support.

We are so grateful to Amanda Fielding, our intrepid and always timely Senior Editor at McGraw-Hill, and to our long-time McGraw-Hill advisor, Jim Shanahan. Additional thanks go to Kim Davis, Managing Editor; Richard Ruzycka, Senior Production Supervisor; and Madhulika Jain, Project Manager. All contributed considerably to making this a very readable and professional book.

There are two groups of people without whom none of our work would be possible. We mention them together because they are intimately linked: our residents and their patients with mental disorders. The residents, with never a suggestion of resistance, joined us in embarking on this new direction in mental health education, and their mental health patients, many of whom were underserved, willingly participated, and greatly valued their care—and the improvement that followed.

Equally important, two friends and colleagues deserve our deepest thanks for reading and critiquing drafts of the book—and providing input to greatly improve its content and presentation: Patrick Hemming, an internist at Duke and Steve Frankel, a psychiatrist at UC San Francisco.

Finally, the research basis for our work would never have materialized without Judi Lyles, who was always one step ahead in overseeing many of our research projects, and the book itself would not have been possible but for the admirable efforts of Jinie Shirey and Ellyssa Knaggs in the day-to-day work of preparing it.

Three Axioms of Mental Health Care for Medical Settings

As outlined in the Preface, there are compelling reasons for all clinicians to become familiar with mental and addiction disorders: they provide the vast majority of all care!

To provide effective guidelines for clinicians, we need a different approach to teaching about mental disorders than has typically been used. We define mental disorders as both mental and substance use disorders.[1] Psychiatry textbooks typically focus on psychological symptoms, such as feeling sad or worried, to make a mental disorder diagnosis, for example for depression or panic disorder. In medical settings, however, a far more complex job emerges. You must address physical as well as psychological symptoms. While you are already familiar with physical symptoms related to diseases, their role in mental health disorders is less often considered.

To guide you, Chapters 1 and 2 are devoted to the key role physical symptoms play in mental health diagnoses in medical settings. In this chapter, we begin by presenting **3 axioms** for mental health care. They will help you identify the group of patients in whom you most likely will find mental disorders.

- *Axiom 1*: **Mental and medical disorders often coexist**. Such co-occurrence of disorders is called *comorbidity*; one disorder is comorbid with the other. Successfully addressing one requires effectively addressing both disorders.[2,3]
- *Axiom 2*: **Many mental health disorders present with chronic and disabling physical symptoms.** Patients with mental health disorders in medical settings often do not present with psychological symptoms. Rather, physical symptoms typically predominate and can obscure the psychological symptoms of the mental disorder. There are no specific physical symptoms associated with mental disorders, and they may involve any body system. However, there is 1 unique feature: the more severe, chronic, and disabling the physical symptoms, the more likely there is an associated mental disorder.[4] *While psychological symptoms are always essential in diagnosing mental disorders, they are not a sufficient initial presenting symptom to rely on for identifying many mental and substance use disorders.* Often, the psychological symptoms (and the mental disorders they represent) become apparent only when providers with an index of suspicion inquire directly about them.[4]

- *Axiom 3*: **There are 2 common types of chronic physical symptom presentations of a mental disorder: medical disease and medically unexplained symptoms (MUS).**

  - Many mental disorders pair with a *chronic medical disease*, at least in part because of its adverse psychological impact; for example, the dyspnea of severe heart failure may produce depression because the patient can no longer play golf, do housework, go to church, or rake the yard. In this situation, the severe physical symptoms and disability of a chronic medical disease can be considered a "red flag" for an associated mental disorder.

- Many mental disorders present with *chronic MUS*, defined as physical symptoms that have little or no identifiable disease or pathophysiologic basis.[5,6] Chronic unexplained physical symptoms, such as severe chronic pain or disabling chronic fatigue, also are closely associated with mental disorders, such as depression or anxiety, and are another "red flag" indicating an associated mental disorder.

Why don't patients immediately express psychological symptoms in addition to their physical symptoms? The stigma of having a mental disorder is a common explanation.[7-9] Additionally, patients may think that medical clinicians are not interested in their psychological symptoms or they simply may not be accustomed to discussing their psychological symptoms in medical settings. Also, they may not be fully aware of their psychological symptoms. *In all patients presenting with chronic physical symptoms, therefore, careful inquiry about associated psychological symptoms usually must occur to identify the mental health disorder.*

Now let's examine these axioms in greater detail.

COMORBIDITY OF MENTAL AND MEDICAL DISORDERS

Comorbidity, the co-occurrence of 2 or more diagnoses, is the rule in medicine whether involving mental disorders, medical disorders, or both,[10] for example depression and cancer, depression and anxiety, or diabetes and angina pectoris. Although current medical practices often focus on just the disease, it has been well demonstrated that treating the comorbid mental health problem improves the medical problem beyond the impact of medical treatment alone.[11-13] For example, treating comorbid depression in patients with diabetes improves control beyond just treating the diabetes because, for example, as they become less depressed, patients are better able to control their medications and diet.[14]

Medical clinicians encounter many comorbid mental disorders. Prevalence data indicate the following: (1) 25% of clinic patients will have a major mental disorder[15] and 68% of these will have a comorbid disease of some type; and (2) 58% of clinic patients will have a disease, 29% of whom have a comorbid mental disorder.[16] *The more severe and chronic the medical disease, the more likely there is an associated mental disorder.*[17]

Rarely do the mental disorder and the associated disease act independently. Rather, they almost always interact. Consider the following examples:

1. **Chronic disease leads to a mental disorder**; for example, immobility and inability to work due to cancer or angina pectoris leads to new or worsening depression.
2. **Mental disorder leads to a chronic disease**; for example, alcoholism leads to cirrhosis of the liver, and depression leads to poor adherence to diabetes treatment and, in turn, poor control.
3. **Disease treatment leads to a mental disorder**; for example, corticosteroid or thyroid medications lead to anxiety, and β-blockers lead to depression. (See Table 1-1.)
4. **Mental disorder treatment leads to a chronic disease**; for example, an antidepressant or atypical antipsychotic increases the QT interval in a patient with heart disease. (See Table 1-2.)
5. **Disease itself directly causes a mental disorder**, for example depression from hypothyroidism, Cushing's disease, or hyperparathyroidism, and anxiety from a pheochromocytoma. (See Table 1-3.)

TABLE 1-1. Disease Treatment Causing Mental Disorders

DISEASE TREATMENT	MENTAL DISORDER
Steroids β-Blockers HRT/OCPs Clonidine Digoxin Metoclopramide Opiates	Depression
Steroids HRT/OCPs Digoxin Dicyclomine Metoclopramide Albuterol	Anxiety

HRT = hormone replacement therapy; OCP = oral contraceptive pill.

TABLE 1-2. Mental Disorder Treatment Causing Physical Disease

MENTAL DISORDER TREATMENT	DISEASE
SSRI	Obesity Tremor Sexual dysfunction Nausea
SNRI	Hypertension Tachycardia Sexual dysfunction
Bupropion	Lower seizure threshold Anxiety
Mirtazapine	Sedation (lower doses) Obesity
Lithium	Thyroid disorder ECG changes
Lamotrigine	Hepatitis Skin changes
Antipsychotics	Obesity Metabolic disturbance (hyperlipidemia)
Stimulants	Hypertension Insomnia Myocardial infarction

ECG = electrocardiogram; SNRI = serotonin-norepinephrine reuptake inhibitor; SSRI = selective serotonin reuptake inhibitor.

TABLE 1-3. Diseases Causing Mental Disorders

DISEASE PROCESS	MENTAL DISORDER
Hypothyroidism Myocardial Infarction Stroke Various electrolyte disturbances Dementia Multiple sclerosis Normal pressure hydrocephalus Autoimmune disorders Severe anemia	Depression
Asthma/COPD Pheochromocytoma Hyperthyroidism	Anxiety
Neurosyphilis	Psychosis

COPD = chronic obstructive pulmonary disease.

MEDICALLY UNEXPLAINED SYMPTOMS

In the preceding section on comorbidity, we assumed that a patient presents with psychological symptoms reflecting a mental disorder and physical symptoms representing a comorbid medical disorder. However, diagnosing and treating mental disorders becomes more complex when we incorporate the very common problem of chronic medically unexplained symptom (MUS) presentations. While the patient still has psychological symptoms of a mental disorder, their physical symptoms do not reflect a medical disorder. Rather, the physical symptoms are "unexplained,"[5,6] for example chronic back pain, headaches, or chronic fatigue with no explanation following a careful laboratory and consultative investigation. Thus there is no comorbid medical disease; rather, there is a mental health disorder where its psychological symptoms often are less prominent than the unexplained, chronic physical symptoms.

While there is debate about why MUS occurs,[17] there is no debate about this fact: chronic MUS is a "red flag" for an associated mental disorder.[4,5,17]

It is apparent that a vicious circle may develop. Further complicating the problem, there are often more than 1 mental and medical disorder. Data from our medical clinics demonstrate that patients referred for mental health care had an average of 2.3 DSM-5 (*Diagnostic and Statistical Manual of Mental Disorders, 5th Edition*) mental disorders and 3.3 medical disorders.[18]

In sum, to diagnose and treat mental disorders, you must be intimately familiar with the complexities of disease comorbidity.

For example, we found a 94% prevalence of major or minor depression in a chronic, high-utilizing group of MUS patients.[19] Consider the physical symptom(s) of chronic MUS to be symptoms of a possible associated mental disorder. Research demonstrates that the greater the number and severity of unexplained chronic symptoms, the more likely there is an associated mental disorder.[4]

The physical symptoms of chronic MUS make both diagnosis and treatment of mental disorders more difficult. For *diagnosis*, MUS can distract the clinician from seeking an associated mental disorder by seeming to demand more and more workup to find a (nonexistent) disease explanation.[5] Also, *treatment* must address the disabling physical symptoms themselves as well as the psychological symptoms of the mental disorder, with the former typically being far more difficult to treat.[20]

SUMMARIZING THE PHYSICAL AND PSYCHOLOGICAL SYMPTOM PRESENTATIONS OF MENTAL DISORDERS IN MEDICAL SETTINGS

Many patients with a mental disorder will have both physical and psychological symptoms, although the latter are often less prominent and may require active inquiry to identify them. To suspect a mental disorder, you will want to be alert to several different symptom presentations:

1. Psychological symptoms of a mental disorder in isolation
2. Psychological symptoms of a mental disorder associated with more prominent disabling physical symptoms of a chronic comorbid medical disease
3. Psychological symptoms of a mental disorder associated with more prominent disabling physical symptoms of chronic MUS

As summarized in Figure 1-1, this means that in many cases, to diagnose a mental disorder, you will first need to sort through chronic, disabling physical symptoms to decide whether they are due to a disease and/or MUS. You then seek a possible associated mental disorder. Table 1-4 shows an example of a common mental disorder profile in a medical setting.

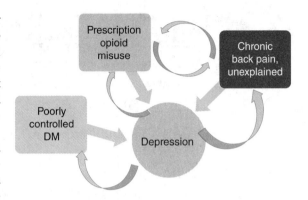

FIGURE 1-1. Interactions of medical, mental health, and unexplained symptom diagnoses. Blue = documented organic disease; gray = mental disorder; black = MUS. All three dimensions may adversely interact; consider also how treatment of one disorder may have adverse effects on another.

In sum, to provide good mental health care, focus on patients with chronic physical symptoms, whether due to MUS and/or a comorbid medical disease. Chronic, severe, and disabling physical symptoms of either type are "red flags" for an associated mental disorder. The more severe the physical symptoms, the more likely there is a mental disorder. Thus alerted, we then inquire carefully to identify the unique psychological symptoms that define the specific comorbid mental disorder, for example major depression, posttraumatic stress disorder, and panic disorder. In Chapter 2, we describe the diagnostic approach to physical symptoms in medical settings, which is often the first step to diagnosing and treating a mental disorder.

TABLE 1-4. Example of a Common Mental Disorder Profile in a Medical Setting

*1. Major depression

*2. Prescription opioid misuse

**3. Congestive heart failure, mild

**4. Diabetes mellitus, poorly controlled

***5. Chronic, severe low back pain after non-explanatory workup

* = mental disorder; ** = documented organic disease; *** = MUS.

Note: All 5 diagnoses may adversely interact; consider also how treatment of 1 disorder may have adverse effects on another.

REFERENCES

1. Peek C. A consensus lexicon or operational definition: integrated behavioral health and primary care. In: *Agency for Healthcare Research and Quality*. Washington, DC: AHRQ; 2012.

2. Kroenke K. Studying symptoms: sampling and measurement issues. *Ann Intern Med*. 2001;134(9 Pt 2):844-853.

3. Kroenke K, Jackson JL, Chamberlin J. Depressive and anxiety disorders in patients presenting with physical complaints: clinical predictors and outcome. *Am J Med*. 1997;103:339-347.

4. Kroenke K. The interface between physical and psychological symptoms. Primary care companion. *J Clin Psychiatry*. 2003;5(suppl 7):11-18.

5. Smith RC, Dwamena FC. Classification and diagnosis of patients with medically unexplained symptoms. *J Gen Intern Med*. 2007;22(5):685-691.

6. Sharpe M. Somatic symptoms: beyond 'medically unexplained'. *Br J Psychiatry*. 2013;203:320-321.

7. National Academies of Sciences, Engineering, and Medicine. Ending discrimination against people with mental and substance use disorders: the evidence for stigma change. In: *The National Academies of Sciences, Engineering, and Medicine*. Washington, DC: National Academies Press; 2016.

8. World Organization of Family Doctors. *Companion to Primary Care Mental Health*. New York, NY: Wonca (World Organization of Family Doctors) and Radcliffe Publishing; 2012.

9. Eisma MC. Public stigma of prolonged grief disorder: an experimental study. *Psychiatry Res*. 2018;261:173-177.

10. Melek S, Norris D. *Chronic Conditions and Comorbid Psychological Disorders. Millman Research Report*. Seattle, WA: Millman; 2008:19.

11. Thorpe K, Jain S, Joski P. Prevalence and spending associated with patients who have a behavioral health disorder and other conditions. *Health Aff (Millwood)*. 2017;36(1):124-132.

12. Gallo JJ, Hwang S, Joo JH, et al. Multimorbidity, depression, and mortality in primary care: randomized clinical trial of an evidence-based depression care management program on mortality risk. *J Gen Intern Med*. 2016;31(4):380-386.

13. Katon WJ, Lin EH, Von Korff M, et al. Collaborative care for patients with depression and chronic illnesses. *N Engl J Med*. 2010;363(27):2611-2620.

14. Agency for Healthcare Research and Quality. Behavioral programs for type 2 diabetes mellitus: current state of the evidence. AHRQ Pub. No. 16(17)-EHC031-3EF, November 2016.

15. Norquist GS, Regier DA. The epidemiology of psychiatric disorders and the de facto mental health care system. *Annu Rev Med*. 1996;47:473-479.

16. Druss B, Reisinger-Walker E. Mental disorders and medical comorbidity. In: *The Robert Wood Johnson Foundation*. Synthesis Project: National Library of Medicine; 2011.

17. Katon W, Sullivan M, Walker E. Medical symptoms without identified pathology: relationship to psychiatric disorders, childhood and adult trauma, and personality traits. *Ann Int Med*. 2001;134:917-925.

18. Dwamena F, Laird-Fick H, Freilich L, et al. Behavioral health problems in medical patients. *J Clin Outcomes Manag*. 2014;21:497-505.

19. Smith RC, Gardiner JC, Lyles JS, et al. Exploration of DSM-IV criteria in primary care patients with medically unexplained symptoms. *Psychosom Med*. 2005;67(1):123-129.

20. Smith RC, Lein C, Collins C, et al. Treating patients with medically unexplained symptoms in primary care. *J Gen Intern Med*. 2003;18:478-489.

2

Evaluating Physical Symptoms

In Chapter 1, we presented 3 axioms of mental health care for medical settings: (1) The comorbidity of medical and mental disorders is frequent; (2) chronic physical symptoms are a common presentation in patients with a mental disorder; and (3) chronic physical symptoms may be due to medical disease and/or medically unexplained symptoms (MUS).

Because physical symptoms are prominently associated "red flags" for mental disorders, we now address the diagnostic approach to them, with the understanding that all physical disease problems are not associated with a mental disorder. One caveat is that patients occasionally present only with psychological symptoms. In that case, we of course proceed directly to develop the details needed to establish a mental disorder diagnosis, as outlined in later chapters. In most instances, however, physical symptoms are so common that they usually are considered first, then inquiring about psychological symptoms when you can better focus on a possible mental disorder.

You may say that you already know medical diagnostics; after all, that's what has been emphasized throughout your medical training. Here's the problem. There can be diagnostic uncertainties when the symptoms are difficult to explain in MUS. Consequently, we will provide guidelines for evaluating physical symptoms that will allow you to comfortably expand your evaluation to the psychological realm without worrying that you have missed some physical disease. We now address the medical diagnostic approach in the presence of prominent physical symptoms. In later chapters, we address how to diagnose the

psychological symptoms needed to make a specific mental health diagnosis.

DEFINITIONS

We have defined a *mental disorder* as a mental or substance use disorder. We define a *disease* as a disorder included in current classifications of diseases (eg, editions of the International Classification of Diseases).[1,2] These are the diseases you might find listed in medical textbooks, characterized by a unique pathophysiologic basis.

Medically unexplained symptoms are the opposite—physical symptoms with little or no disease or pathophysiologic explanation, also referred to as somatization or somatoform disorders. Patients who have an organic disease can also have MUS when the symptoms are not attributable to the disease or are out of proportion to what would be expected. MUS poses a far greater diagnosis problem for clinicians, so we address it in detail.

The *Diagnostic and Statistical Manual of Mental Disorders* (DSM) has provided an influential classification. DSM-4 defined the following MUS disorders in the somatoform category: somatization disorder, undifferentiated somatoform disorder, conversion disorder, pain disorder, hypochondriasis, body dysmorphic disorder, and somatoform disorder not otherwise specified.[3] While useful for research, none had sufficient validity to use clinically nor were they comprehensive enough to capture more than a few of the chronic MUS patients commonly seen in medical settings.[4,5] Widespread dissatisfaction led to a change where many of the DSM-4 disorders were combined into what is now called *somatic symptom disorder* in DSM-5.[6] Not validated, it has been criticized for being too sensitive and lacking specificity.[7-11] Moreover, the complex criteria of both DSM-4 and DSM-5 have further discouraged the use of these diagnoses by medical clinicians. Rather, clinicians have developed medical names for MUS syndromes, for example chronic pain (low back, neck, head), fibromyalgia, irritable bowel syndrome, nonulcer dyspepsia, and chronic fatigue syndrome.[12] Indeed, almost every body system has one or more disorders characterized by its specific type of MUS. Multiple efforts to demonstrate that some of these MUS subsets are actually a true disease (with a pathophysiological basis) have been unsuccessful, and the various entities also lack validity because of overlapping criteria.[13]

DIAGNOSIS OF MEDICALLY UNEXPLAINED SYMPTOMS

Because you already are well trained in physical diseases, we do not address medical diagnosis (or treatment) here. We assume this familiarity in our frequent references to integrating mental health and disease care. That is, you conduct your diagnostic approach to making a disease diagnosis the same way you always do.

We focus here on evaluating the physical symptoms of chronic MUS. We have not found the somatic symptom disorder criteria of DSM-5 or the multiple DSM-4 somatoform diagnoses helpful for the reasons given previously. We do, however, embrace the DSM-4 approach requiring exclusion (ruling out) of a disease explanation before making a diagnosis of MUS. Because of Western medicine's long use of a disease-based classification system, we believe the only logical way to diagnose chronic MUS is to first exclude (rule out) disease.[14,15]

CHRONIC MEDICALLY UNEXPLAINED SYMPTOMS

Chronic MUS is extraordinarily prevalent. Approximately 10% of clinic patients have chronic MUS.[14,16] Their clinical picture (and diagnostic evaluation) is summarized in Table 2-1.

TABLE 2-1. The Important Features of Chronic MUS

Clinical profile

1. Any symptoms, but usually involve musculoskeletal, GI, cardiopulmonary, or nervous systems; typically pain (head, low back, neck, muscular, joints); and which do not usually fit a standard disease pattern
2. Symptoms are chronic, multiple, disabling; not precipitated by stress but worsened by it
3. Some patients with a prior disease, will subsequently develop the same symptom as MUS, eg, chest pain postmyocardial infarction without evidence of further heart damage
4. History of abuse in childhood—as high as 70% in chronic MUS
5. High health care utilization behaviors—number of visits is proportional to the severity and disability of an underlying mental disorder. Health care seeking is driven by anxiety

Diagnosis

1. Requires lab investigation/consultation to first rule out possible underlying true diseases except in low-risk patients with chronic low back pain
2. Workup should not be repeated

Differential diagnosis

1. Any disease
2. Also need to consider some mental disorders sometimes confused as MUS:
   - Factitious disorder—self-induced disease; extreme = Munchausen syndrome
   - Malingering—deliberately faked symptoms for financial/other gain

Mental disorders are present in up to 100% of chronic MUS patients. They are more likely the greater are the number and duration of MUS symptoms, the greater their severity and disability
   - Depression (Chapter 4)
   - Anxiety (Chapter 5)
   - Prescription Substance Misuse (Chapter 6)

Screening: PHQ-15

Prevention: Only a 3-7-day supply of opioids for acute pain and close follow-up to ensure resolution

GI = gastrointestinal; MUS = medically unexplained symptoms; PHQ-15 = Physical Health Questionnaire-15.

Physical Symptom Profile

Most commonly, symptoms are ill defined and are related to the musculoskeletal, gastrointestinal, cardiopulmonary, and nervous systems, although any system may be involved.[14,17-20] Pain often is the most prominent symptom and can occur anywhere but is most likely in the low back, neck, head, pelvis, chest, and joints.[19] Nonpain complaints include fatigue, constipation, diarrhea, and bloating. Symptoms often occur in combination and may fit published patterns of known syndromes, for example fibromyalgia, chronic fatigue syndrome, or irritable bowel syndrome. Importantly, worrisome symptoms suggesting an organic disease, such as fever, sciatica, angina, or weight loss, are usually not present. While the physical symptoms may be intermittent in less severe instances and occur only in relationship to stressful events, most of the time symptoms are continuous and independent of life stresses, although often worsened by a new stress. In obtaining the longitudinal history, patients may report what seemed initially to be a minor illness, but one that did not clear and became chronic MUS. A common history is acute back pain that did not remit, often continuing to receive prescription opioids for the pain and eventuating with chronic, progressively more severe MUS. On other occasions, chronic MUS may follow a respiratory infection or gastroenteritis. Especially troubling to the clinician who fears missing a disease diagnosis are patients who have had a serious disease and who, once resolved, continue having the same symptoms without recurrence of the actual disease, for example recurrent chest pain not due to coronary insufficiency following a myocardial infarction.[14]

Psychological Symptom Profile

While we have emphasized that psychological symptoms may not be prominent, they are nonetheless usually present and typically bespeak an underlying mental disorder. Outlined in detail in later chapters, symptoms of depression and anxiety are frequent and almost universal in the high care-utilizing and disabled MUS patient.[4] In many, prescription substance misuse also occurs. Also, symptoms of posttraumatic stress disorder (PTSD) may be present, especially in patients who have a history of some type of abuse.[21-23] Similarly, family structures may have been insecure, current relationships are often frayed, and lifestyles are sometimes chaotic.[22] Further, because of the severity of their disability, job performance may be spotty and many are not employed, often on disability support.

Finally, many chronic MUS patients are very unhappy with the medical system for a host of reasons, for example not curing them, not believing their symptoms, not giving them the medications they want, or believing that treatments provided do not work.[24] In general, this lack of satisfaction has led to considerable doctor-shopping, frequent hospitalizations and emergency room visits, and high overall health care utilization.[14] Thus, an unhappy patient often faces the clinician, making the latter's skills in establishing a strong relationship paramount if they are to be effective.[25] We will address this situation in detail in Chapter 3 when we introduce the Mental Health Care Model.

Diagnostic Evaluation

While the history and physical examination continue to be important,[16] they are alone not sufficient in diagnosing chronic MUS. Rather, to rule out a possible explanatory disease, *most of these patients require carefully focused investigative and/or consultative evaluation relative to their particular symptom presentation; see the later exception to this rule for chronic low back pain where evaluation beyond the history and physical examination often is not required.* That is, before one makes a diagnosis of chronic MUS, first exclude reasonable disease possibilities that could explain the symptoms, even in the absence of clear-cut objective data from the history and physical examination.

While you need to provide a good diagnostic evaluation, you do *not need to repeat studies* that have already been performed; rather they are reviewed as part of the workup.[26-29] The habit of repeated testing "just to be sure nothing has changed" has not proven valuable. Rather, it has been demonstrated that once the diagnosis of chronic MUS is made, an explanatory disease rarely supervenes.[16,30] Nevertheless, one continues to be observant via careful history and physical examination for a complicating disease.[18] One suspects this possibility if there is a distinct change in symptom pattern, especially if there are objective changes on physical examination. Then it is appropriate to evaluate for a complicating disease.

Some have opposed a rule-out diagnostic approach, advocating instead that we use physical and/or psychological symptom criteria of various disorders (eg, irritable bowel syndrome, fibromyalgia, chronic fatigue syndrome, or somatic symptom disorder) to make the diagnosis. Consider, for example, the temptation to diagnose chronic MUS with no investigation at all when the physical symptom profile does not fit any disease and there are many psychological symptoms of distress. This must be chronic MUS and no further workup is required, right? Wrong—for the most part. For example, in patients whose clinical symptom criteria suggest *irritable bowel syndrome* (eg, chronic abdominal pain, altered bowel habits, or both), 35% of patients had an underlying disease explanation.[31] Also, *chronic pelvic pain* often is believed to be "psychological" after a negative pelvic examination in a distressed woman with many psychological symptoms. However, from 41% to 75% of these women have a disease explanation such as pelvic inflammatory disease, endometriosis, and adhesions.[32] Definitive investigation is required to exclude these possible underlying disorders.[33]

Evolving data, however, indicate that low-risk patients with *chronic low back pain* do not require imaging or other investigation. Indeed, recalling that unnecessary surgery often follows imaging, clinical trials demonstrate that those who have received imaging have worse outcomes than those who did not; the indication for imaging in chronic low back pain is evidence of neurologic impairment, particularly where surgery is a possible need.[16,34] The data are less clear in high-risk patients (older, soft neurologic signs, history of fever, associated systemic illness), and you must decide that on an individual basis using carefully focused testing.

Researchers have worked hard to refine and systematize physical and psychological symptom criteria to diagnose chronic MUS syndromes. While many have had moderate-high sensitivity, they consistently suffer from low specificity. A test for MUS with low specificity, as you know, means that its false positives represent a true disease we would not want to miss.[31,35-37]

There is another important reason for a definitive but focused approach. The first step in treatment is to alleviate the concern in both clinician and patient that there may be some explanatory disease. Both clinician and patient must dismiss concerns about a disease explanation before treatment can be effective.[12,14]

Differential Diagnosis

One always keeps in mind that certain rare diseases (eg, porphyria) or that more common diseases with atypical presentations (eg, Lyme disease, multiple sclerosis) may present with physical symptoms suggesting MUS, even when the workup for a more likely differential diagnosis is negative. If there is a good, objective reason to suspect an unusual diagnosis, we of course extend the investigation. However, we warn against the practice of ordering test after test, when likely to be negative, "just being sure" there is no physical disease. Rather, relying on prevalence and objective clinical data is the best guide. Ordinarily, there is little reason to extend the initial workup.

There also are some uncommon psychiatric disorders that may present with prominent physical symptoms that we must not mistake for MUS: factitious disorder and malingering.[22,38] Patients with *factitious disorder* present with physical symptoms that have a pathophysiologic basis that the patient surreptitiously produces, for example injecting themselves with feces to produce a fever and taking excessive doses of anticoagulants to induce bleeding. When extreme, this condition is called *Munchausen syndrome*. *Malingering* patients have physical symptoms with no explanatory disease but do not have MUS. They consciously seek to deceive clinicians, insisting that they have disabling physical symptoms to obtain some type of monetary or other gain.[38] They are uncommon and differ from MUS in that they are consciously seeking to deceive us. While MUS patients may receive some apparent benefit from their disorder, so-called secondary gain, they are not consciously setting out to deceive.[38]

Screening

A well-validated, brief screening tool, the Patient Health Questionnaire-15 (PHQ-15), has been developed and can be useful in medical settings for identifying MUS patients;[39] see Table 2-2. A recently developed abbreviated version of the PHQ-15, the Somatic Symptom Scale-8 (SSS-8) appears promising. It has 8 items, strong psychometrics, correlates well with the PHQ-15, and is sensitive to clinical improvement.[40] The PHQ-15 is recommended along with the Patient Health Questionnaire-9 (PHQ-9) for depression and the Generalized Anxiety Disorder Questionnaire-7 (GAD-7).[41,42] Depression and anxiety, discussed in detail in later chapters, are often comorbid with chronic MUS.

Prevention

While it has not been conclusively established, many believe that better addressing acute problems, such as low back pain, tension headaches, or pain following dental surgery, can prevent what should have been

TABLE 2-2. The Physical Health Questionnaire (PHQ-15)			
PHYSICAL SYMPTOMS (PHQ-15)			
During the *past 4 weeks*, how much have you been bothered by any of the following problems?	Not bothered at all (0)	Bothered a little (1)	Bothered a lot (2)
a. Stomach pain	❑	❑	❑
b. Back pain	❑	❑	❑
c. Pain in your arms, legs, or joints (knees, hips, etc)	❑	❑	❑
d. Menstrual cramps or other problems with your periods WOMEN ONLY	❑	❑	❑
e. Headaches	❑	❑	❑
f. Chest pain	❑	❑	❑
g. Dizziness	❑	❑	❑
h. Fainting spells	❑	❑	❑
i. Feeling your heart pound or race	❑	❑	❑
j. Shortness of breath	❑	❑	❑
k. Pain or problems during sexual intercourse	❑	❑	❑
l. Constipation, loose bowels, or diarrhea	❑	❑	❑
m. Nausea, gas, or indigestions	❑	❑	❑
n. Feeling tired or having low energy	❑	❑	❑
o. Trouble sleeping	❑	❑	❑
			Total Score = _____
Scoring: 5-9 = mild; 10-14 = moderate; 15+ = severe.			

a self-limited illness from becoming a chronic MUS problem. Overprescribing of opioids for such problems is common and doing so seems to reinforce the pain, suggesting a possible breeding ground for opioid-dependent chronic pain.[43,44]

The common approach of routinely and indiscriminately providing a 1-month supply of opioids for many different problems has been discouraged by the Centers for Disease Control and Prevention, which recommends no more than a 3- to 7-day course

of opioids for any acute problem.[45] If the acute pain has not resolved, the patient should be evaluated and nonpharmacologic measures advised, such as limited exercise or physical therapy. We discuss the use of opioids in detail in Chapter 6.

SUMMARY

You have seen that the clinician seeking to make a mental health diagnosis will often need to address the patient's presenting physical symptoms of severe chronic MUS or a disabling comorbid medical disease. The physical complaints of both are highly associated with, and should be considered "red flags" for, an associated mental disorder. While one can evaluate psychological symptoms (of a mental disorder) and physical symptoms (of a medical disease or MUS) concurrently, the clinician often first performs a diagnostic evaluation of the presenting physical symptoms. Then, upon recognizing chronic MUS and/or a chronic medical disorder, they can be more comfortable in exploring the associated comorbid mental disorder.

You are now familiar with how to work through the physical symptom presentations of a mental health disorder. However, before addressing the specific psychological symptoms of a mental disorder—and their treatments—we first present in Chapter 3 an overarching treatment model, the Mental Health Care Model, that applies to all mental health disorders we discuss.

REFERENCES

1. Department of Health and Human Services. Generic ICD-9-CM. Reno, Nevada: Channel Publishing; 1994.
2. World Health Organization. The ICD-10 Classification of Mental and Behavioral Disorders—Clinical Descriptions and Diagnostic Guidelines. Geneva, Switzerland: World Health Organization; 1992.
3. American Psychiatric Association. *Diagnostic and Statistical Manual of Mental Disorders—DSM-IV*. 4th ed. Washington, DC: American Psychiatric Association; 1994.
4. Smith RC, Gardiner JC, Lyles JS, et al. Exploration of DSM-IV criteria in primary care patients with medically unexplained symptoms. *Psychosom Med*. 2005;67(1):123-129.
5. Douzenis A, Seretis D. Descriptive and predictive validity of somatic attributions in patients with somatoform disorders: A systematic review of quantitative research. *J Psychosom Res*. 2013;75(3):199-210.
6. American Psychiatric Association. *Diagnostic and Statistical Manual of Mental Disorders*. 5th ed. Washington, DC: American Psychiatric Association; 2013.
7. Frances AJ, Nardo JM. ICD-11 should not repeat the mistakes made by DSM-5. *Br J Psychiatry*. 2013;203:1-2.
8. Kraemer HC. Validity and psychiatric diagnoses. *JAMA Psychiatry*. 2013;70(2):138-139.
9. Dimsdale JE, Creed F, Escobar J, et al. Somatic symptom disorder: an important change in DSM. *J Psychosom Res*. 2013;75(3):223-228.
10. Cloninger CR. Establishment of diagnostic validity in psychiatric illness: Robins and Guze's method revisited. In: Robins LN, Barrett JE, eds. *The Validity of Psychiatric Diagnoses*. New York, NY: Raven Press; 1989:9-16.
11. Robins LN, Barrett JE. *The Validity of Psychiatric Diagnoses*. New York, NY: Raven Press; 1989.
12. Smith RC, Lein C, Collins C, et al. Treating patients with medically unexplained symptoms in primary care. *J Gen Intern Med*. 2003;18:478-489.
13. Wessely S, Nimnuan C, Sharpe M. Functional somatic syndromes: one or many? *Lancet*. 1999;354:936-939.
14. Smith RC, Dwamena FC. Classification and diagnosis of patients with medically unexplained symptoms. *J Gen Intern Med*. 2007;22(5):685-691.
15. Sharpe M. Somatic symptoms: beyond 'medically unexplained'. *Br J Psychiatry*. 2013;203:320-321.
16. Kroenke K. A practical and evidence-based approach to common symptoms: a narrative review. *Ann Intern Med*. 2014;161(8):579-586.
17. Kroenke K. The interface between physical and psychological symptoms. Primary care companion. *J Clin Psychiatry*. 2003;5 (suppl 7):11-18.
18. Smith RC. Somatization disorder: defining its role in clinical medicine. *J Gen Intern Med*. 1991;6:168-175.
19. Kroenke K, Price RK. Symptoms in the community—prevalence, classification, and psychiatric comorbidity. *Arch Intern Med*. 1993;153:2474-2480.
20. Fink P, Toft T, Hansen MS, Ornbol E, Olesen F. Symptoms and syndromes of bodily distress: an exploratory study of 978 internal medical, neurological, and primary care patients. *Psychosom Med*. 2007;69(1):30-39.
21. Katon W, Sullivan M, Walker E. Medical symptoms without identified pathology: relationship to psychiatric disorders, childhood and adult trauma, and personality traits. *Ann Int Med*. 2001;134:917-925.
22. Levenson J. *Textbook of Psychosomatic Medicine*. Washington, DC: American Psychiatric Association; 2005.
23. Woodruff RA, Goodwin DW, Guze SB. *Psychiatric Diagnosis*. New York, NY: Oxford University Press; 1974.
24. Groves JE. Taking care of the hateful patient. *N Engl J Med*. 1978;298:883-887.
25. Kroenke K. Unburdening the difficult clinical encounter. *Arch Intern Med*. 2009;169(4):333-334.
26. Escobar JI, Gara M, Silver RC, Waitzkin G, Holman A, Compton W. Somatisation disorder in primary care. *Br J Psychiatry*. 1998;173:262-266.
27. Escobar JI, Waitzkin H, Silver RC, Gara M, Holman A. Abridged somatization: a study in primary care. *Psychosom Med*. 1998;60:466-472.
28. Frymoyer JW. Back pain and sciatica. *N Engl J Med*. 1988;318:291-300.

29. Verbrugge LM, Ascione FJ. Exploring the iceberg—common symptoms and how people care for them. *Med Care.* 1987;25:539-569.

30. Eikelboom EM, Tak LM, Roest AM, Rosmalen JG. A systematic review and meta-analysis of the percentage of revised diagnoses in functional somatic symptoms. *J Psychosom Res.* 2016;88:60-67.

31. Smith RC, Greenbaum DS, Vancouver JB, et al. Psychosocial factors are associated with health care seeking rather than diagnosis in irritable bowel syndrome. *Gastroenterology.* 1990;98(2):293-301.

32. Hopkins MP, Smith DH. Chronic pelvic pain: profile of a resident teaching clinic. *Am J Gynecol Health.* 1989;3:25-29.

33. Cashman S, Biers S. Chronic pelvic pain in benign and functional urological conditions: a review and comparison of the UK and European guidelines. *J Clin Neurol.* 2018;11(2):115-121.

34. Deyo RA. Can parsimonious practice please patients and practitioners? The case of spine imaging. *J Gen Intern Med.* 2016;31(2):140-141.

35. Horwitz BJ, Fisher RS. The irritable bowel syndrome. *N Engl J Med.* 2001;344:1846-1450.

36. Tibble JA, Sigthorsson G, Foster R, Forgacs I, Bjarnason I. Use of surrogate markers of inflammation and Rome criteria to distinguish organic from nonorganic intestinal disease. *Gastroenterology.* 2002;123:450-460.

37. Vanner SJ, Depew WT, Paterson WG, et al. Predictive value of the Rome criteria for diagnosing the irritable bowel syndrome. *Am J Gastroenterol.* 1999;94:2912-2917.

38. Schneider RK, Levenson JL. *Psychiatry Essentials for Primary Care.* Philadelphia, PA: American College of Physicians; 2008.

39. Kroenke K, Spitzer RL, Williams JB. The PHQ-15: validity of a new measure for evaluating the severity of somatic symptoms. *Psychosom Med.* 2002;64(2):258-266.

40. Gierk B, Kohlmann S, Hagemann-Goebel M, Lowe B, Nestoriuc Y. Monitoring somatic symptoms in patients with mental disorders: sensitivity to change and minimal clinically important difference of the Somatic Symptom Scale-8 (SSS-8). *Gen Hosp Psychiatry.* 2017;48: 51-55.

41. Korber S, Frieser D, Steinbrecher N, Hiller W. Classification characteristics of the Patient Health Questionnaire-15 for screening somatoform disorders in a primary care setting. *J Psychosom Res.* 2011;71(3):142-147.

42. Kroenke K, Spitzer RL, Williams JB, Lowe B. The Patient Health Questionnaire Somatic, Anxiety, and Depressive Symptom Scales: a systematic review. *Gen Hosp Psychiatry.* 2010;32(4):345-359.

43. Deyo RA, Hallvik SE, Hildebran C, et al. Association between initial opioid prescribing patterns and subsequent long-term use among opioid-naive patients: a statewide retrospective cohort study. *J Gen Intern Med.* 2017;32(1):21-27.

44. Barnett ML, Olenski AR, Jena AB. Opioid-prescribing patterns of emergency physicians and risk of long-term use. *N Engl J Med.* 2017;376(7):663-673.

45. Centers for Disease Control and Prevention. *Prescribing Opioids for Chronic Pain.* Washington, DC: CDC; 2016.

3

Mental Health Care Model

Let's summarize where we have been and where this chapter is going. From Chapters 1 and 2, you learned that mental disorders often occur in patients presenting with the physical symptoms of chronic medical disorders and/or chronic medically unexplained symptoms (MUS). This means that, in any patient with severe, disabling physical symptoms, we must also actively inquire about the associated psychological symptoms that can lead us to a diagnosis of a comorbid mental disorder.

In this chapter, before presenting the specific mental disorders and their treatment, we introduce the **Mental Health Care Model** (MHCM), an overarching model for the treatment of the mental disorders we will consider. The MHCM identifies aspects of treatment that are common across all mental disorders. As we progress to later chapters, we will show how pharmacologic and other treatments of specific mental disorders are integrated into the MHCM. (While the MHCM actually applies to all health care interactions, we label it "mental" because these problems are far more complex and require this overarching framework.)

THE MENTAL HEALTH CARE MODEL

The MHCM has 5 dimensions addressing a wide range of often overlooked needs in treating patients with mental health disorders:

1. Establish *communication* and an effective *clinician-patient relationship*
2. *Educate* the patient

3. Obtain the patient's *commitment* to treatment
4. Determine the patient's *goals*
5. *Negotiate* a specific treatment plan

The pharmacologic and other treatments specific to each mental disorder that we present in Chapters 4 to 6 are integrated into the last dimension—negotiating a treatment plan. Treating mental disorders, however, is far more complex than simply prescribing medications. Rather, it also requires the other 4 measures we now discuss in detail.

The MHCM has a wide-ranging conceptual background in self-determination theory,[1,2] shared decision making,[3-7] motivational interviewing,[8-10] social cognitive theory,[11,12] and the chronic care model.[7,13,14] The overarching theoretical backdrop is the general systems-based biopsychosocial (BPS) model,[15,16] and the patient-centered approaches required to operationalize it.[17-19] The BPS model contrasts with the current biomedical/biotechnical model and its isolated focus on diseases. It integrates the patient's psychological and social life to complement the biological or disease aspects of the biomedical model. Instead of describing the patient just in disease terms, the BPS model describes them from disease (biological), psychological, and social perspectives. One elicits this multifactorial database, using PCI rather than the isolated physician-centered interview used when focusing only on diseases.[20]

The MHCM values patient autonomy[21,22] and emphasizes that while the clinician is the expert on disease and treatment, the patient is the expert on their life experience, needs, limitations, and priorities.[22,23]

With the MHCM focus on self-management,[7] fostering patients' self-efficacy (confidence) is paramount.[11,12] Finally, the MHCM emphasizes a negotiated (rather than prescribed) approach with a focus on the partnership with the patient,[24] thus emphasizing the centrality of the clinician-patient relationship.[3,25] Applicable to all mental health disorders, the specific way in which the MHCM is applied depends on the types and numbers of mental disorders and on the specific, unique problems they present.

Figure 3-1 graphically depicts the MHCM. Its centerpiece is the patient-centered interaction (**PCI**), and the following 4 principles are integrated with it: **E**ducating the patient, obtaining a **C**ommitment to treatment, establishing **G**oals for treatment, and **N**egotiating a specific treatment plan. The mnemonic **ECGN** is useful in recalling them. Now let's discuss these 5 principles in more detail and how you can incorporate them into your practice.

I. Patient-Centered Interactions

Patient-centered skills are the single most critical aspect of treatment in mental disorders. In the various mental disorders we'll consider in the chapters that follow, PCI are always at the center of treatment.[3,25] Here, we describe exactly how to conduct them.[26] PCI skills emphasize how to be empathic, the key variable in all interactions.[27] PCI skills also maximize communication and the clinician-patient relationship.[28] We know from an extensive literature in both medicine and psychiatry that PCI is associated with improved health outcomes as well as increased patient satisfaction and medication adherence and with decreased doctor-shopping and malpractice suits.[26,29,30] Indeed, data demonstrate a greater treatment effect from the relationship with the clinician than from pharmacotherapy for mental disorders.[31]

We present a PCI model that is unique in having 4 controlled research studies that demonstrate it is evidence-based.[32-36] The PCI model is summarized in Table 3-1 and presented in detail in *Smith's Patient-Centered Interviewing—An Evidence-Based Method*[26]; several demonstration videotapes of the PCI accompany the book and are easily viewed from McGraw-Hill's Access Medicine website (www.accessmedicine.com/SmithsPCI).

Each interaction with a new or follow-up mental health patient begins with the PCI, summarized here:

Steps 1 and 2, respectively, set the stage and develop the agenda for an interaction. They prepare for the patient-centered parts to follow in steps 3 and 4. See Table 3-1 for the specific substep items to address in steps 1 and 2. In step 2, it is especially important to elicit the full agenda, often asking, "What else?" or "Anything else? I want to be sure we cover all you want to address today." After completing the agenda, the clinician transitions to steps 3 and 4 by saying, "Tell me more about (the chief complaint, such as chest pain or worry)." In the mental health patient with many complaints, especially when first seen, carefully setting the agenda will almost always prevent the frustrating occurrence of new items arising at the end of the interaction.

Steps 3 and 4 generate *the patient's story* comprising[26]:

- The physical symptom story reflects chronic MUS and/or comorbid disease and is applicable in patients with only a disease as well as those with MUS or mental disorders. The clinician repeatedly uses *open-ended skills* (eg, "expand on the chest pain") for a minute or so to develop the physical symptom story in the patient's own words. This is where you first learn about mental health patients' chronic physical symptoms. You may not get all of them here, and any unclear details are

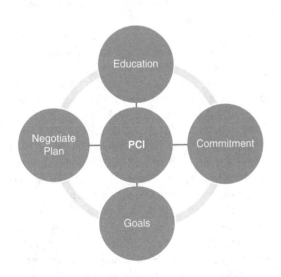

FIGURE 3-1. The Mental Health Care Model (MHCM). PCI = patient-centered interaction.

TABLE 3-1. The Patient-Centered Interviewing Model

PATIENT-CENTERED INTERVIEWING METHOD
(5-STEPS, 21-SUBSTEPS)

STEP 1—Setting the Stage for the Interview
1. Welcome the patient
2. Use the patient's name
3. Introduce yourself and identify your specific role
4. Ensure patient readiness and privacy
5. Remove barriers to communication (sit down)
6. Ensure comfort and put the patient at ease

STEP 2—Chief Concern/Agenda Setting
1. Indicate the time available for the visit
2. Forecast what you would like to have happen in the interview; for example, check blood pressure
3. Obtain a list of all issues the patient wants to discuss; for example, specific symptoms, requests, expectations, understanding
4. Summarize and finalize the agenda; negotiate specifics if there are too many agenda items

STEP 3—Opening the History of Present Illness (HPI)
1. Start with open-ended beginning question focused on the Chief Concern
2. Use "non-focusing" open-ended skills (attentive listening): silence, neutral utterances, nonverbal encouragement
3. Obtain additional data from nonverbal sources: nonverbal cues, physical characteristics, autonomic changes, accouterments, and environment

STEP 4—Continuing the Patient-Centered History of Present Illness (HPI)
1. Elicit physical symptom story—obtain a description of the physical symptoms using focusing open-ended skills
2. Elicit personal and social story—develop the more general personal/social context of the physical symptoms using focusing open-ended skills
3. Elicit emotional story—develop an emotional focus using emotion-seeking skills
4. Respond to feelings/emotions—address the emotion(s) using emotion-handling skills
5. Expand story—continue eliciting further personal and emotional context, address feelings/emotions using focusing open-ended skills, emotion-seeking skills, emotion-handling skills

STEP 5—Transition to the Clinician-Centered History of Present Illness (HPI)
1. Give a brief summary of your understanding
2. Check its accuracy
3. Indicate that both content and style of inquiry will change if the patient is ready

revisited later in the clinician-centered parts of the interaction.

- The personal story reflects the psychological and social context of the physical symptom story. Repeatedly employing *open-ended skills* over the next 1 to 2 minutes, the clinician facilitates a focus on the personal dimensions that arose when the patient told the physical story (eg, "tell me more about losing your job because of the pain" or "you said your wife was upset"). During this part, you will hear the psychological

symptoms and other dimensions of the patient's mental health problem, again pinning down additional details later when clinician centered.

- The emotional story reflects the emotions related to both physical and personal stories.[26] Using a new set of skills, the *emotion-seeking skills*, the clinician inquires directly about emotions[37]; for example, "how did that feel emotionally when you lost your job?" If no emotion is elicited after 2 to 3 tries with this direct inquiry, the clinician probes indirectly, asking what impact the illness has had on them and/or on their family or asks what the patients thinks is causing the situation. The clinician even can suggest others might be "upset" in this situation as a way to encourage emotion; for example, "I think I'd be upset if that happened to me." The idea here is to elicit emotion. Once an emotion is obtained, it is essential to have a good understanding of it, so a few open-ended questions are required to achieve this understanding. *Responding to the emotion:* We now have the full biopsychosocial story, comprising the physical or disease story and the psychological and social stories, including the patient's emotional reactions. What now? Have we tapped into your greatest fear, a patient expressing emotions? While teachers often told you to "be empathic," they seldom indicated exactly how to do that. Yet many clinicians feel helpless or confused when their patients become emotional, for example, wondering with discomfort, "What do I do? He's crying." Consequently, we have devised an effective way to deal with this.

In our model, we identify *four empathic skills*, sometimes descriptively called emotion-handling skills,[37] that help you respond to a patient's emotions:

Name the emotion
Understand the emotion

Respect the emotion
Support the emotion

- They are recalled by the mnemonic **NURS**.[26] For example, the clinician might say,

"You were pretty angry (naming)
I can understand that (understanding) after all you have been through (respecting)
Thanks for sharing that (respecting)
This helps me to better meet your needs (supporting)."

Thus, a provider will "***NURS the emotion***" after they elicit and understand it. One does this repeatedly as new emotions arise or old ones resurface. You can see how the NURS skills are especially needed in tension-laden conversations, for example, around disagreements on using opioids or fear of taking antidepressants; alternatively, they're equally helpful with someone who is depressed because they are dying of

lung cancer. Usually taking no more than 3 to 5 minutes to get to this point, one then transitions to step 5.

Step 5 is very brief and signals to the patient that a change in style of questioning will occur, one where the clinician will ask many more questions designed to pin down necessary details of the story in the clinician-centered part of the interview. For example, starting with a NURS comment, the step 5 transition might be, "… you've had this back pain for 5 years and it's worse, that's been really difficult (respecting), so let's see what we can do working together here (supporting). I'd like to switch gears now and ask some questions to get the details I need on the chest pain and the high blood pressure you mentioned. Is that okay?" Alternatively, if you have already heard about the patient's mental health issues, such as depression, you include that in the summary, "…switch gears … details of your feeling depressed."

Clinician-centered interview: Using closed-ended skills, one elicits significant details of, say, the pain, medications, suicidality, prior depression treatment, and other important data needed to complete the HPI for both mental and physical disorders. As you know, we also obtain a great deal of routine information, such as the patient's past medical history and social history. It is also at this point that you pin down necessary details of the mental health story; for example, ask about depression if suspected but not yet mentioned, medications used, suicidal thoughts, prior hospitalizations, or abuse. In Chapters 4 to 6, you will hear the details of the information needed for mental health patients, and in Chapter 7 we present the format for the entire psychiatric interview, including both patient-centered and clinician-centered dimensions.

While the PCI to this point occurred at the start of the interview, we continue using its open-ended and empathic skills (NURS) periodically throughout the clinician-centered and treatment phases. It is at the conclusion of the interaction, when outlining treatment, that we implement the remainder of the MHCM, which we now describe.

See the Table 3-2 overview for the remaining parts of the MHCM.

II. Educate the Patient

Educating the patient is the first step in treatment. Simply providing information and telling patients

TABLE 3-2. Mental Health Care Model (MHCM)

Education
1. *ASK*—"What's Your Understanding"
   a. Their problem/diagnosis, why they have it, its outcome
   b. What they want done
2. *TELL*
   • "I Have Good News"
      a. Clarify misunderstandings and what needs to be done
      b. Ominous conditions not found (from prior workup)
      c. More testing/consultation not now necessary
         i. You will follow-up for any change
      d. You know diagnosis; eg, depression, anxiety, chronic pain, prescription substance disorder, alcoholism (and comorbid medical problem)—name/explain it
   • "You Need Better Treatment"
      e. Depression (anxiety) makes pain (other symptom) worse → needs medication
         i. Problem is "real" or "not in head" (not a "psych case")
      f. Addicting prescription medications (opioids, benzodiazepines, stimulants) make pain and depression worse → need to slowly taper and discontinue
      g. Need to stop or cut down alcohol use
3. *ASK*—"To be sure I've not been confusing, please summarize what you've heard"

Commitment
1. ASK—"Are you committed to treatment?"
2. TELL—"You need to be active, I can't do it by myself "
3. ASK—"Please summarize your commitment"

Goals
1. Obtain *long-term goals*

Negotiate Plan
1. *ALL plans are scheduled*—nothing is "as needed"
2. *Medications*—details of the following examples to follow in next 3 chapters
   a. *Antidepressant*—for depression or anxiety
   b. *Trazodone*—for sleep
   c. *Naltrexone*—for alcohol withdrawal
3. *Addicting medications* (prescription opioid, benzodiazepine and amphetamine detoxification often require referral)
   a. Determine present dose
   b. Regularize dose schedule—no PRN dosing regimens
   c. Start taper at 1 pill/day each week
   d. Ask them to think about which pill in their dosing schedule they can stop at the next visit
4. *Symptomatic and other medication for medical problem*
5. *Exercise* program—determine present level → prescribe small increase
6. *Social activity*—determine present level → prescribe small increase
7. *Regular follow-up visits*
8. Have *patient summarize* treatment plan
9. *Praise* patient for commitment
10. *Other aspects of treatment* plan (relaxation, diet, PT, OMT)—later
11. Do not advise more tests or consultation (other than PT or OMT)

ASK for EMOTIONS and use NURS at each step

what they need to do is not adequate education. To properly educate the patient, we first *determine their present understanding*, their thoughts and concerns about their diagnosis and treatment, how they think their diagnosis should be labeled, and what treatment they prefer. Upon learning what they already know and think should happen, we can *clarify any misunderstanding and inform them* of our recommendation. Finally, we *ask their understanding* of what we have discussed and recommended. This so-called **"ask-tell-ask"** format has proven very effective.

Let's now take a closer look at these different facets.

Determine Patient's Understanding. (ASK) We already may have some information about the patient's interests from the earlier, patient-centered and clinician-centered parts of the interview. We now delve more deeply into their beliefs and understandings about their problem and what they think should be done. They sometimes know almost everything, while, at other times, they may not know some very basic facts and/or have some mistaken understandings. We must understand their so-called explanatory model.[38] We might begin the treatment phase by saying, "So, what's your understanding of your problem, what do you think needs to happen?" Asking such a simple question usually easily gets the patient to share their understanding about treatment, but if it does not we continue to use open-ended questioning until we are clear on their perspective of what their treatment should be.

Specifically, it can be important to obtain the patient's understanding of the disease, MUS, or mental health problem, the treatment options, and the prognosis with and without treatment.[23] For example, a study demonstrated that patients more often prefer counseling to medications for depression, viewing the latter as addicting and the former as better addressing the root of the problem.[39] We also uncover other potential disagreements this way; for example, the patient thinks that narcotics are useful for chronic pain.

Inform Patient Where Necessary and Make a Recommendation for Treatment. (TELL)

INFORM. Once you have an understanding of the patient's explanatory models, you need to provide the information needed to correct any gaps in their knowledge or any misunderstandings they may have. It is at this point that you should also clarify your rationale for any disagreements, using NURS to enhance your relationship with the patient during what can be a tense interaction. Always indicate you understand their point of view even though you may not agree or be able to comply—and acknowledge their difficult situation and express that you want to work with them.

RECOMMEND. You now provide your recommendation, making the most important point first using short clear statements and avoiding medical jargon. Other issues can be addressed after the patient understands the first one. Disagreements may again occur and threaten the clinician-patient relationship; for example, they want narcotics and you think another approach is better. Elicit their emotion, develop an understanding of it, and NURS it—emphasizing that you want always to do what is best for them and that giving narcotics does not help. Remain respectful, clear, and firm—and don't argue.

Determine Patient's Understanding of Your Input. (ASK) We now determine if the patient has understood the recommendations. It works best to frame this effort in a way that does not question their memory, typically saying something like, "We've talked about a lot and I want to be sure I haven't been confusing. Can you tell me what you've understood about our discussion?" If there are still misunderstandings, they must be corrected, again continuing to use NURS skills with emotion-laden material.

Some examples where we often need to correct a misunderstanding about the health condition and/or the treatment recommended include

- For chronic MUS (chronic pain)—explain that ominous conditions were not found; that surgery, further testing, and consultation are not needed; that the problem is physical and real and not "in their head"; what their somatic diagnosis is (eg, irritable bowel) and its mechanism; that stress, depression, and anxiety are part of the problem and can be helped with medications; and that cure is not likely but they can expect to improve and to better manage their symptoms.

- For prescription substance misuse—explain that narcotics and tranquilizers aggravate the pain problem and cause depression; that they need to be slowly tapered and discontinued; that if the medications are slowly withdrawn while better medications are used they will not suffer withdrawal reactions; that you do not advise sudden "cold turkey" discontinuation.

- For depression and/or anxiety—explain that they are not a "psych case"; that they are not "allergic" to antidepressants and that their prior negative experiences most likely reflect simple side effects that can be controlled by reducing the dose or using a different antidepressant; that side effects usually clear after a week or so; that antidepressants are not addicting; why one takes antidepressants for anxiety; why the patient might not feel better after 1 week of treatment.

III. Commitment to Treatment

The second spoke of the MHCM wheel, essential for self-management, goes more quickly. For treatment to be effective, the patient must take responsibility and become a partner in it.[7,24] During the education phase above, the clinician will have recommended the treatment approach; for example, reducing narcotics, taking an antidepressant, and exercising. It is essential here that the patient *agree explicitly* with the recommendation. The clinician facilitates commitment by indicating that they will be working with the patient regularly and will fulfill their obligations, such as providing medications, but that they need also to hear an explicit commitment to the treatment plan from the patient.[40-42] For example, the clinician could say, "… so, that's what I'll do, but I need to hear that you are on board. You'll also have a lot to do here to make our work successful; are you committed?" It is important that patients verbalize this commitment, and hear themselves say that they are committed to the treatment. Frequently, significant others are involved and their agreement is also important. The clinician may later experience problems with nonadherence to medications or other aspects of the treatment, and commitment must be reestablished, sometimes at each visit.

If patients will not commit or later prove refractory to adhering to the treatment plan despite reinforcing the need for their commitment, clinicians first evaluate themselves to be sure they are not adversely affecting their relationship with the patient; for example, being impatient, appearing disinterested, or being too lenient. Then, assuming the patient's resistance is not due to the clinician's role, the clinician needs to indicate to the patient that they cannot continue to fulfill their part if the patient does not comply with theirs; for example, the patient does not take antidepressant prescribed, does not follow exercise program prescribed, and does not come for follow-up visits as scheduled but continues to want narcotics refilled by phone. If not done already, a written contract is signed, including agreement on criteria for discharge from the clinician's care. While, in our experience, discharging the patient from care is uncommon, there are occasional times when it is necessary. Chapter 6 provides more detail on contracts and other aspects of prescription opioid misuse.

IV. Goals of Treatment

The third spoke of the MHCM wheel focuses on goals. Setting goals is important to effective mental health management and change.[7,23] Often patients can be overwhelmed by the magnitude of their illnesses; for example, diabetes, depression, heart failure, prescription opioid dependence, or any combinations of such serious health problems. This emotional overload can obscure recognition of the positive aspects of their lives and what things are important to them. While the clinician-patient relationship itself helps to address this, we must also encourage recognition of what makes life worth living, what is important in the future, and what has been important to them that they have had to give up. While goals should be generated by the patient, the clinician facilitates the process of goal setting. Common goals include decreased symptoms, better functioning, improved relationships, getting back to work/school, seeing a grandchild graduate, and going to the ball park or church. These long-term goals of the patient are operationalized by the following treatment plan, which will include several short-term goals following each visit ("homework").

V. Negotiate a Treatment Plan

In the fourth spoke of the MHCM wheel, specific treatment plans occur. It is here that the medications you will learn in Chapters 4 to 6 are discussed and implemented. The following overview contains examples for each category and is not specific to any one condition, nor is it exhaustive. In general, the more things we can get patients to do that are healthy, the greater success they will have with symptom management or abatement.

For treatments that apply to many mental health disorders, we expand on our discussion here. The more abbreviated entries are by no means complete and, rather, are limited examples, some expanded upon later in the text.

Medications (initial and later visits)

- Mental disorders (common pharmacological approaches used)

  - Antidepressants
  - Antipsychotics
  - Tapering schedule for narcotics and/or benzodiazepines

- Medical disorders (common examples)

  - Hydrochlorothiazide
  - Atorvastatin
  - Beta-blocker

Nonpharmacologic Treatments (initial and later visits)

- Mental disorders

  - Medication contract for narcotics or benzodiazepines
  - Drug screens for narcotics or benzodiazepines
  - Referral to psychiatry or counseling specialist; for example, for desensitization in panic disorder or ECT in severe depression or psychotherapy

- Medical disorders

  - Paracentesis
  - Colonoscopy
  - Allergy testing

Increased Physical Activity (initial and later visits)

- *Physical exercise program:* This is a good idea for most mental health patients, including those who are quite disabled and deconditioned. The clinician identifies what the patient's baseline physical activity is and then negotiates what they can do on a regularly scheduled basis. On each follow-up visit, an increase is negotiated when possible, gently pushing but not insisting. Cautions to adhere to the specific schedule are important because some will overdo it in their eagerness to improve and this will create new muscular strains that set them back. Many patients will be quite deconditioned and exercise plans may seem miniscule; for example, walk to mailbox once daily, walk upstairs once daily. Important even at these low levels, the program is progressively increased, asking the patient to decide what more they can do at the next visit, such as climb the stairs twice a day and walk to the mailbox 3 times a day. Healthier patients will of course begin with higher levels; for example, walk around the block 3 times daily; jog 3 times weekly.

- *Physical therapy referral:* Physical therapy is not an alternative to a home exercise program but can be an adjunct for those who are severely deconditioned and/or disabled, of course matching recommendations to the patient's condition and desires.

- *Osteopathic manipulative therapy:* We have found osteopathic manipulative therapy, not to be confused with chiropractic treatments, to be very useful but its availability is not widespread.

Increased Social Activity (initial and later visits).

Many patients will have greatly curtailed their social activities as a result of their health problems. Because social activities are critical for mental health and well-being, it is important to explore what activities patients have given up that they would resume if able. By asking them to decide, with your support, what they could do now as part of their treatment to return to a better life, the patient becomes more motivated to resume their social activities. For example, your patient might initially suggest that they would like to return to going to church weekly; at each subsequent visit, find what additional activities they might do, such as playing bridge once a week in addition to church. As they achieve these small steps, they can later add visits with close relatives, going to the movies, and attending concerts or plays as possible activities that get them out of the house and/or socializing with people.

You may find it more effective to address these activities after getting the earlier treatments underway.

As with exercise, the MHCM model follows this approach: learn their current level of activity, negotiate a specific schedule of new social activities the patient is comfortable with, and then gradually increase over time.

Sleep Hygiene (initial and later visits).

Sleep is critical to life and one's happiness,[43] but insomnia is very common and quite disruptive in many mental disorders. We discuss the medication management in Chapter 4. To complement pharmacological approaches, we outline several measures of sleep hygiene that often benefit patients in Table 3-3.

TABLE 3-3. Sleep Hygiene Measures

1. Address obvious causes; eg, snoring partner, pet animals in the bed, large amounts of fluid before bedtime, any caffeine products at all during the day (caffeine should be discontinued completely before concluding insomnia is refractory), drinking alcohol for sleep or just before bedtime (while it may enhance going to sleep, it disrupts later restful sleep), exercising or meditating or eating a large meal before going to bed, blinking lights or unnecessary noises (radio, TV) nearby (quiet, soothing, and rhythmic noises may help), conducting stressful work or conversations or planning the next day's work just before bedtime, uncomfortable bedroom temperature (generally a cool temperature is best).
2. Establish a regular sleeping pattern each day and do not take naps during the day—get up and go to bed at the same time each day.
3. Use the bed only for sex and sleep—no TV, reading, talking, Internet surfing, or eating.
4. Remove clocks from line of vision to prevent the urge to look when awake.
5. If awake for than 30-60 min, get up and do something nonstimulating, such as an unpleasant task like ironing or cleaning.

Importantly, if the insomnia does not resolve with these and nonaddicting medications, you must be certain there are no other causes that could require a different treatment, for example, obstructive sleep apnea, periodic limb movement disorder/restless legs syndrome, circadian rhythm sleep disorders, medications, or a medical disorder. Often, a sleep laboratory consultation is required for refractory insomnia for conduct of a nocturnal polysomnogram.[44]

Relaxation Techniques (later visits)

- Regularly scheduled relaxation procedures are helpful; for example, breathing focused meditation, progressive muscular relaxation, yoga.
- In Table 3-4, we include a simple relaxation exercise.[45-47]

Dietary, Tobacco, and Alcohol Counseling (later visits)

- Patients adopting healthy habits often become ready to address other more difficult health hazards they engage in, especially as their motivation

and self-confidence increase with treatment of their mental disorder.

- This topic is discussed extensively in *Smith's Patient-Centered Interviewing: An Evidence-Based Method*.[26]

Visit With Significant Other (initial and later visits)

- It is important at some early point to have the spouse, parent, or other close family member or friend join the patient at one of your visits.[23] We have observed that some partners or family members will inadvertently undercut what the clinician and the patient are trying to accomplish; for example, "…he can't do that exercise, it'll make his back worse." These companions need to hear the treatment program that has been outlined for the patient and its rationale. It is crucial to get them on your side, otherwise, they may work against you despite your and their best intentions.
- With a more receptive companion, often signaled by their impatience and frustration with the patient, we often can engage them as a "comanager."

Identify Community Resources (later visits)

- These resources will vary according to the particular community where you work but may involve counseling, psychiatry, exercise and relaxation programs, Alcoholics Anonymous, smoking cessation groups, weight loss groups, church groups, and the like.[8] Specific resources are provided with each later chapter.

Set Specific Follow-Up Visit (every visit)

- Follow-up visits are almost always scheduled, and never left on an as-needed basis.[7] Early on, in most mental health problems, the initial visits are at 1- to 2-week intervals, although sometimes telephone contact suffices. As well, if available, a skilled office person or a case manager can monitor patients' progress as long as the patient is improving. Frequent visits or other contacts are necessary in cementing a strong, caring relationship as well as for adjusting medications and other negotiated treatments.
- As part of each visit, it is important to also briefly examine the patient regarding any physical complaint they may have, reassuring the patient when there has been no change.

TABLE 3-4. Breathing Meditation for Patients

1. In a quiet room where you will not be disturbed, sit on a chair or cross-legged on a pillow on the floor. Try to sit straight but be comfortable.
2. Close your eyes and pay attention to your breathing, focusing on each breath, saying to yourself, "In" with each inhalation and "Out" as you exhale. Breathe as you normally would, likely taking breaths of various depths. Beginning with a deep breath or two often helps get the process going, but don't hyperventilate.
3. Start counting your breaths, as "In…Out-1" → "In-Out-2" → (continue; you may want to start over or count backwards once you hit 100).
4. Continue focusing on your breathing, trying to "breathe from the stomach"—this means push your abdomen out to inhale and let it come back as you exhale; try not to move your chest up and down when you breathe. As you count, stay focused on the movement of your abdomen, in and out.
5. As you do this, your mind will likely wander to other thoughts, such as a task you need to do. This is perfectly ok. Once you realize it, though, simply drop the thought and return your focus to the breathing, the abdomen moving in and out, continuing to count.
6. (If you have problems falling asleep, keep your eyes open and proceed the same way. Keep a constant focus of your eyes on, say, your shoelaces or a door knob.)

When you first meditate, stop after 10 min, or so. When you stop, slowly open your eyes, stretch your muscles, and get your bearings. Then gradually resume your regular day. You will feel quite relaxed and peaceful. As you become more accustomed to meditating, you can extend the meditations to 15 or 20 min, even meditating 2 times a day. Also, during a busy day, you can get a similar effect at, say, a meeting, by focusing on the breath for just a couple breaths, beginning with 1 deep breath or 2.

There is a variation of this technique you can try, called progressive muscular relaxation. After you've begun the breathing meditation, change your focus to your muscles. You are going to tense a specific muscle area of your body for 10 s (to feel what tension is like) and then relax it, staying focused on just that small area of your body, to feel what a completely relaxed muscle group feels like. You then move to the next adjacent area. Most people begin by tensing and relaxing 1 foot, then the calf, the thigh, the buttocks (do the right side first and then the left), the abdomen, the chest, the back, the neck, the shoulders, the arms (right then left), and the face. When you finish this sequence, return to the breathing for a few minutes before you stop.

- It is helpful to provide a print-out of what you have found and are recommending. Sometimes in providing much complex information or information loaded with emotion, it is helpful to audio-record the interaction so they can review it later and share it with significant others.[48] These activities are necessary because patients forget up to 40% of routine information provided and even more of emotion- and stress-laden information.[49] We also know that while clinicians believe they provide adequate information, many patients disagree.[50,51]

INITIATING THE MENTAL HEALTH CARE MODEL

While you will likely implement many of the above measures over time, *the initial approach often focuses on such steps as starting antidepressants (for anxiety as well as for depression), opioid tapering, and exercise.* Revisited in detail later in their respective chapters, the following is an overview of how this might play out.

At the initial visit, begin antidepressants at low doses to avoid adverse reactions. Because many patients have insomnia, this also is treated. Rather than prescribing addictive benzodiazepines, better sleep often can be achieved using trazodone or an antidepressant like mirtazapine; you'll learn doses in Chapter 4. As well, if the patient is taking opioids, establish a regularized (non-prn) dose schedule and give just enough pills to last until the next visit. Ask the patient to be thinking about which tablet can be reduced at the next visit, say, from 6 to 5 tablets per day of oxycodone. In almost all cases, it is a good idea to try to negotiate some type of exercise program that is reasonable to the patient, again in a scheduled fashion.

At the next visit, say, 1 week or 2 later, follow-up on all the above facets of the treatment. In addition to ensuring that the patient has not become suicidal, which is a rare reaction to beginning antidepressants,[52] inquire about the patient's comfort with the medications and address side effects. If none, consider increasing the antidepressant dose to a low-normal therapeutic range. If the patient is too sleepy or is still not sleeping through the night, make adjustments in the dose of medication used to enhance sleep. If opioids are being tapered, learn which pill the patient wants to reduce at this visit and provide sufficient numbers of pills to last until the next appointment, again asking the patient to decide which pill they would like to remove from their schedule at the next visit. Similarly, be sure to follow-up on progress with the exercise program and see if you can negotiate a small increase in it.

At the next visit, you might further increase the dose of an antidepressant and may need to further adjust medications according to the success with insomnia. Patients are sometimes uncomfortable with reducing opioids at every visit, and you may accommodate that by changing to every other visit. We encourage reductions at least every 2 to 3 weeks. Similarly, you do not need to be rigid about the exercise program, as you focus more on achieving cooperation and success over the long term.

By the next visit, patients with insomnia should be sleeping through the night and be on full doses of an antidepressant, and, if you are tapering opioids, they should have made some reductions in dose and be on an increasing exercise program. According to the specific situation, many of the other therapeutic approaches above in the MHCM may also have been introduced, and you may begin to introduce others, such as increased social activities, visits with a significant other, or meditation.

As the patient both accommodates to the treatment program and improves, visits can be extended to every 2 to 4 weeks. Critically, however, as you'll learn in Chapters 4 and 5, decisions need to be made about achieving complete remissions of depression and anxiety. The decisions are usually made from 8 to 12 weeks after achieving a full dose of the antidepressant. If there is a full remission, you can continue seeing the patient every 4 to 6 weeks. If there is not a full remission, however, changes in medications and other treatment will be needed as you'll learn. For now, we just want to give you an overview of how the MHCM is initiated and how the treatment plan can work over time.

SUMMARY

You now have a good understanding of the overall treatment approach for mental disorders. You will be providing patient education and reorienting patients to their disease process, getting their commitment to proceed with the treatment, setting goals, and negotiating a treatment plan—using patient-centered and NURS skills throughout.

Now that you know how these fit into the MHCM, we move to the specific diagnosis and treatment issues for mental disorders, particularly addressing the medications required for treatment. In Chapters 4 to 6, we will review the specific psychological symptom criteria for making diagnoses of what we propose to be the core mental disorders all medical clinicians can master: depression, anxiety, and prescription substance misuse. We also will present the pharmacological and other treatments unique to each disorder.

REFERENCES

1. Deci EL, Ryan RM. The support of autonomy and the control of behavior. *J Pers Soc Psychol.* 1987;53:1024-1037.
2. Williams GC, Cox EM, Hedberg VA, Deci EL. Extrinsic life goals and health-risk behaviors in adolescents. *J Appl Soc Psychol.* 2000;30:1756-1771.
3. Trevena L, Barratt A. Integrated decision making: definitions for a new discipline. *Patient Educ Couns.* 2003;50:265-268.
4. Joosten EA, Defuentes-Merillas L, de Weert GH, Sensky T, van der Staak CP, de Jong CA. Systematic review of the effects of shared decision-making on patient satisfaction, treatment adherence and health status. *Psychother Psychosom.* 2008;77(4):219-226.
5. Cegala DJ, Chisolm DJ, Nwomeh BC. Further examination of the impact of patient participation on physicians' communication style. *Patient Educ Couns.* 2012;89(1):25-30.
6. Bauer AM, Parker MM, Schillinger D, et al. Associations between antidepressant adherence and shared decision-making, patient-provider trust, and communication among adults with diabetes: diabetes study of Northern California (DISTANCE). *J Gen Intern Med.* 2014;29(8):1139-1147.
7. Battersby M, Von Korff M, Schaefer J, et al. Twelve evidence-based principles for implementing self-management support in primary care. *Jt Comm J Qual Patient Saf.* 2010;36(12):561-570.
8. Spencer JC, Wheeler SB. A systematic review of motivational interviewing interventions in cancer patients and survivors. *Patient Educ Couns.* 2016;99(7):1099-1105.

9. Miller W, Rollnick S. *Motivational Interviewing—Helping People Change*. 3rd ed. New York: The Guilford Press; 2013.

10. Kusurkar RA, Croiset G, Mann KV, Custers E, Ten Cate O. Have motivation theories guided the development and reform of medical education curricula? A review of the literature. *Acad Med*. 2012;87(6):735-743.

11. Bandura A. Self-efficacy: toward a unifying theory of behavioral change. *Psychol Rev*. 1977;84:191-215.

12. Bandura A. Social cognitive theory: an agentic perspective. *Annu Rev Psychol*. 2001;52:1-26.

13. Glasgow RE, Emmons KM. How can we increase translation of research into practice? Types of evidence needed. *Annu Rev Public Health*. 2007;28:413-433.

14. Miller CJ, Grogan-Kaylor A, Perron BE, Kilbourne AM, Woltmann E, Bauer MS. Collaborative chronic care models for mental health conditions: cumulative meta-analysis and metaregression to guide future research and implementation. *Med Care*. 2013;51(10):922-930.

15. Engel GL. The need for a new medical model: a challenge for biomedicine. *Science*. 1977;196:129-136.

16. von Bertalanffy L. *General System Theory: Foundations, Development, Application, Revised*. New York, NY: George Braziller; 1968.

17. Levenstein JH, McCracken EC, McWhinney IR, Stewart MA, Brown JB. The patient-centered clinical method. 1. A model for the doctor-patient interaction in family medicine. *J Fam Pract*. 1986;3:24-30.

18. McWhinney I. The need for a transformed clinical method. In: Stewart M, Roter D, eds. *Communicating with Medical Patients*. London: Sage Publications; 1989:25-42.

19. Rogers CR. *Client-Centered Therapy*. Boston: Houghton Mifflin Company; 1951.

20. Smith R, Fortin AH VI, Dwamena F, Frankel R. An evidence-based patient-centered method makes the biopsychosocial model scientific. *Patient Educ Couns*. 2013;90:265-270.

21. Gruen A. *The Betrayal of the Self—The Fear of Autonomy in Men and Women*. New York, NY: Grove Press; 1986.

22. deBronkart D. From patient centred to people powered: autonomy on the rise. *BMJ*. 2015;350:h148.

23. Quill TE, Holloway RG. Evidence, preferences, recommendations—finding the right balance in patient care. *N Engl J Med*. 2012;366(18):1653-1655.

24. Quill TE. Partnerships in patient care: a contractual approach. *Ann Intern Med*. 1983;98:228-234.

25. Matthias MS, Salyers MP, Frankel RM. Re-thinking shared decision-making: context matters. *Patient Educ Couns*. 2013;91(2):176-179.

26. Fortin AH VI, Dwamena F, Frankel R, Lepisto B, Smith R. *Smith's Patient-Centered Interviewing—An Evidence-Based Method*. 4th ed. New York, NY: McGraw-Hill, Lange Series; 2018.

27. de Waal FB. The antiquity of empathy. *Science*. 2012;336(6083):874-876.

28. Watzlawick P, Bavelas JB, Jackson DD. *Pragmatics of Human Communication: A Study of Interactional Patterns, Pathologies, and Paradoxes*. New York, NY: WW Norton & Company; 1967.

29. Stewart M. Evidence for the patient-centered clinical method as a means of implementing the biopsychosocial approach. In: Frankel R, Quill T, McDaniel S, eds. *The Biopsychosocial Approach: Past, Present, Future*. Rochester, NY: Univeristy of Rochester Press; 2003:123-132.

30. Stewart MA. Effective physician-patient communication and health outcomes: a review. *Can Med Assoc J*. 1995;152(9):1423-1433.

31. Correll CU, Carbon M. Efficacy of pharmacologic and psychotherapeutic interventions in psychiatry: to talk or to prescribe: is that the question? *JAMA Psychiatry*. 2014;71(6):624-626.

32. Smith R, Gardiner J, Luo Z, Schooley S, Lamerato L. Primary care physicians treat somatization. *J Gen Int Med*. 2009;24:829-832.

33. Smith RC, Lyles JS, Gardiner JC, et al. Primary care clinicians treat patients with medically unexplained symptoms—a randomized controlled trial. *J Gen Intern Med*. 2006;21:671-677.

34. Lyles JS, Hodges A, Collins C, et al. Using nurse practitioners to implement an intervention in primary care for high utilizing patients with medically unexplained symptoms. *Gen Hosp Psychiatry*. 2003;25:63-73.

35. Smith RC, Lyles JS, Mettler J, et al. The effectiveness of intensive training for residents in interviewing. A randomized, controlled study. *Ann Intern Med*. 1998;128:118-126.

36. Smith R, Laird-Fick H, Dwamena F, et al. Teaching residents mental health care. *Patient Educ Couns*. 2018; 101:2145-2155.

37. Cole SA, Bird J. *The Medical Interview*. New York: Elsevier-Saunders; 2013.

38. Kleinman A. Explanatory models in health-care relationships: a conceptual frame for research on family-based health-care activities in relation to folk and professional forms of clinical care. In: Stoeckle JD, ed. *Encounters Between Patients and Doctors*. Cambridge: The MIT Press; 1987:273-283.

39. van Schaik DJF, Klijn FJ, van Hout HPJ, et al. Patients' preferences in the treatment of depressive disorder in primary care. *Gen Hosp Psych*. 2004;26:184-189.

40. Prochaska JO, DiClemente CC. Towards a comprehensive model of change. In: Miller WR, Heather N, eds.

Treating Addictive Behaviors: Processes of Change. New York, NY: Plenum Press; 1986:3-27.

41. Sharpe M, Peveler R, Mayou R. The psychological treatment of patients with functional somatic symptoms: a practical guide. *J Psychosom Res.* 1992;36:515-529.

42. Stoffelmayr B, Hoppe RB, Weber N. Facilitating patient participation: the doctor-patient encounter. *Primary Care.* 1989;16:265-278.

43. Walker M. *Why We Sleep—The New Science of Sleep and Dreams.* London: Allen Lane; 2017.

44. Buysse DJ, Rush AJ, Reynolds CF III. Clinical management of insomnia disorder. *JAMA.* 2017;318(20): 1973-1974.

45. Khoury B, Knauper B, Schlosser M, Carriere K, Chiesa A. Effectiveness of traditional meditation retreats: a systematic review and meta-analysis. *J Psychosom Res.* 2017;92:16-25.

46. Kabat-Zinn J. *Wherever You Go, There You Are: Mindfulness Meditation in Everyday Life.* New York, NY: Hyperion; 1994.

47. Benson H. *The Relaxation Response.* New York, NY: William Morrow and Company, Inc.; 1975.

48. Fallowfield LJ, Lipkin M. Delivering sad or bad news. In: Lipkin M, Putnam SM, Lazare A, eds. *The Medical Interview.* New York, NY: Springer-Verlag; 1995: 316-323.

49. Ley P. Doctor-patient communication: some quantitative estimates of the role of cognitive factors in noncompliance. *J Hypertens Suppl.* 1985;3(1):S51-S55.

50. Clever S, Ford D, Rubenstein L, et al. Primary care patients' involvement in decision-making is associated with improvement in depression. *Med Care.* 2006;44:390-405.

51. Young H, Bell R, Epstein R, Feldman M, Kravitz R. Types of information physicians provide when prescribing antidepressants. *J Gen Int Med.* 2006;21: 1172-1177.

52. Friedman RA. Antidepressants' black-box warning—10 years later. *N Engl J Med.* 2014;371(18):1666-1668.

4

Major Depression and Related Disorders

INTRODUCTION

To this point, from Chapters 1 to 3, you have learned about the frequent physical symptom presentation of mental health problems in medical settings. And you have heard about the overarching treatment model, the Mental Health Care Model (MHCM), that guides treatment of all mental disorders. We now begin to provide the details, especially of medications, for the first of the three mental health problems medical clinicians will need to address in the future—depression.

The theme of this book is that all physicians require competence with common mental health problems, such as depression, not to the level of becoming psychiatrists but equivalent to their competence with, for example hypertension, asthma, or diabetes.[1] Given the shortage of psychiatrists,[2] many believe that medical physicians can provide effective treatment for "treatment-responsive" depression, which we will define for you later in this chapter.[3]

This chapter provides you with tools to recognize and manage depression in its many forms.

BACKGROUND

Depression is the leading cause of disease burden, work disability, and death by suicide worldwide and, yet, most patients go untreated.[4,5] An estimated 350 million people are affected. In the United States, approximately 7% of the population has depression, a rate that is even higher in females and young people.[6] One in every 5 women and 1 in every 10 men are affected, and the prevalence increases with each successive birth cohort and progressively with older age,

affecting 9% of the elderly living in the community, and 25% of those living in institutions. Among older adults, the presence of depression also is associated with increased chronic disease burden 10 years later.[7] The economic impact in the United States is estimated at $210 billion per year.[8] There are additional personal costs to families,[9] and research demonstrates that effective treatment can save over $5 for every $1 spent on treatment.[10]

Indeed, treatment has been demonstrated to be very effective in multiple clinical trials, including a recent meta-analysis.[11] Not only do antidepressants help for psychological symptoms, but they also have been demonstrated to improve medical outcomes, for example improved survival following an acute coronary syndrome.[12] Risk factors for depression include economic poverty, being single, a history of abuse (emotional, physical, or sexual), and a family history of depression. Recent data indicate that severe affective disturbances during adolescence are associated with increased premature mortality—indicating the need for early intervention.[13]

Depressive disorders have been recognized since antiquity. In Hippocratic writings, melancholia (black bile) was attributed to disrupted humoral balance. In the 1960s, the amine hypothesis emerged following the discovery of antidepressant medications. Depressed patients had lower levels of urinary metabolites of the indoleamine serotonin and the catecholamine norepinephrine. In the 1980s, it was observed that depressed patients displayed aberrant hypothalamic-pituitary-adrenal (HPA) function: they had higher serum levels of cortisol and a failure to suppress

TABLE 4-1. The Biopsychosocial Dimensions of Depression

	PREDISPOSING	PRECIPITATING	PERPETUATING	PREVENTIVE
Biological	Family history Medical illness	Alcohol misuse Medications	Hypothyroidism Nonadherence Medical illness	Aerobic exercise
Psychological	Learned helplessness			Positive self-talk Mindfulness
Social	Childhood trauma or neglect	Relationship breakup Loss of employment Bereavement		Social networks

cortisol following administration of dexamethasone. The dexamethasone suppression test emerged as a possible biomarker for depression. In the 1990s, the inflammatory model emerged. Patients with depression were found to have elevated levels of inflammatory markers such as C-reactive protein, interleukin-6, and tumor necrosis factor. It was later discovered that these factors impede the synthesis of neurotransmitters, enhance glutamate neurotoxicity, and impede hippocampal neurogenesis. With effective treatment, levels of inflammatory markers decline, and neuroplasticity is restored.

The pathogenesis of depressive disorders is multifactorial and reflects the interplay of many biopsychosocial factors important to treatment. From Table 4-1, for example, you may find that a patient who is depressed has adverse biological predisposing factors (such as a family history of depression and refractory diabetes), psychological factors (learned helplessness), and social contributors (childhood trauma). On the other extreme, such adverse influences could perhaps be offset by aerobic exercise (biological), mindfulness meditation (psychological), and networking (social). This is an example of the biopsychosocial model you learned about in Chapter 3.[14]

DIAGNOSIS AND TREATMENT ISSUES COMMON TO ALL DEPRESSIVE DISORDERS

The Spectrum of Depressive Disorders. There are over a dozen recognized variants of depression in the *Diagnostic and Statistical Manual of Mental Disorders*, 5th ed. (DSM-5) (Table 4-2).[6] We will focus primarily on the most common problem—major depressive disorder. Then we consider briefly the less common disorders. Last, we'll consider bipolar disorder in considerable detail. While it has similarities to other depressive disorders, its differences are greater than among the other depressive disorders.[6,15]

Depression is a heterogenous group of disorders that share hallmark symptoms of low mood, lack of interest, and diminished pleasure. As you know from Chapters 1 and 2, many depressed patients also will present with physical symptoms of an underlying physical disease or as a manifestation of medically unexplained symptoms, with chronic pain being among the most common.

TABLE 4-2. The Spectrum of Depressive Disorders

Major depressive disorder
Persistent depressive disorder (dysthymia)
Adjustment disorder with depressed mood
Bereavement
Female-specific disorders
    Premenstrual dysphoric disorder
    Perimenstrual depressive disorder
    Postpartum depression
Winter depression or seasonal affective disorder
Late age onset and vascular depression
Depression related to a medical illness
Substance/medication-induced depression
Disruptive mood dysregulation disorder
Bipolar disorder, depressed, depression with mixed features

In addition to having common symptom presentations, the depressive disorders have common treatment approaches.

- You've already learned the MHCM in Chapter 3; see Figure 4-1. It applies to all health care disorders but is especially useful in patients with mental disorders. Here is a very brief summary: the centerpiece of the MHCM is the *patient-centered interaction* (PCI),[16] which maximizes communication and the clinician-patient relationship. The first of the four spokes of the model is *education,* which involves determining the patient's understanding of their disorder, clarifying any misunderstandings and providing your general recommendation for treatment. Second, you obtain a *commitment to treatment,* emphasizing the patient's responsibility as well as your own. Third, we develop the patient's *long-range goals* for care, such as what he/she would like to do if they were not ill. The fourth dimension of treatment is *negotiating a treatment plan.* This includes the specific pharmacologic and non-pharmacologic treatments unique to the mental health disorder—which in this chapter is depression.

- Fortunately, the medications and non-pharmacologic approaches for most depressive disorders are the same, and the medications are used in similar doses. As you'll learn in Chapter 5, the medications for anxiety disorders also are much the same as those used for depression—but in lower starting doses. You thus can learn a few of these medications and apply that knowledge to both depression and anxiety disorders. You will need to understand these medications as well as you now understand medications for hypertension and diabetes. We will provide clear instructions to guide you in mastering them.

MAJOR DEPRESSIVE DISORDER

Diagnosis. Major depressive disorder is the most prevalent and serious of the depressive disorders. The diagnosis is characterized by at least 5 of the 9 following depressive symptoms during a 2-week period, which must include 1 of the first 2 criteria listed: (1) a sad or depressed mood; (2) lack of interest or pleasure (anhedonia); (3) insomnia or hypersomnia; (4) lack of energy and tiredness; (5) loss of appetite or excessive appetite; (6) guilt or self-loathing; (7) difficulty concentrating; (8) psychomotor agitation or retardation; and (9) feelings of hopelessness or thoughts of dying or self-harm.

To make the diagnosis of major depressive disorder, the symptoms must create *significant dysfunction* and not be otherwise explainable by medications or a medical disorder. Table 4-3 summarizes the DSM-5 diagnostic criteria.[6]

What exactly might the clinician say to identify these symptoms of depression if they don't arise spontaneously in the patient-centered portion of the interaction. One uses the physician-centered skills of direct inquiry, relying on closed-ended questioning. For example, in a patient with chronic pain who has mentioned nothing about depression, you can explore with very direct and specific questions. Here are some examples.

- "How's your mood, you know, have you felt depressed?"

- "Have you been feeling sad or having crying spells with all this pain?"

- "What do you like to do for fun, the things you do for pleasure?" (This key question gets at the criterion for lack of pleasure in one's life, so-called anhedonia.)

- "How's your sleep been? How long does it take to get to sleep? Do you waken and are unable to get back to sleep?"

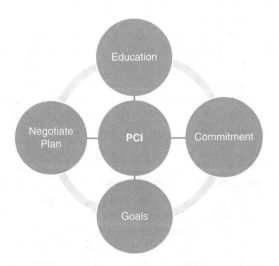

FIGURE 4-1. The Mental Health Care Model (MHCM). PCI = patient-centered interaction.

TABLE 4-3. DSM-5 Diagnostic Criteria for Major Depressive Disorder

A. Five (or more) of the following symptoms have been present in the same 2 weeks, and represent a change from previous functioning, at least 1 of the symptoms is either (1) depressed mood or (2) loss of interest or pleasure.
   1. Depressed mood most of the day, nearly every day, as indicated by either subjective report or observation made by others
   2. Markedly diminished interest or pleasure in all, or almost all activities most of the day, nearly every day
   3. Significant weight loss when not dieting or weight gain
   4. Insomnia or hypersomnia
   5. Psychomotor agitation or retardation
   6. Fatigue or loss of energy
   7. Feelings of worthlessness or excessive or inappropriate guilt
   8. Diminished ability to think or concentrate, or indecisiveness
   9. Recurrent thoughts of death, recurrent suicidal ideation without a specific plan, or a suicide attempt or a specific plan for committing suicide
B. The symptoms cause clinically significant distress or impairment in social, occupational, or other important areas of functioning.
C. The episode is not attributable to the physiological effects of a substance or to another medical condition.

Source: Reprinted with permission from the *Diagnostic and Statistical Manual of Mental Disorders,* Fifth Edition, (Copyright ©2013). American Psychiatric Association. All Rights Reserved.

- "What's your energy level, is it up to par, can you do as much as in the past when you felt well?"
- "How's your appetite and weight with all this trouble?"
- "When you awaken at night or at other times, what kinds of thoughts go through your mind, do you feel guilty or are you critical of yourself?"
- "How's your ability to concentrate on something when you need to?"
- "Do you get agitated or the opposite when you just can't get the energy to do anything?"
- "Do you ever feel like there's just no hope?"
- "How solid are your relationships with...spouse...children...friends?"

- "Have you ever thought of harming or injuring yourself, or does taking your life ever cross your mind?"

Screening. Shown in Table 4-4, the Patient Health Questionnaire-9 (PHQ-9) is a reliable, valid, and well established measure that represents the 9 DSM-5 diagnostic criteria for Major Depressive Disorder. There is a minimum score of 0 and a maximum score of 27. Normal = 0 to 4; mild depression = 5 to 9; moderate depression = 10 to 14; severe depression = 15 to 19; very severe depression = 20 or more.[17] Thus, easier to remember cut-points are 5, 10, 15, and 20. Many clinics use the PHQ-9 routinely to identify depressed patients, and it should be performed in all patients where there is suspicion of depression; it's useful for following patients' progress as well as for diagnosis. Some guidelines recommend annual screening for depression in all adults.[18]

The Patient Health Questionnaire-2 (PHQ-2) comprises just the first 2 items of the PHQ-9, and can be self-administered via a patient portal or by the clinician during the visit. A score of 3 or more has a sensitivity of greater than 80% for the diagnosis of major depressive disorder. A patient who endorses a positive response with either item on the PHQ-2 scale should complete the PHQ-9.

Treatment. In Table 4-5, we present commonly used antidepressants, the starting and therapeutic doses used, and the side effects. Effective in all age groups and all levels of depression severity,[19] they are classified as selective serotonin reuptake inhibitors (SSRI), serotonin-norepinephrine reuptake inhibitors (SNRI), and a miscellaneous group of various mechanisms labeled "other." You'll see how we use medications from each of these pharmacological classes.

Despite the different mechanisms of action, all antidepressants are equally effective in alleviating the core symptoms of depression. This means that selecting which one to use depends on the other factors we now review.

1. *Side effects:* It is important to avoid adverse side effects (see Table 4-5), especially if they may aggravate a preexisting medical condition. For instance, you might avoid mirtazapine because it can increase appetite and weight and impair glycemic control in an obese patient with diabetes. Conversely, the side effects of increased appetite and sedation associated with mirtazapine may benefit patients receiving cancer chemotherapy who have lost appetite, become cachectic, and experience trouble sleeping. Another

TABLE 4-4. Patient Health Questionnaire (PHQ-9) Scale				
PHQ-9				
Over the *last 2 weeks*, how often have you been bothered by any of the following problems?				
	Not at all (0)	Several days (1)	More than half the days (2)	Nearly every day (3)
1. Little interest or pleasure in doing things	❑	❑	❑	❑
2. Feeling down, depressed, or hopeless	❑	❑	❑	❑
3. Trouble falling or staying asleep, or sleeping too much	❑	❑	❑	❑
4. Feeling tired or having little energy	❑	❑	❑	❑
5. Poor appetite or overeating	❑	❑	❑	❑
6. Feeling bad about yourself—or that you are a failure or have let yourself or your family down	❑	❑	❑	❑
7. Trouble concentrating on things, such as reading the newspaper or watching television	❑	❑	❑	❑
8. Moving or speaking so slowly that other people could have noticed? Or the opposite—being so fidgety or restless that you have been moving around a lot more than usual	❑	❑	❑	❑
9. Thoughts that you would be better off dead or of hurting yourself in some way	❑	❑	❑	❑
Add the score from each column				
Add column scores =			**Total Score = _____**	

example is the orgasmic delay commonly associated with the SSRIs paroxetine and fluoxetine. It may be unacceptable for some patients, but it can be beneficial in men affected by premature ejaculation.

Nocebo effect: Some patients experience adverse effects from low doses of many medications and require special attention. The expectation of an adverse effect is called the nocebo effect, the opposite of a placebo effect.[20-22] It is important to distinguish it from a true adverse effect because it does not require a medication change. The nocebo effect is more commonly observed in patients who have experienced adverse effects with previous drugs of many types ("...I just can't handle medications, I'm allergic to everything...") and in patients with chronic depression or anxiety. The nocebo effect has caused great problems with adherence to antidepressant medications and we work hard to offset

it; this is where the MHCM comes in. Initially anticipating and addressing the problem is key when starting an antidepressant. It works best to start with a low dose and increase the dose more gradually than usual into the therapeutic range. Initially, we explain to the patient that they likely will have some jitteriness, dry mouth, and constipation (expected side effects) but that the symptoms usually clear in a week or so. We then strongly advise them not to stop the medication if they have any problems. Instead, we ask them to call and we typically will reduce the dose.

2. *Possible drug interactions:* Some antidepressants interfere with the metabolism of drugs concurrently prescribed for a physical or psychiatric illness. For instance, as in Table 4-5, the SSRIs fluoxetine and paroxetine taken by a patient on the β-blocker metoprolol for hypertension can lead to a twofold

TABLE 4-5. Use of Antidepressant Medications in Depressive Disorders

	ANTIDEPRESSANT MEDICATIONS					ANTIDEPRESSANT SIDE EFFECTS					
CLASS	INITIAL DOSE[a] (mg/d)	THERAP. DOSE[b] (mg/d)	HALF-LIFE	SEDATION	WEIGHT GAIN	SEXUAL	CARDIAC	ANTICHOLINERGIC	SEIZURES	DRUG INTERACTION[b]
SSRI										
Sertraline Zoloft	50	100-200	Medium	+/−	+	++	−	+	−	2D6 inhibitor +/− At high doses only
Fluoxetine Prozac	20	20-60	Long	−	+/−	++	−	+	−	2D6 inhibitor 4+ Incr. flecainide and β-blocker level
Citalopram Celexa	20	20-60	Short	+/−	+	++	QTc increased	−	−	Incr. flecainide level
Escitalopram Lexapro	10	10-20	Short	−	+	++	QTc increased	−	−	Incr. flecainide level
Paroxetine Paxil	20	20-40	Short	+	++	+++	−	+	−	2D6 inhibitor 4+ Incr. flecainide and β-blocker level
SNRI										
Venlafaxine XR Effexor XR	37.5	75-225	Short	−	+/−	+++	Increased BP & heart rate	−	−	Decr. Indinavir level
Duloxetine Cymbalta	30	30-60	Short	−	+/−	+++	+/−	−	−	2D6 inhibitor 1+

OTHER									
Mirtazapine *Remeron*	15	15–45	++	+++	+	–	–	–	
Bupropion	75–150	300–450	–	–	–	+ Increased BP	+++	+++	2D6 inhibitor 1+
Bupropion SR *Wellbutrin SR*	100 (50 bid)	300–400 (used bid)	–	–	–	+ Increased BP	+++	+++	
Bupropion XL *Wellbutrin XL*	150	300–450	–	–	–	+ Increased BP	+++	+++	

2D6 = P450 2D6 pathway[23-25]; BP = blood pressure; QTc = corrected QT interval on an electrocardiogram where abnormal with increased risk for arrhythmias is > 470 in women and > 450 in men—especially risky when > 500, at which point medication should be discontinued; SNRI = serotonin-norepinephrine reuptake inhibitor; SSRI = selective serotonin reuptake inhibitor.

[a]For patients with *anxiety disorders* use **one-half the starting dose for depression.** For patients *older than 60 years*, the **therapeutic dose is reduced by one-half in the table above.**

[b]The following antidepressants should be avoided or used with great caution for the conditions listed because they often interact to increase the levels of medications commonly used for the condition[23-25]:

1. All SSRI/SNRI: (1) patients on anticoagulation; (2) patients using centrally acting appetite suppressants, eg, sibutramine, migraine taking 5HT agonists. *Use mirtazapine or bupropion to treat depression in these situations*

2. Paroxetine: patients on medications for constipation, for ADHD

3. Venlafaxine: patients at risk for arrhythmia, hypertension, on anticoagulation

4. Duloxetine: patients with difficult to control hypertension, on anticoagulation

5. Fluoxetine: patients with ADHD on stimulants

Also, be aware of need for dosage reductions in patients with comorbid liver and renal disease.

increase in serum levels of metoprolol, resulting in postural hypotension; this, in turn, may then be inadvertently attributed to the SSRI.[23-25] The full effect of a drug inhibitory interaction also may not be fully realized until it achieves a steady state. Since fluoxetine has a prolonged half-life, the peak effect on blood pressure may only be apparent 1 to 2 weeks following its initiation.

3. *Patient preference:* Even a patient who has never previously received a prescription for an antidepressant medication may have strong opinions about the efficacy and side effects of one drug over another.[3] As you recall from the MHCM, we need first to understand the patient and their concerns for a treatment to be successful. For example, direct-to-consumer advertising and personal stories about benefits and adverse effects may convey an understanding counter to scientific evidence. Also, some patients voice a strong preference for a nonsedating or weight sparing compound. Others express a preference for a medication that does not produce sexual dysfunction.

4. *Past history or family history of antidepressant response:* Make a detailed inventory of previous medications: duration, dosage, adverse effects, and response. It is reasonable to reinstitute an antidepressant that has worked in the past. However, if the patient has tried numerous drugs and failed to respond to any, or has experienced adverse effects, it is wise to choose a different agent from a different therapeutic class. For instance, a patient who has failed to respond to previous trials of the SSRIs fluoxetine, paroxetine, and citalopram, may benefit from an SNRI such as duloxetine or venlafaxine, rather than an alternative SSRI such as sertraline. Antidepressant responses are heritable and a history of response to a specific antidepressant in a first-degree relative may suggest an initial choice.

5. *Presence of concurrent psychiatric or medical disorders* (eg, panic disorder, neuropathic pain, hypertension): While we've said antidepressants are equally effective in the management of depression, they may vary somewhat in the spectrum of therapeutic activity. Food and Drug Administration (FDA) approval reflects this variation and it may be reasonable to begin with a medication they approve. For instance, while all SSRIs are commonly prescribed for panic disorder, only sertraline, paroxetine, and fluoxetine are approved for this indication. In addition to the depression spectrum, several of these medications have therapeutic impacts on various medical disorders. The SSRI paroxetine is approved for managing vasomotor symptoms in perimenopausal women. Bupropion is approved for smoking cessation and winter depression. In addition, it has demonstrated efficacy in the management of ADHD. SNRIs may be more effective in managing musculoskeletal and neuropathic pain syndromes. Duloxetine specifically has been reported effective in the treatment of stress urinary incontinence. Conversely, at high doses, the SNRI venlafaxine is associated with an elevation of blood pressure and should not be an initial choice in the patient with poorly controlled hypertension. Table 4-6 summarizes the current FDA approval status of several commonly used antidepressants.[26]

6. *Safety in overdose:* The old tricyclic antidepressants (TCA) fell into disfavor following the introduction of less toxic SSRIs, SNRIs, and the other new antidepressants. The medical consequences of a TCA drug overdose are more serious than overdose with the newer antidepressant compounds. For this reason, although of equivalent antidepressant effect, TCAs are not considered first-line agents any longer and are reserved for patients who fail to respond to several trials of newer and safer compounds. Similarly, the old monoamine oxidase inhibitors have severe side effect profiles, and we recommend that you never use them.

7. *Cost:* Considering that all antidepressants are equally effective it is reasonable to initiate treatment with an inexpensive generic formulation. All the SSRIs, the majority of SNRIs, mirtazapine, and bupropion are available in inexpensive generic formulations. There is no evidence that the newer, expensive antidepressant compounds are superior to generic agents.

8. *Gender:* Women are more susceptible to depression than men and experience more recurrences and treatment resistance. A variety of psychosocial and biological (neuroendocrine) factors have been implicated in this gender discrepancy. Treating depression during pregnancy and lactation requires knowledge of teratogenicity and fetal toxicity and the excretion of compounds in breast milk. Prenatal exposure to the SNRI venlafaxine is associated with an increased risk of hypertensive

TABLE 4-6. FDA Approval Status of Commonly Prescribed Antidepressants

	FDA INDICATIONS OTHER THAN MDD[a]
SSRIs	
Citalopram (Celexa)	
Escitalopram (Lexapro)	GAD
Sertraline (Zoloft)	OCD, PD, PTSD, PMDD, SAD
Fluoxetine (Prozac)	OCD, BN, PD
Paroxetine (Paxil)	OCD, PD, SAD, PTSD, GAD, PMDD,
SNRIs	
Venlafaxine (Effexor)	GAD, SAD, PD
Duloxetine (Cymbalta)	DNP, FM, GAD, CMP
Other New Antidepressants	
Bupropion (Wellbutrin, Zyban)	WD, SC
Trazodone (Desyrel)	
Mirtazapine (Remeron)	

BN = bulimia nervosa; CMP = chronic musculoskeletal pain; DNP = diabetic neuropathic pain; FDA = Food and Drug Administration; FM = fibromyalgia; GAD = generalized anxiety disorder; OCD = obsessive compulsive disorder; PD = panic disorder; PMDD = premenstrual dysphoric disorder; PTSD = posttraumatic stress disorder; SAD = social anxiety disorder; SC = smoking cessation; SNRI = serotonin-norepinephrine reuptake inhibitor; SSRI = selective serotonin reuptake inhibitor; WD = winter depression.

[a]All antidepressants are approved for major depressive disorder (MDD).

disorders of pregnancy. Paroxetine is associated with a higher risk of cardiovascular malformations as compared to other SSRIs. The pharmacokinetic profiles of breast milk excretion have been defined, and SSRIs sertraline and paroxetine are first line choices, but other medications also can be used because the effect on the infant is small. Mothers need not discontinue either breastfeeding or taking an antidepressant.[27]

Initial Medication Treatment. There are 3 essential considerations at the outset of treatment:

1. Avoiding early discontinuation
2. Reaching a therapeutic dose
3. Managing insomnia

In Table 4-7, we outline an initial medication treatment cycle using two different examples in patients with the common pattern of depression associated with insomnia. It highlights ensuring adherence, achieving a therapeutic dose, and managing insomnia. Finally, it indicates an endpoint of the treatment cycle at 8-12 weeks, as discussed later.

A critical first treatment goal is achieving adherence to medications. Following a diagnosis of depression, rates of early discontinuation exceed 30% for specialists as well as medical clinicians.[28] Adverse effects and the nocebo effect commonly lead patients to discontinue the medication, as does a poor clinician-patient relationship.[29]

A second major task of initial treatment is to ensure that you achieve a therapeutic dose of the antidepressant you selected. Research indicates that most clinicians fail to prescribe full therapeutic doses.[5,30] Table 4-5 depicts starting and therapeutic doses of the antidepressants, and Table 4-7 provides specific examples for ensuring full therapeutic doses of two different medications. We generally start with a subtherapeutic dose to reduce side effects and, consistent with its toleration, gradually increase to a full therapeutic dose.

A third important focus of initial management is insomnia, defined as needing more than 30 minutes to fall asleep (initial insomnia) or to get back to sleep after awakening (maintenance insomnia) or being unable to return to sleep after awakening (terminal insomnia). Insomnia is present in most depressed patients and is terribly debilitating. We need to get them sleeping through the night. This achievement alone makes patients feel much better, well before the antidepressant takes effect, and greatly enhances their trust in you and their cooperation with other aspects of treatment. As in the two examples in Table 4-7, we recommend 2 ways for addressing insomnia in addition to the sleep hygiene measures outlined as part of the MHCM in Chapter 3.

■ Mirtazapine has prominent sleep-promoting side effect and is a good choice for patients with prominent insomnia. You also may achieve lesser sedation with SSRIs sertraline, citalopram, and paroxetine.

TABLE 4-7. Initial Medication Treatment Issues

VISIT[a]	PHQ-9	KEY ISSUES[b]	DOSING EXAMPLE 1	DOSING EXAMPLE 2
Initial	≥ 10	Insomnia Explain adverse effects[c]	Sertraline 50 mg (subtherapeutic dose) Trazodone 50 mg	Mirtazapine 15 mg (low therapeutic dose)
Week 1	≥ 10	Insomnia Adverse effects (reduce dose)	Sertraline 75 mg (still subtherapeutic dose) Trazodone[d]: increase if not sleeping through night; reduce dose if too sleepy	Mirtazapine 15 mg: if too sleepy, change to SSRI or SNRI and use trazodone for sleep
Week 2	≥ 10	Insomnia Adverse effects	Sertraline 100 mg (low therapeutic dose) Adjust trazodone for sleep	Mirtazapine 30 mg (average therapeutic dose) (if sleepy, stay at 15 mg)
Week 3 or 4	Falling, rising Unchanged	Improvement? Nondrug treatment	Sertraline 100 mg (increase to 150 mg if no response) Adjust trazodone for sleep	Mirtazapine 30 mg (if sleepy, stay at 15 mg)
Week 5 or 6	Falling, rising Unchanged	Improvement? Nondrug treatment	No change unless need to adjust trazodone	No change unless need to adjust mirtazapine for sleep
Week 8-12[e] _decision time!_	1. < 10 2. ≥ 10 3. No change	1. Full remission 2. Partial remission 3. Nonremission	1. Continue present regimen 2. Increase sertraline to 200 or add "Other" medication 3. Completely change medication regimen	1. Continue present regimen 2. Increase mirtazapine to 45 mg or add SNRI or SSRI 3. Completely change medication regimen

PHQ-9 = Patient Health Questionnaire-9; SNRI = serotonin-norepinephrine reuptake inhibitor; SSRI = selective serotonin reuptake inhibitor.

[a]Office visits initially but phone calls may be used if the patient is stable; skilled office personnel can sometimes be helpful for stable patients.

[b]Always ask if suicidal and address immediately at any visit if present (see end of chapter).

[c]Tell patients the specific symptoms they likely will have, that they are transient, and to call if too bothersome so you can reduce the dose; tell them not to stop the medication.

[d]If too sleepy in mornings, take trazodone at supper instead of bedtime before reducing the dose.

[e]Decisions are made 8-12 weeks after achieving full antidepressant doses.

- Alternatively, you may want to avoid the weight gain that can occur with mirtazapine. In this case, we recommend trazodone. It is an atypical antidepressant with a sleep-promoting side effect so strong that trazodone cannot be used in antidepressant doses. It is useful, however, as a "sleeping pill" when used in conjunction with an SSRI or SNRI. We typically begin at 50 mg at bedtime and increase the dose once or twice weekly by 25 to 50 mg increments until the patient is sleeping through the night, seldom needing more than 100 to 150 mg. Trazodone sometimes can cause sleepiness in the mornings, and we address this by moving the dose from bedtime to several hours before bedtime, say, at supper time. Trazodone is given concurrently with the antidepressant you have selected to treat the depression.

We recommend weekly (or biweekly if the situation demands) contact until a full therapeutic dose is achieved, the patient is sleeping through the night, and there are no problems with adverse drug effects. Over the next 6 to 12 weeks, we advise contact every 2 weeks and then every 3 weeks for follow-up to monitor progress. Once stability is established, you can use the telephone for alternating contacts. Further, well-trained office personnel or professional care managers can sometimes handle visits and/or phone contacts in stable patients. Because depression is often comorbid with medical diseases, these must also be addressed, watching carefully for adverse impacts of the disorders and/or their medications on the depression.[3] At each contact, you must always check for suicidality and act immediately in its presence; see the end of this chapter on how to identify and manage the suicidal patient.

Recalling from Chapter 2 that depression is often comorbid with other psychiatric disorders,[3] we briefly mention the following, addressed in greater detail in Chapters 5 and 6, respectively.

Comorbid Anxiety. Managing concurrent anxiety in the depressed patient begins with determining whether the patient meets diagnostic criteria for an anxiety disorder, such as Generalized anxiety or panic disorder. Although SSRIs and SNRIs are also treatment for anxiety, they take 3 to 4 weeks to have an anti-anxiety (and anti-depressant) effect. To address the anxiety occurring in depression, you can combine the antidepressant with a brief course (2-4 weeks) of an adjunctive antianxiety agent. Benzodiazepines such as clonazepam (0.5 mg 2 times a day) produce a rapid anxiolytic effect, but have the limitations of sedation, tolerance, withdrawal, dependence, and misuse—if used chronically. Alternatives to benzodiazepines are preferred in patients with comorbid substance use disorders. Hydroxyzine, diphenhydramine, gabapentin, and pregabalin also may be effective and are not associated with tolerance, withdrawal, or misuse although gabapentin may potentiate opioid highs and has some street value. β-Blockers are also useful, particularly in patients with performance anxiety. Buspirone, which has an antidepressant effect as well, is approved also for managing generalized anxiety disorder (but not for panic disorder). Adjunctive anti-anxiety agents can be prescribed around the clock to prevent panic attacks, or as needed upon the earliest signs of anxiety. Prescribing them initially on a regular schedule is more effective, since the anticipation of panic often contributes to anxiety.

Comorbid Chronic Pain and Prescription Opioid Misuse. Chronic pain, is observed in many patients with depression.[31] The comorbidity of depression and chronic pain decreases the likelihood of response to treatment of either condition and decreases patient satisfaction with care. Adverse effects of opioid analgesics such as somnolence and cognitive dysfunction may confound symptoms commonly observed in depression—and opioids themselves cause depression with chronic use. Chapter 6 describes in detail how you first establish a scheduled (non-prn) dosing regimen of the opioid and then taper slowly by, say, one tablet per day every 1 to 2 weeks, for example from 4 tablets per day to 3 tablets per day of oxycodone. Often presenting primarily as a patient with a pain complaint, the associated depression is treated as outlined here—as one also attends to other aspects of the MHCM, especially the clinician-patient relationship and physical exercise. Resistance exercise training, for example, has been demonstrated to significantly reduce depressive symptoms.[32]

While we worked to prevent and educate the patient about adverse medication effects, we must also address them when they arise.

1. *Weight gain:* Weight gain is a common side effect with mirtazapine, but it may also occur with SSRIs and SNRIs. If life style interventions, such as physical exercise and diet, are ineffective, weight gain often requires changing to another antidepressant.

2. *Sexual dysfunction:* Sexual dysfunction is a leading cause of antidepressant nonadherence. Among all antidepressants, bupropion and mirtazapine have the lowest incidence. The sexual response cycle includes three phases: interest (libido), arousal (erection/lubrication) and orgasm. Depression itself impairs interest. Antidepressants can impair all phases of the sexual response cycle. Women often experience diminished arousal, while men complain of diminished libido and orgasm. Among SSRIs, paroxetine has the highest incidence of sexual dysfunction. Dose reduction and 48-hour drug holidays may help decrease these effects. Antidotes for drug-induced sexual dysfunction include buspirone, bupropion, and phosphodiesterase inhibitors sildenafil and tadalafil. We ordinarily try the latter group.

3. *Treatment-emergent activation syndrome:* Poorly defined, many perceive that patients placed on an antidepressant may experience an activation

syndrome from the antidepressant.[33] Symptoms include hyperactivity, irritability, agitation, and panic attacks. This condition is more commonly observed with SNRIs and is thought to be associated with enhanced noradrenergic activity. The presence of hypomanic features during an episode of major depression, which suggest an alternative diagnosis of bipolar disorder, increases the risk of inducing a treatment-emergent activation syndrome. Antidepressant-induced panic attacks and other anxiety manifestations can be managed with reducing the dose, later titrating slowly back into the therapeutic range. Induction of hypomanic features may require switching to a mood stabilizer and considering a diagnosis of bipolar disorder, discussed later in this chapter.

4. *Serotonin syndrome:* This side effect occurs from excessive doses of serotonin-containing antidepressants, usually when given together or sequentially without an adequate washout period (see Table 4-8 for switching antidepressants). Although it is uncommon, it can be life-threatening with hyperthermia, seizures, loss of consciousness, arrhythmias, and hypertension following myriad symptoms: nausea/vomiting, altered mental status with irritability and confusion, myoclonus and hyperreflexia, and ataxia. Management is supportive and often requires admission to the hospital intensive care unit. There is also overlap with the hypertensive crisis occurring when monamine oxidase inhibitors (MAOI) are combined with an SSRI or SNRI that has not had an adequate washout (eg, 2 or more weeks) before starting the MAOI; long-acting drugs like fluoxetine need a 6 to 8 week washout. Although it is important to know about this effect, we continue to recommend that you not use a MAOI. Non-antidepressant medications containing serotonin (triptans, tramadol, cocaine) also can cause serotonin syndrome when combined with an SSRI or SNRI.

5. *Discontinuation/withdrawal syndrome:* Do not stop antidepressants abruptly—and warn patients not to do so—when patients have been taking them for more than 4 to 6 weeks. With SSRIs and SNRIs (especially those with a short half-life and few metabolites, eg, venlafaxine, paroxetine) and with tricyclics, the following withdrawal syndrome may occur: depressed and anxious mood, nausea, vomiting, diarrhea, paresthesia, insomnia, headaches, vertigo,

TABLE 4-8. Switching Antidepressants

SWITCHING FROM	SWITCHING TO	
Tricyclic	SSRI or SNRI	Taper over 5-7 d; start new drug 2-3 d later
SSRI	SNRI	Taper over 2-5 d, then start SNRI; use lower dose if switch from fluoxetine; longer taper if high doses fluoxetine; monitor serotonin syndrome
SSRI	Different SSRI	Taper over 2-5 d, then start SSRI; use lower dose if switch from fluoxetine; longer taper if high doses fluoxetine; monitor serotonin syndrome
SNRI	SSRI	Taper over 2-5 d; then start SSRI
SNRI	Different SNRI	Taper over 2-5 d; then start new
Mirtazapine	Other drugs	Taper over 2-5 d; then start new
Other drugs	mirtazapine	Taper over 2-5 d; then start new
Bupropion	Other drugs	Taper over 1 *wk*; start new drug as usual the same time starting taper
Other drugs	Bupropion	Taper over 1-2 *wk* (2-3 for SNRI); gradually increase dose of bupropion during this time

SNRI = serotonin-norepinephrine reuptake inhibitor; SSRI = selective serotonin reuptake inhibitor.

tremor, ataxia, and sweating. While unpleasant, it is not life-threatening, unlike the serotonin syndrome above. Supportive treatment and/or reinstitution of the antidepressant resolves the withdrawal.

Determining Future Treatment at the 8- to 12-Week Endpoint. In summary, from Table 4-7, to this point, you have learned that we see patients every 1 to 2 weeks initially, extending later to 2- to 3-week intervals if they are improving and stable. At the initial visit, we start at a subtherapeutic or low therapeutic dose of an antidepressant and soon increase to full therapeutic doses.

What's the endpoint? We seek **full remission by 8 to 12 weeks.**[3] *Full remission* means complete clearing of symptoms and return to full functional status, signaled by a PHQ-9 less than 10 and often less than 5. A *partial remission* is defined as a PHQ-9 that has fallen by 5 to 15 points but not to 10 or lower. *Nonremission* means there has been no clinical improvement and little change, if any, on the PHQ-9. Based on the extensive research findings of the STAR*D trial, we do the following at 8 to 12 weeks, summarized in the last row of Table 4-7.[3,34,35]

1. *Full remission:* Continue the same regimen and follow every 2 to 6 weeks, depending on continued improvement and stability and the needs of comorbid problems. Data indicate that about 35% to 40% will achieve full remission after a trial with a full dose of one antidepressant.

2. *Partial remission:* In the presence of an incomplete response, one first ensures that the following are not responsible: nonadherence to medications, substance use problem, an alternative diagnosis (especially bipolar disorder); a causative medical disorder and/or its treatments.

   - With a partial remission, if not already at maximum therapeutic doses, you can increase the present antidepressant to that level. Alternatively, if at maximum or near maximum therapeutic dose range, add a second antidepressant from another class—*but do not combine an SNRI with an SSRI.* That is, satisfactory combinations are SSRI-Other and SNRI-Other. One then proceeds in a similar fashion as in the first 8 to 12 weeks by adding the new antidepressant, continuing to monitor response and side effects.
   - If there has been no further improvement over the second 8 to 12 weeks, we recommend referral to a psychiatrist for consultation regarding medications and/or alternative treatments, such as antipsychotics or electroshock. One also would consider this referral sooner in very depressed

patients who have responded only partially, particularly if elderly and/or if there is any question of suicidality. As discussed later, all depressed patients also should be offered psychotherapy initially, from a psychologist or other counselor, and it would be especially appropriate if there has been no remission on medications if the patient had not already begun counseling.

3. *Nonremission:* Again, first ensuring there is no alternative explanation for failure to respond, we discontinue the initial medication, following the schedule in Table 4-8 and then begin with a medication from a different class. We follow the patient as outlined in the first 8- to 12-week treatment course. Nonremission or partial remission at the next 8- to 12-week point indicates the need for consultation from a psychiatrist for medications and/or alternative treatments. As before, we make referrals sooner in the more severe and minimally responsive patients.

Data indicate that we can expect another 15% to 20% to have responded after the second trial of an antidepressant, for a total full remission rate at 16 to 24 weeks of 50% to 60%.[3,34,35] Unfortunately, this rate does not include relapses, so that the relapse-free rate is only 43%.[35]

Long-Term Treatment. For those who have responded, data indicate that with a first bout of depression, you can stop the medication from 4 to 12 months after achieving full remission. However, recurrence is common. About 50% to 60% of those will recur with a second episode, one-third of them within 12 months. In this case, you retreat as described above. If you and the patient decide to discontinue medications again following a second remission, the recurrence rate is now higher, in the range of 80% to 90%. If there is another recurrence, most recommend lifelong treatment with the antidepressant.

Additional Measures. There are augmentation strategies you can use to supplement your treatment, particularly if you cannot obtain consultation with a psychiatrist for medication suggestions or alternative treatments. These treatments are summarized in Table 4-9.

How Your Psychiatry Consultant Can Help You. The indications for referral are summarized in Table 4-10.[18] Patients who experience nonresponse

TABLE 4-9. Augmentation Strategies

1. Anxiety and chronic pain—see earlier discussion
2. Atypical antipsychotics (AAP)—for refractory depression; doses discussed later in this chapter for bipolar disorder. AAP are not used primarily in treating depression.
3. Fatigued, immobilized—stimulants like thyroid, low-dose amphetamines
4. Perimenopausal—estrogen
5. Male hypogonadism—testosterone

to 2 consecutively adequate trials of antidepressants in 2 different drug classes are considered *treatment-resistant*.[3,35] Of patients with major depression, 30% to 40% have treatment-resistance—especially high with comorbid medical and/or psychiatric disorders.[3,34,35]

■ *Pharmacogenetic testing*: A growing consensus suggests that pharmacogenetic testing may be useful in guiding treatment choice in resistant cases. It can identify ultrarapid metabolizers, who may require doses of antidepressants that exceed the recommended range, as compared to poor metabolizers, who may develop adverse effects from conventional doses and require lower than usual doses.

■ *Addressing comorbid addiction problems*: It is not uncommon that patients with addiction problems require referral for detoxification, either inpatient or outpatient. Indeed, the presence of depression is a risk factor predicting chronic opioid use.[36] Alternatively, chronic opioid use is associated with treatment resistant depression[37] and new onset depression.[38] Not surprising, removing addictive substances may cure the depression and other mental health disorders. Addiction specialists also may conduct detoxification clinics with methadone or buprenorphine. Unless specifically trained, medical clinicians cannot undertake these activities.

TABLE 4-10. Indications for Referral to Psychiatry

1. Treatment-resistance
2. Suicidal ideation
3. Psychotic symptoms, including Bipolar Disorder-I
4. Substance use disorder
5. Neuromodulation, such as electroconvulsive therapy (ECT)
6. Patient's request

■ *Neuromodulation*: Patients that fail to achieve remission with medication combinations and psychotherapy (see next) may benefit from neuromodulation therapy.

a. *Electroconvulsive therapy (ECT)*: Electroconvulsive therapy is the most effective treatment for managing treatment-resistant mood disorders, and it is the most effective approach in patients who have failed to respond to 2 consecutive antidepressant trials.[39] As well, recent data indicate it is cost-effective after failure of 2 or more lines of other treatment.[40] It is also more effective than other available neurostimulation procedures such as vagal nerve stimulation and repetitive transcranial magnetic stimulation. When performed under accepted protocols it is safe. It involves the application of a modified electric pulse, between 2 scalp electrodes, that induces a generalized convulsive seizure, which is suppressed with a muscle relaxant. Contrary to a belief that ECT produces brain damage, it appears to enhance neurogenesis and neural plasticity. Considering the worldwide prevalence of disabling treatment-resistant depression, it is troublesome that the most effective treatment is seldom considered.[39] In patients with severe depression who are not treatment resistant, the response rate in 70%, while in treatment resistant patients, the response rate is 58%.[41]

b. *Vagal nerve stimulation* is also approved by the FDA for the management of depression that has failed to respond to at least 2 consecutive antidepressant trials. A permanent neurosurgical procedure, it involves the stimulation of the afferent vagal nerve, indirectly altering the neural circuits involved in the pathophysiology of depression. Despite its efficacy and safety, it is not widely used, largely because of restricted insurance payment for this surgical procedure.

c. *Repetitive transcranial magnetic stimulation* (RTMS) is well-established as an effective treatment for medication resistant depression. It uses alternating magnetic fields to induce an electric current in the brain and immediately induces activation in subcortical limbic regions, as well as cortical areas directly beneath the coil. Unlike ECT, RTMS does not require anesthesia. This modality is used infrequently, largely because of limited availability and limited insurance coverage.

    d. *Transcranial direct current stimulation* is an investigational procedure that is increasingly used by patients given its easy availability and low cost.

How Nonpsychiatry Mental Health Professionals Can Help You. We have been highlighting the use of the MHCM and medications as your primary avenue for caring for depressed patients. We then indicated how psychiatry consultation can be helpful in the more difficult patient.

    An additional, powerful treatment modality that is as effective, or more so, than antidepressants is psychotherapy.[3,42] Used in combination with medications, psychotherapy can have a significant additive impact on the outcomes of depression. Indeed, many believe it is more than additive. **All depressed patients should be offered psychotherapy at the outset** because of its powerful impact. For patients who refuse, we offer it regularly during the course of treatment. Therapy is useful not just for difficult problems. It also can play a role in patients who respond to medications by helping them address problematic personal issues that may play a role in their depression. Consider its potential impact in addition to using the MHCM and medications.

    Importantly, we do not advise you to conduct psychotherapy yourself without specific training. There are many other skilled mental health professionals (MHPs) who can provide this treatment, for example psychologists, medical social workers, psychiatric social workers, and other counselors trained specifically for certain situations, for example grief, adolescence, substance abuse, or end of life. In Table 4-11, we summarize the indications for referral.[18]

    The form of therapy proven to be of most benefit and used by many therapists is cognitive-behavioral therapy (CBT). There are, however, many other forms

---

TABLE 4-11. Indications for Referral to Nonpsychiatry Mental Health Professionals

1. Depression, refer initially or later in treatment
2. Prominent interpersonal problems
3. Comorbid substance use disorder
4. Prolonged grief
5. Comorbid panic disorder
6. Medically unexplained symptoms and chronic pain
7. The patient's request

---

of proven value, for example grief therapy, insight psychotherapy, supportive psychotherapy, family therapy, mindfulness therapy, and interpersonal therapy. It is outside the scope of this text to review them, but it is important to know about the role of psychotherapy in depression management and encouraging patients to accept a referral.

    Then, once the patient is in therapy, continue seeing the patient and inquire about how the consultation is proceeding. Stay in touch with the consultant and let your patient know you are interested in that aspect of treatment as well.

OTHER DEPRESSION SYNDROMES

This group of disorders is characterized by depression, but each has unique features diagnostically.[6] While treatment is much the same as already outlined, there also are some unique modalities that can be helpful. We review them here briefly.

Persistent Depressive Disorder (Dysthymia)

Dysthymia, sometimes called chronic depression, is characterized by a depressed mood that occurs for most of the day for at least 2 years. The 12-month prevalence of this condition in the United States is estimated at 0.5%. Treatment is as outlined for major depressive disorders, but it often is less effective. Refractory cases merit referral.

Adjustment Disorder With Depressed Mood

In these patients, the depressive syndrome begins within 3 months of an identifiable stressor of any type and, characteristically, is out of proportion to the apparent magnitude of the stressor. Treatment with antidepressants and psychotherapy (to address the stressor) is indicated.

Persistent Complex Bereavement Disorder

Previously described as prolonged or pathological grief, this depressive syndrome lasts 12 months or longer after the death of a loved one. Unique symptoms include (1) intense sorrow and emotional pain, (2) yearning for the deceased, (3) preoccupation with the deceased, (4) a desire to die to be with the deceased, and (5) impairment of social or occupational function. Treatment with antidepressants has been helpful, and counseling targeting the grief reaction is indicated.

Premenstrual Dysphoric Disorder

The essential features include mood lability, irritability, dysphoria, and anxiety symptoms that occur during the premenstrual phase of the cycle and remit upon the onset of menses. The 12-month prevalence of premenstrual dysphoric disorder is between 1.8% and 5.8% in menstruating women. Many patients with this condition also experience major depressive disorder, at which point antidepressant treatment is effective.

Perimenopausal Depression

As many as 70% of perimenopausal women report depressive symptoms. Changes in hormones, psychosocial stress, and the burden of physical illness have all been implicated. Estrogen is known to enhance levels of neurotransmitters and the antidepressant effects of supplemental estrogen are comparable to those of antidepressants—if the woman also meets criteria for depression. We are not, however, suggesting use of estrogen alone for treatment of perimenopausal depression. Estrogen is not a mood enhancer in depression-free women or in postmenopausal women.

Late-Age Onset Depression and Vascular Depression

An emerging body of literature implicates coronary risk factors, such as hypertension, diabetes, dyslipidemia, cigarette smoking, and obesity, in the pathogenesis of "vascular" depression. The vascular depression hypothesis initially emerged with the discovery that depression with an onset in late life is commonly associated with subcortical and periventricular white matter hyperintensity lesions visualized on magnetic resonance imaging, suggesting microvascular pathology. This is a condition distinguished by apathy, executive function deficits, and resistance to antidepressant treatment. At least one promising study has suggested that lowering blood pressure reduces the progression of white matter lesions. Whereas the vascular depression hypothesis has focused exclusively on depression with an onset in late life, vascular risk factors may be equally relevant in the pathogenesis and course of depression in younger individuals.

Seasonal Affective Disorder (Winter Depression)

The 2 variants of seasonal affective disorder include (1) seasonal exacerbation of long-standing major depressive disorder or persistent depressive disorder (dysthymia), and (2) isolated winter depression that emerges in the fall and resolves in the spring. The condition is related to advanced or delayed circadian rhythms induced by seasonal changes. Winter depression is distinguished by a low mood, hypersomnia, excessive appetite, and weight gain. Patients benefit from consultation to obtain light therapy as well as from melatonin and bupropion. Alternatively, the clinician can recommend patients buy the light box (does not require consultation) and instruct them to work in front of it for about 30 minutes each morning.

Postpartum Depression and Blues

A spectrum of mood disorders is observed in the months following childbirth or pregnancy loss. *Postpartum blues* is a transient state, characterized by heightened emotional reactivity, tearfulness, emotional lability, and irritability. It occurs in 50% of women, following childbirth. *Nonpsychotic postpartum depression* occurs in 10% to 20% of women. *Psychotic postpartum depression*, is often associated with impulses to harm the infant. Depression also often occurs following pregnancy loss. In 50% of cases, postpartum depression has its onset during pregnancy. This provides an opportunity to intervene during pregnancy. See earlier section on treatment during pregnancy and lactation.

Depression Related to a Medical Illness

Depression is commonly associated with medical illness and the medications used to treat it; see Table 4-12. Seventy-five percent of patients with persistent depressive disorder (dysthymia) have a chronic physical illness.

Substance/Medication-Induced Depression

This is a pervasive and persistent disorder of mood or markedly diminished interest or pleasure, caused by intoxication with, chronic use of, or withdrawal from many addicting substances. Most of these patients will require referral for detoxification, if your efforts fail. Chapter 6 describes your initial approach.

Disruptive Mood Dysregulation Disorder

Disruptive mood dysregulation disorder is a childhood onset depressive disorder characterized by (1) frequent temper outbursts and (2) chronic and

TABLE 4-12. Physical Conditions and Medications Commonly Associated With Depressive Symptoms

DISEASES	MEDICATIONS
Hypothyroidism	Hormonal agents (corticosteroids, tamoxifen)
Anemia	
Chronic obstructive airways disease	Antiviral agents (efavirenz)
Chronic pain	Immunologic agents (interferon)
Chronic kidney disease	
Cancer	Antimigraine (triptans)
Cardiovascular diseases	Retinoic acid derivatives (isotretinoin)
Neurologic diseases (Parkinson disease, stroke, dementia)	Opioids
Obstructive sleep apnea	
Diabetes	

persistent irritability or angry mood between severe temper outbursts. The overall 12 month prevalence of disruptive mood dysregulation disorder among children and adolescents is 2% to 5%. It is more common among males than females.

BIPOLAR DISORDER

Bipolar disorder is an episodic and recurrent disorder, characterized by manic or hypomanic episodes in addition to depression. While included in a chapter on depression, recent genetic evidence suggests it may be more closely related to schizophrenia.[6,15] Subdivided into 2 categories, bipolar I disorder has a lifetime prevalence of 1.0% and is defined by the patient having experienced at least 1 *manic episode*. Bipolar II disorder has a lifetime prevalence of 0.8% and is defined by patients having at least 1 *hypomanic episode*. The depressive phase of either type of bipolar disorder is indistinguishable from that of major depression and typically precedes the first hypomanic or manic episode.

Diagnosis. You need to identify hypomanic and manic episodes to make a diagnosis of bipolar disorder. Bear with us here on an important but complex definition.[6] A **manic episode** is a distinct period of abnormally and persistently elevated, expansive, or irritable mood and abnormally and persistently increased goal-directed activity or energy that lasts *at least 7 days* and is present most of the day nearly every day with impairment

of occupational and/or social functioning. It may be of shorter duration if severe enough to result in hospitalization. Mania is characterized by (1) inflated self-esteem or grandiosity, (2) decreased need for sleep, (3) pressured speech or more talkative than usual, (4) racing thoughts (flight of ideas), (5) distractibility, (6) hyperactivity with increased goal-directed actions (social, work, school, sexual) or agitation with purposeless non-goal directed actions, and (7) excessive involvement in activities with painful consequences such as extravagant spending, sexual indiscretion, or ill-advised business investments. A DSM-5 diagnosis requires three or more of these behaviors.

A **hypomanic episode** is defined similarly except the duration of symptoms need only be *4 days*, and it is less severe, does not cause the marked impairment in occupational and social functioning of a manic episode, and does not require hospitalization or have psychotic features.

In general, bipolar I disorder will be easier to recognize because of its more florid, psychotic presentation and dysfunction. Bipolar II has been more difficult to recognize and often goes untreated. Both, however, are equally disruptive to patients from a functional perspective and one should not be viewed as more severe than the other. Failure to make a diagnosis can have grave consequences not only for work and social functioning but also because of high suicide rates of 1% annually, 20 times the general population rate.[43]

Screening Diagnostic Tools. Screening tools for bipolar disorders can be helpful in medical settings. We have found the screener in Table 4-13, reproduced graphically in Figure 4-2, to be very useful in our clinics and that it takes no more than 3 to 4 minutes once you become familiar with it.[44] It is not as complicated as it appears. The 2-stem questions ask about emotions or feelings of euphoria and/or irritability, while the criterion B screening question asks about thoughts and behaviors associated with 1 or both of the first 2. Only if there is a "YES" score on 1 (or 2) of the first 2 and on number 3, the Criterion B Screening Question, do you proceed to ask the later Criterion B Symptom Questions. The number of the latter then provides the score that gives us the risk of a bipolar disorder. Importantly, this questionnaire stems from the reliable, valid World Health Organization Composite International Diagnostic Interview (WHO-CIDI), which, in turn, is closely related to actual clinical evaluations by experts.[44]

TABLE 4-13. Screening for Bipolar Disorders

Stem Questions

1. EUPHORIA STEM QUESTION.

   Some people have periods lasting several days when they feel much more excited and full of energy than usual. Their minds go too fast. They talk a lot. They are very restless or unable to sit still and they sometimes do things that are unusual for them, such as driving too fast or spending too much money.

   Have you ever had a period like this lasting several days or longer?

   If this question is endorsed, the next question (the irritability stem question) is skipped and the respondent goes directly to the criterion B screening question.

2. IRRITABILITY STEM QUESTION.

   Have you ever had a period lasting several days or longer when most of the time you were so irritable or grouchy that you either started arguments, shouted at people or hit people?

   If neither question is endorsed, stop questioning.

Criterion B Screening Question

3. People who have episodes like this often have changes in their thinking and behavior at the same time, like being more talkative, needing very little sleep, being very restless, going on buying sprees, and behaving in many ways they would normally think inappropriate. Did you ever have any of these changes during your episodes of being excited and full of energy or very irritable or grouchy?

   Respondents who fail to endorse this question after endorsing one of the first 2 stem questions (above) are skipped out of the remaining questions.

   Respondents who endorse this question are then administered the 9 additional symptom questions.

Criterion B Symptom Questions

Think of an episode when you had the largest number of changes like these at the same time. During that episode, which of the following changes did you experience?

- Were you so irritable that you either started arguments, shouted at people, or hit people?
  - *This first symptom question is asked only if the euphoria stem question (#1 above) is endorsed.*
- You became so restless or fidgety that you paced up and down or couldn't stand still?
- Did you do anything else that wasn't usual for you—like talking about things you would normally keep private, or acting in ways that would usually find embarrassing?
- Did you try to do things that were impossible to do, like taking on large amounts of work?
- Did you constantly keep changing your plans or activities?
- Did you find it hard to keep your mind on what you were doing?
- Did your thoughts seem to jump from one thing to another or race through your head so fast you couldn't keep track of them?
- Did you sleep far less than usual and still not get tired or sleepy?
- Did you spend so much more money than usual that it caused you to have financial trouble?

Scoring

Add the number of positive (YES) responses on the symptom questions 1-9 (or 8)

     9 YES—very high risk (80% or more)

     7-8 YES—high risk (50%-79%)

     6 YES—moderate risk (25%-49%)

     5 YES—low risk (5%-24%)

     0-4 YES—very low risk (>5%)

Differential Diagnosis

1. *Major depressive disorder*, also called "unipolar" depression to denote the absence of mania or hypomania in a diagnosis of bipolar disorder, is the most important differential. Making this distinction is not easy because most patients with either type of bipolar disorder present initially with depression. Until they have a manic or hypomanic episode, the bipolar diagnosis cannot be made, and they are diagnosed and treated almost always as major depressive disorder.

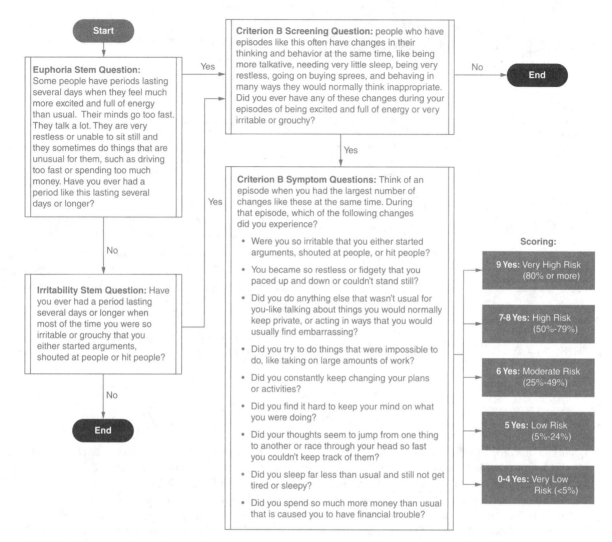

FIGURE 4-2. Screening for bipolar disorders.

There are some clues that will raise your suspicion for bipolar depression in patients who seem to have a diagnosis of unipolar depression. Table 4-14 outlines these. For example, be suspicious of any unipolar depression diagnosis in: young people with the sudden onset of depression, especially if there is a family history of bipolar disorder or any other psychiatric disorder, including a "nervous breakdown." Be even more suspicious if there have been multiple episodes and treatment with antidepressants has not been effective—or seemed to make them worse. Recent data also indicate that diagnoses of ADHD and anxiety disorders may predispose

to a subsequent bipolar diagnosis, particularly if both are present.[45]

How common is this problem? In one study, from 16.1% to 47% of patients diagnosed as having major depressive episodes had multiple symptoms of bipolar disorders.[46] If you are effectively diagnosing depression, you will see patients with bipolar disorders, particularly in the younger population.

2. *Other considerations* in patients with mood swings and irritability. When you have concerns about these alternative psychiatric diagnoses, psychiatric consultation is almost always needed.

TABLE 4-14. Distinguishing Unipolar and Bipolar Depressive Disorders

	UNIPOLAR DEPRESSION	BIPOLAR DEPRESSION
Age onset	30 and older	Teens to 30s
Family history	Sometimes	Very often (includes other psychiatric disorders also)
Type of onset	Gradual	Abrupt
Number of episodes	Less frequent	Many
Response to antidepressants	Good	Poor
Gender	Females > males	Females = males
Sleep	Insomnia primarily	May have hypersomnia. May be sleepless for many days

a. *Substance use disorder*—including delirium and other manifestations of withdrawal. Addictions are highly prevalent in bipolar disorders and have a tremendous impact on outcome.[47] Indeed, it is difficult to conclusively make a diagnosis of a bipolar (or unipolar) disorder until substances, such as alcohol, illicit drugs, and prescription drugs (opioids, benzodiazepines, amphetamines) have been excluded as the cause. If they are potential contributors to symptoms, as they often are, the diagnosis of a bipolar disorder is most accurately made only after complete tapering and discontinuation of the substance involved for 3 to 6 months.

b. *Other psychiatric disorders*
   - *Borderline personality disorder*—mood swings here typically are much briefer and do not meet criteria for a bipolar disorder; see Chapter 10 on personality disorders.
   - *Adult attention-deficit/hyperactivity disorder* (ADHD)—this almost always begins in childhood and this history is required before making an ADHD diagnosis.[48] Again, these patients typically do not meet the duration of symptoms criteria for a bipolar disorder. See Chapter 8.
   - *Schizophrenia and schizoaffective disorders*—bipolar I disorder with psychotic manifestations can provide confusion. Noted earlier, these are closely related disorders, especially genetically.[6,15] See Chapter 9.
   - *Major depression with psychotic features*—this disorder also can pose difficult diagnostic problems and requires a psychiatrist to make the distinction.

c. *Medical conditions*—underlying medical conditions are uncommon but important considerations, for example uncontrolled hyperthyroidism including thyrotoxic storm, frontal lobe disorders; medications such as thyroid, corticosteroids, isoniazid, and levodopa.

Treatment. Medical clinicians will not usually be handling bipolar I patients during the manic phase. This disorder requires psychiatric consultation and inpatient management. As well, most of these patients require subsequent outpatient management by a psychiatrist. You will be able to co-manage the medical issues and monitor for recurrence and deterioration. Because bipolar I disorder typically presents with an apparent unipolar depression, however, your most important role for these patients is diagnosing the manic episode that heralds an onset of the bipolar disorder.

Your focus will be more on the patients with bipolar II disorder, those with hypomania. Not only will you be able to diagnose these patients but, given the dearth of psychiatrists for consultation,[2] you will also often need to treat them and follow them long-term.[49] We now outline a treatment plan.

Treatment must address three overarching dimensions: (1) hypomania, (2) depression, and (3) maintaining a symptom-free state once achieved. We do not recommend lithium because of its narrow therapeutic window and the need for extensive laboratory monitoring. Instead, we recommend treatment using other mood stabilizers and atypical antipsychotics:

- *Atypical antipsychotics (AAPs)*: AAPs are used to control the hypomanic symptoms. As well, some agents, such as quetiapine, also address depressive symptoms and can be used for maintenance. Table 4-15 summarizes the key pharmacological information

TABLE 4-15. Use of Atypical Antipsychotic Medications for Bipolar Disorders

	INDICATIONS	STARTING DOSE (mg/d)	SCHEDULE OF UPTITRATION	TARGET DOSE (mg/d)	EPS[b]	ORTHOSTATIC HYPOTENSION	METABOLIC EFFECT	SEDATION
Quetiapine XR *Seroquel XR*	Mania/hypomania Depression Maintenance	100 at bedtime	Increase every 2-3 d as BP tolerates	300-800 300-600 (for depression)[a]	+/−	+++	++	+++
Risperidone[c] *Risperdal*	Mania/hypomania	2 at bedtime	Increase 1 mg/d as tolerated	4-6	++	++	++	++
Aripiprazole *Abilify*	Mania/hypomania	10 in AM	Increase by 5-10 every 2 d as tolerated	10-30	+	+	+	+
Ziprasidone[d] *Geodon*	Mania/hypomania	20 twice/day with food	Increase by 20 mg every 2 d as tolerated	160	+	+	+	++
Olanzapine *Zyprexa*	Mania/hypomania Maintenance	5 at bedtime	Increase 5 mg/ wk as tolerated	10-20	+	+/−	+++	++

BP = blood pressure; EPS = extrapyramidal syndrome.

Note: Elderly patients and those with comorbid renal or hepatic disease should be started at one-half the above dose recommendations.

[a]When quetiapine is used to augment unipolar depression, the target dose is 150-300 mg/d.

[b]See Chapter 9 for details of the side effects.

[c]May have marked prolactin increase; if clinical suspicion, obtain levels.

[d]May prolong QTc (corrected QT interval on baseline ECG); if rises above > 500 ms, discontinue medication.

for various AAPs: their indication (for mania/hypomania, depression, maintenance), starting dose, uptitration of dose, target dose, and side effects. With the starting doses indicated, you can rather quickly up-titrate to the target dose. We recommend you target the lower therapeutic dose and observe for effective control of the hypomanic symptoms. If incomplete control of symptoms (look especially for irritability, depression, racing ideas, and insomnia), then increase the dose gradually. Because of prominent metabolic effects from many of the AAPs, we recommend careful observation, beginning with baseline weight and BMI, lipid profile, and blood sugar/glycohemoglobin. We follow these parameters every 4 weeks for the first 3 months, then annually; also obtain prolactin levels if there is a clinical indication. See Chapter 9 for a full review of side effects of AAPs and their management.

■ *Mood stabilizer:* A mood stabilizer is often administered concurrently with the AAP during the initial hypomanic phase to initiate maintenance treatment. Some agents, like lamotrigine, are also used to manage the depressive component. Table 4-16 summarizes the important pharmacological information you will need: indications, starting dose, uptitration of dose, target dose, and side effects. Rare side effects are the reason for the slow uptitration.

Antidepressants should not be used for treatment of bipolar disorders except as noted later. If the patient is already on them, which is often the case, it is best to reduce the dose or taper and discontinue them altogether.

TABLE 4-16. Use of Mood Stabilizing Medications for Bipolar Disorders

	INDICATIONS	STARTING DOSE (mg/d)	TITRATION	TARGET DOSE	SIDE EFFECTS	COMMENT
Lamotrigine *Lamictal*	Depression Maintenance	25 daily	25/d × 2 wk; then 50/d × 2 wk; then 100/d × 2 wk, then 200/d	200-300 per day	Stevens-Johnson syndrome "Rash" Hepatitis Anemia, leukopenia, thrombocytopenia	Instruct patients to report any rash immediately
Divalproex sodium *Depakote*	Mania/ hypomania Maintenance	500-1000 twice daily	Reaches steady state in 5 d; can increase 500-1000/d as tolerated	Serum valproic acid level of 85-125 µg/mL	Encephalopathy Increased ammonia Thrombocytopenia Hepatitis, pancreatitis Sedation, weight gain, tremor	Obtain at baseline and every 3 mo: valproic acid level, liver functions, and CBC
Carbamazepine *Tegretol*	Mania/ hypomania Maintenance	200 ER twice daily	Reaches steady state in 3-4 d; increase by 200/d as tolerated; maximum = 1600/d		Stevens-Johnson syndrome Hyponatremia Hepatitis Pancytopenia Vertigo, somnolence	Obtain at baseline and every 3 months: carbamazepine level, serum sodium, liver functions, and CBC

Patients are followed initially at weekly intervals, increasing the intervals as improvement and stability of hypomania and depression are established. Managing side effects carefully, you increase the AAP until the hypomania is controlled. You are simultaneously increasing the mood stabilizer so that the maintenance impact is beginning. But it also is essential to treat the depression. You will see from the tables that quetiapine and lamotrigine both have antidepressant effects as well.

Because of this, we recommend beginning treatment for most type II bipolar disorder patients with these two medications using the doses in the tables. Acutely, patients will be receiving good anti-hypomania and antidepressant coverage with the quetiapine. At the same time, you can gradually increase the lamotrigine dose, as outlined, while the slow uptitration enables you to offset the potential of serious adverse effects like the Stevens-Johnson syndrome. Because the quetiapine provides maintenance coverage as well, there is no hurry in getting the lamotrigine dose to target levels. After 3 to 4 months of control of the hypomania and depression, the quetiapine can be tapered and discontinued, consistent with continued control. The lamotrigine will now be at full dose and can be counted on to handle both the antidepressant and maintenance functions. If hypomania or depression recurs, resume the quetiapine and continue the lamotrigine. These can be continued indefinitely or another attempt can be made to taper and discontinue the quetiapine. If used indefinitely, try to lower the doses of both agents, consistent with continued control.

If depression persists, an antidepressant can be used, raising the risk of provoking a switch from depression to hypomania; this is less likely in the bipolar II disorder patient. Bupropion or an SSRI have had the lowest likelihood of triggering a hypomanic episode. It is at this point, however, that you should consider psychiatric referral for medication consultation and possible ECT.

Long-term management can be a challenge with many patients experiencing relapses, often associated with prominent non-adherence to medications and to follow-up visits. For maximizing adherence and maintenance of control, the MHCM and its principles apply particularly well. As well, psychotherapy has been a powerful adjunct to management using therapists familiar with bipolar disorder. Often, multiple providers are involved in monitoring successful control.

All must watch carefully for evidence of relapse—and inform the patient and their family to do so also—particularly any signs of increased irritability, racing thoughts, depression, and sleep difficulties. During visits with various providers, we check for medication adherence and side effects, substance use, suicidality, insomnia, any mood change, and the status of their present life and stresses. We always strongly urge that the patient observe careful sleep hygiene because lack of sleep can induce hypomania. Just as important is avoidance of addicting substances.

In ending this section on bipolar disorders, it is important to remind you of the key role played by the MHCM. Its focus on a strong clinician-patient relationship, educating the patient, obtaining a commitment to treatment, establishing their goals, and respectful negotiation of the treatment plan is the key to successfully managing patients with the bipolar disorders.

SUICIDE

There are more than 40,000 deaths by suicide in the United States each year, a rate so high that suicide is the tenth leading overall cause of death in this country, and it continues to increase.[50] Men, using deadlier means, are about twice as likely as women to commit suicide, although women make more attempts. The greatest number of deaths by suicide are in the 75+ range for men and the 45 to 64 age range for women. Just as alarming, suicide is the second leading cause of death in the 15 to 34 age range. The highest rates of suicide are Native Americans and Alaskan Natives > non-Hispanic whites > Hispanics > African Americans.[51] Worldwide, there are more than 800,000 deaths yearly, amounting to 1.4% of all deaths.[52] Many, however, believe these data are considerably underestimated.[53] There are about 20 to 30 times as many attempts as completed suicides.[52] Approximately 5% of any community will have an attempted suicide at least once.[54] Recent increases in the suicide rate are concerning and preferentially have involved young adults with less formal education[55] and those with antisocial personality disorder, anxiety disorders, depressive disorders, and a history of violence.[50] These risk factors (mental health disorders) are present in greater than 90% of people who commit suicide.[18] About 45% of patients dying of suicide have seen a medical clinician in the month beforehand, and as many as three-fourths saw one in the preceding year, suggesting that increased awareness on the part of health care providers could have a powerful preventive impact.[18,56]

Fortunately, there is mounting evidence, compared to 2005, for the effectiveness of interventions that can prevent death by suicide. These include (1) restricting access to lethal means; (2) using antidepressants for depressed patients—especially the elderly, children, and adolescents; (3) using ECT early rather than as a last resort; (4) providing psychotherapy; (5) careful follow-up of those making an attempt; (6) making mental health services available; and (7) implementing school-based mental health and suicide awareness efforts.[52]

The National Institute of Mental Health (NIMH) has summarized the *risk factors* for suicide that should raise your concerns whenever present in your patients, especially when more than 1 is present (Table 4-17).[51] Notice that mental disorders are listed first. The greatest risk occurs in patients with major depressive disorder and bipolar disorder—the subjects of this chapter. They are 20 times more likely, compared to people with no mental disorder, to commit suicide.[43] Indeed, the rate for patients with a psychiatric disorder of lifetime suicidal attempts as high as 29%, and the mortality rate from suicide is 2% to 15% in those with depressive disorders, and up to 15% to 20% in those who ever have been hospitalized for a mental disorder.[54]

Consider the impact then of some common *precipitating factors*: recent loss (spouse, job), worsening of mental and substance use disorders, and worsening medical disease. Suicide rates are high in substance use disorders, especially with adverse acute events, sometimes occasioned by patients' substance use. There are, however, some well-recognized *protective factors*: social support, religious affiliation, being married, and children in the household. This points to the therapeutic value of providing support yourself to patients with a mental health disorder. Many have become very isolated, and you may be the only person relating to them.

Let's look now at how to make a diagnosis and manage suicidality.

Screening. For brief screening purposes, the P4 screening inventory can be useful for clinicians, as outlined in Table 4-18.[57] It provides an algorithm for assessing the four Ps: **p**ast suicide attempts, suicide **p**lan, **p**robability of completing suicide, and **p**reventive factors.

Diagnosis and Management. First, be assured that asking about suicidality does not provoke it! This is a common, understandable fear of providers. Using your clinician-patient relationship and communication skills to their maximum, we must be aware of symptoms that can suggest suicidal potential, clues that we must probe more deeply because patients often will not simply volunteer that they are having suicidal thoughts. The NIMH also provided the key signs and symptoms you will need to recognize as a clue to inquire about suicidality (Table 4-19), especially in patients who display any of the risk factors in Table 4-17.[51] However, even in the absence of the features in either table, we always screen for suicidality at each visit or telephone contact in patients with or suspected of having a mental disorder.

Patients will not acknowledge suicidality if you ask a cursory question like, "You're not suicidal are you?" Using your empathic skills to establish a noncritical, supportive relationship and a safe atmosphere, you will be more successful following these guidelines in the order given:

1. *Normalize and screen for thinking about death:* This is just the introduction to the topic of death, and we first normalize the conversation because these patients already feel isolated, different, and scared. For example, "I've seen lots of people with similar problems and some, not all, have thoughts

---

TABLE 4-17. Risk Factors for Suicide

1. Depression, other mental disorders, or substance abuse disorder
2. Chronic medical conditions
3. Chronic pain
4. A prior suicide attempt
5. Family history of a mental disorder or substance abuse
6. Family history of suicide
7. Family violence, including physical or sexual abuse
8. Having guns or other firearms in the home
9. Having recently been released from prison or jail
10. Being exposed to others' suicidal behavior, such as that of family members, peers, or celebrities

TABLE 4-18. P4 Screener

Have you had thoughts of actually hurting yourself?

                  NO   YES

Four Screening Questions	←

1. Have you ever attempted to harm yourself in the past?

       NO   **YES**

2. Have you thought about how you might actually hurt yourself?

       NO   **YES** → [How? _____]

3. There's a big difference between having a thought and acting on a thought. How likely do you think it is that you will act on these thoughts about hurting yourself or ending your life some time over the next month?
    a. Not at all likely   _____
    b. Somewhat likely   _____
    c. Very likely   _____

4. Is there anything that would prevent or keep you from harming yourself?

       NO   **YES** → [What? _____]

* P4 is a mnemonic for the 4 screening questions:
   → *past* history, *plan*, *probability*, *preventive* factors

SCORING

Risk Category	Shaded ("Risk") Response	
	Items 1 and 2	**Items 3 and 4**
Minimal	Neither is shaded	Neither is shaded
Lower	At least one item is shaded	Neither is shaded
Higher		At least one item is shaded

that bother them, thoughts that life is not worth living." See where the patient goes with this. You can probe further with, "Did you ever think you'd be better off dead, or even wish it?" If you still are not sure about death thoughts, follow with, "Did you ever hope you'd just not wake up in the morning?"

- If you are convinced there are no thoughts of death, you don't need to pursue suicidality further at this visit.
- If you do have evidence of thinking about death, proceed with the next phase. Remember to use your empathic skills (NURS) throughout, naming any emotion that arises, expressing understanding,

TABLE 4-19. Signs and Symptoms in Suicidal Patients

1. Talking about wanting to die or wanting to kill themselves
2. Talking about feeling empty, hopeless, or having no reason to live
3. Making a plan or looking for a way to kill themselves, such as searching online, stockpiling pills, or buying a gun
4. Talking about great guilt or shame
5. Talking about feeling trapped or feeling that there are no solutions
6. Feeling unbearable pain (emotional pain or physical pain)
7. Talking about being a burden to others
8. Using alcohol or drugs more often
9. Acting anxious or agitated
10. Withdrawing from family and friends
11. Changing eating and/or sleeping habits
12. Showing rage or talking about seeking revenge
13. Taking great risks that could lead to death, such as driving extremely fast
14. Talking or thinking about death often
15. Displaying extreme mood swings, suddenly changing from very sad to very calm or happy
16. Giving away important possessions
17. Saying goodbye to friends and family
18. Putting affairs in order, making a will

acknowledging their plight, praising them for sharing, and explicitly noting your support.

2. *Ascertain reasons to live:* With your concern that the patient could be suicidal (though you don't know that yet), you want to establish what in their life is worth living. This will be a key in management if the patient is suicidal, and it also gives you important contextual and risk information. You might follow with, "Thanks for sharing that, I can see it's been hard for you, and it's scary, I'm here to help. I'm curious, what's in your life you might want to stay alive for, you know, family or church or dog or something like that?" Again, see where this goes, drawing the conversation out open-endedly and empathically, as in the example above. This is how you facilitate a difficult, painful discussion, it's the patient-centered process that's critical to detecting suicidality. You can also inquire more about religion because some religions frown on suicide and this can be an important resource when you begin management.

- At this point, you know death has been on their mind and you have some idea of what they have to live for, so you are ready to determine what the balance of life-death forces is, whether they are suicidal or not.

3. *Ask about specific suicidal ideas—or harming oneself:* It now is time to be specific. You need to know if they have thought of killing or harming themselves, for example, "You told me you've had thoughts of death, have you thought about actually ending your life?"

- If the answer is no, and it often is, you don't need go further, for example, having heard, "Oh no, my goodness, who'd take care of my (spouse, dog)?" or "No, I don't want to go to hell." On the other hand, probe more deeply if you think the patient may be reluctant to be truthful, for example, saying "No, not really."
- If the answer is yes, you have identified suicidal ideation or thinking. You now need to find out, asking directly, the following: (1) how long the thoughts have been occurring, (2) how often they occur, (3) how long they last, and (4) how pervasive they are; for example, "Do you have problems getting rid of the thoughts or do they just pop in every now and then?"
- You next need to determine if the patient has an actual plan; if present, a plan greatly increases the risk, and it is a key decision node in your management.

4. *Ask about specific plan:* You now continue to be specific, if there is a plan, what is it? Continuing to use empathic skills, for example, you might say, "I can see that's bothered you, what exactly would you do to kill yourself? Have you thought about that, you know, taking an overdose of pills or using a gun or breathing your car's exhaust fumes?"

- If the answer is no, many still recommend immediate referral to psychiatry or at least to another MHP trained in suicidal management—and this referral is preferable if available.
  - If psychiatry or other qualified professionals are not available, as often is the case, we recommend that **you manage these patients who do not have a specific plan.**[58,59] This means identifying the correct mental health diagnosis and implementing treatment as

outlined in this chapter, including daily contact to ensure stability and that no plan has developed. This depends on a cooperative patient. You also advise the patient and family that if a plan develops, to go directly to the emergency department. Determining the patient's support system is essential because an informed, caring family can provide around the clock supervision and support. On the other hand, if the patient is not able to cooperate and there is little or no support structure, the patient should be sent to the emergency department or admitted to the hospital as outlined for patients who do have a plan. With a dire shortage of psychiatry specialists, you may need to admit them to the medical wing of the hospital and place them on suicide precautions until a psychiatrist can see them. Err on the side of overreacting.

- If the answer is yes, you determine (1) specific method, (2) exact plans and timing, (3) expectation of what will happen (death, someone find them, throw up the pills), and (4) likelihood they will do it. You may know already but, if not, determine any recent use of substances.

  - You must ensure that the patient sees a psychiatrist immediately, which often means going to the emergency department, some of which have on-site psychiatry services. If they do not, the patient should be admitted to the medicine service and placed on suicide precautions until a psychiatrist can see them. See Chapter 11 for the referral process in an emergency, including how to actually get them to the emergency room and use of the police if necessary.

5. *A caveat:* Many suicidal patients have become withdrawn emotionally, and this can make it very difficult to recognize suicidal intent. Once again, the relationship, sensitivity, and repeated inquiry are in order.

CONCLUSION

You have now learned how to diagnose and manage the most common depressive disorders. While many medications are involved, the therapeutic effects differ little. We encourage you to learn to work with a couple of drugs in each category, and we have highlighted in our examples some common ones we find useful, those with low side effect profiles.

We now transition to Chapter 5 to the closely related anxiety disorders. You'll find that much of your learning from this chapter applies there also.

APPENDIX

Self-Help Resources

1. Wright JH, McCray LW. *Breaking Free From Depression: Pathways to Wellness.* New York, NY: The Guilford Press; 2012.
2. Burns DD. *The Feeling Good Handbook.* Plume Publications; 1999.
3. Griffiths K, Christensen H. *The MoodGym: Overcoming Depression With CBT and Other Effective Therapies.* Ebury Digital; 2011.
4. Williams M, Penman D. *Mindfulness: An Eight Week Plan for Finding Peace in a Frantic World.* New York, NY: Rodale; 2011.
5. Greenberger D, Padesky CA. *Mind Over Mood: Change How You Feel by Changing the Way You Think.* New York, NY: The Guilford Press; 2016.
6. Williams M, Teasdale J, Segal Z, Kabat-Zinn J. *The Mindful Way Through Depression—Freeing Yourself From Chronic Unhappiness.* New York, NY: The Guilford Press; 2007.

Self-Help Websites

www.ecouch.anu.edu.au
www.getselfhelp.co.uk
www.marc.ucla.edu
www.moodgym.anu.edu.au

Depression Self-Help Smartphone Apps (source www.psyberguide.org)

Depression CBT Self-Help
My3
Pacifica
Headspace
Mindshift
Virtual Hope Box

Depression Self-Help Support Groups

Depression Bipolar Support Alliance: www.dbsalliance.org
National Alliance on Mental Illness: www.nami.org

REFERENCES

1. Sederer LI. What does it take for primary care practices to truly deliver behavioral health care? *JAMA Psychiatry*. 2014;71(5):485-486.

2. Cunningham PJ. Beyond parity: primary care physicians' perspectives on access to mental health care. *Health Aff (Millwood)*. 2009;28(3):w490-w501.

3. Rush AJ. STAR*D: What have we learned? *Am J Psychiatry*. 2007;164(2):201-204.

4. Thornicroft G, Chatterji S, Evans-Lacko S, et al. Undertreatment of people with major depressive disorder in 21 countries. *Br J Psychiatry*. 2017;210(2):119-124.

5. Olfson M, Blanco C, Marcus SC. Treatment of adult depression in the United States. *JAMA Intern Med*. 2016;176(10):1482-1491.

6. American Psychiatric Association. *Diagnostic and Statistical Manual of Mental Disorders*. 5th ed. Washington, DC: American Psychiatric Association; 2013.

7. Poole L, Steptoe A. Depressive symptoms predict incident chronic disease burden 10 years later: findings from the English Longitudinal Study of Ageing (ELSA). *J Psychosom Res*. 2018;113:30-36.

8. Greenberg PE, Fournier AA, Sisitsky T, Pike CT, Kessler RC. The economic burden of adults with major depressive disorder in the United States (2005 and 2010). *J Clin Psychiatry*. 2015;76(2):155-162.

9. Ray GT, Weisner CM, Taillac CJ, Campbell CI. The high price of depression: family members' health conditions and health care costs. *Gen Hosp Psychiatry*. 2017;46:79-87.

10. Chisholm D, Sweeny K, Sheehan P, et al. Scaling-up treatment of depression and anxiety: a global return on investment analysis. *Lancet Psychiatry*. 2016;3(5):415-424.

11. Parker G. The benefits of antidepressants: news or fake news? *Br J Psychiatry*. 2018;213(2):454-455.

12. Kim JM, Stewart R, Lee YS, et al. Effect of escitalopram vs placebo treatment for depression on long-term cardiac outcomes in patients with acute coronary syndrome: a randomized clinical trial. *JAMA*. 2018;320(4):350-358.

13. Archer G, Kuh D, Hotopf M, Stafford M, Richards M. Adolescent affective symptoms and mortality. *Br J Psychiatry*. 2018;213(1):419-424.

14. Engel GL. The need for a new medical model: a challenge for biomedicine. *Science*. 1977;196:129-136.

15. Gandal MJ, Haney JR, Parikshak NN, et al. Shared molecular neuropathology across major psychiatric disorders parallels polygenic overlap. *Science*. 2018;359(6376):693-697.

16. Fortin AH VI, Dwamena F, Frankel R, Lepisto B, Smith R. *Smith's Patient-Centered Interviewing—An Evidence-Based Method*. 4th ed. New York, NY: McGraw-Hill, Lange Series; 2018.

17. Kroenke K, Spitzer RL, Williams JB, Lowe B. The Patient Health Questionnaire Somatic, Anxiety, and Depressive Symptom Scales: a systematic review. *Gen Hosp Psychiatry*. 2010;32(4):345-359.

18. McCarron RM, Vanderlip ER, Rado J. Depression. *Ann Intern Med*. 2016;165(7):ITC49-ITC64.

19. Gibbons RD, Hur K, Brown CH, Davis JM, Mann JJ. Benefits from antidepressants: synthesis of 6-week patient-level outcomes from double-blind placebo-controlled randomized trials of fluoxetine and venlafaxine. *Arch Gen Psychiatry*. 2012;69(6):572-579.

20. Moayedi M, Davis KD. Theories of pain: from specificity to gate control. *J Neurophysiol*. 2013;109(1):5-12.

21. Mitsikostas DD, Mantonakis L, Chalarakis N. Nocebo in clinical trials for depression: a meta-analysis. *Psychiatry Res*. 2014;215(1):82-86.

22. Tabor A, Thacker MA, Moseley GL, Kording KP. Pain: a statistical account. *PLoS Comput Biol*. 2017;13(1):e1005142.

23. British Psychological Society. Appendix 16. Table of drug interactions. In: National Collaborating Centre for Mental Health (UK). NICE Clinical Guidelines N, ed. Depression in Adults with a Chronic Physical Health Problem. Leicester, UK: The British Psychological Society; 2010.

24. Ayano G. Psychotropic medications metabolized by cytochromes P450 (CYP) 2D6 enzyme and relevant drug interactions. *Clin Pharmacol Biopharm*. 2016;5:4.

25. Spina E, Santoro V, D'Arrigo C. Clinically relevant pharmacokinetic drug interactions with second-generation antidepressants: an update. *Clin Ther*. 2008;30(7):1206-1227.

26. Food and Drug Administration 2013; https://www.cms.gov/Medicare-Medicaid-Coordination/Fraud-Prevention/Medicaid-Integrity-Education/Pharmacy-Education-Materials/Downloads/ad-adult-dosingchart.pdf. Accessed February 21, 2018.

27. Berle JO, Spigset O. Antidepressant use during breastfeeding. *Curr Womens Health Rev*. 2011;7(1):28-34.

28. Lewis E, Marcus SC, Olfson M, Druss BG, Pincus HA. Patients' early discontinuation of antidepressant prescriptions. *Psychiatr Serv*. 2004;55(5):494.

29. Bauer AM, Parker MM, Schillinger D, et al. Associations between antidepressant adherence and shared decision-making, patient-provider trust, and communication among adults with diabetes: diabetes study of Northern California (DISTANCE). *J Gen Intern Med*. 2014;29(8):1139-1147.

30. Kessler R, Stafford D. Primary care is the de facto mental health system. In: Kessler R, Stafford D, eds. *Collaborative Medicine Case Studies—Evidence in Practice*. New York, NY: Springer; 2008:9-21.

31. Ohayon MM, Schatzberg AF. Chronic pain and major depressive disorder in the general population. *J Psychiatr Res*. 2010;44(7):454-461.
32. Gordon BR, McDowell CP, Hallgren M, Meyer JD, Lyons M, Herring MP. Association of efficacy of resistance exercise training with depressive symptoms: meta-analysis and meta-regression analysis of randomized clinical trials. *JAMA Psychiatry*. 2018;75(6):566-576.
33. Sinclair LI, Christmas DM, Hood SD, et al. Antidepressant-induced jitteriness/anxiety syndrome: systematic review. *Br J Psychiatry*. 2009;194(6):483-490.
34. Menza M. STAR*D: the results begin to roll in. *Am J Psychiatry*. 2006;163:1123-1125.
35. Nelson J. The STAR*D study: a four-course meal that leaves us wanting more. *Am J Psychiatry*. 2006;163:1864-1866.
36. Sullivan MD. Why does depression promote long-term opioid use? *Pain*. 2016;157(11):2395-2396.
37. Scherrer JF, Salas J, Sullivan MD, et al. The influence of prescription opioid use duration and dose on development of treatment resistant depression. *Prev Med*. 2016;91:110-116.
38. Scherrer JF, Salas J, Copeland LA, et al. Prescription opioid duration, dose, and increased risk of depression in 3 large patient populations. *Ann Fam Med*. 2016;14(1):54-62.
39. Sackeim HA. Modern electroconvulsive therapy: vastly improved yet greatly underused. *JAMA Psychiatry*. 2017;74(8):779-780.
40. Ross EL, Zivin K, Maixner DF. Cost-effectiveness of electroconvulsive therapy vs pharmacotherapy/psychotherapy for treatment-resistant depression in the United States. *JAMA Psychiatry*. 2018;75(7):713-722.
41. van Diermen L, van den Ameele S, Kamperman AM, et al. Prediction of electroconvulsive therapy response and remission in major depression: meta-analysis. *Br J Psychiatry*. 2018;212(2):71-80.
42. AHRQ. Nonpharmacological versus pharmacological treatment for patients with major depressive disorder: current state of the evidence. In: Agency for Healthcare Research and Quality, ed. Bethesda, MD: AHRQ; 2016.
43. American Psychiatric Association. Practice guideline for the assessment and treatment of patients with suicidal behaviors. *Am J Psychiatry*. 2003;160(11 Suppl):1-60.
44. Kessler RC, Akiskal HS, Angst J, et al. Validity of the assessment of bipolar spectrum disorders in the WHO CIDI 3.0. *J Affect Disord*. 2006;96(3):259-269.
45. Meier SM, Pavlova B, Dalsgaard S, et al. Attention-deficit hyperactivity disorder and anxiety disorders as precursors of bipolar disorder onset in adulthood. *Br J Psychiatry*. 2018;213(3):555-560.
46. Angst J, Azorin JM, Bowden CL, et al. Prevalence and characteristics of undiagnosed bipolar disorders in patients with a major depressive episode: the BRIDGE study. *Arch Gen Psychiatry*. 2011;68(8):791-798.
47. Stokes PRA, Kalk NJ, Young AH. Bipolar disorder and addictions: the elephant in the room. *Br J Psychiatry*. 2017;211(3):132-134.
48. Sibley MH, Rohde LA, Swanson JM, et al. Late-onset ADHD reconsidered with comprehensive repeated assessments between ages 10 and 25. *Am J Psychiatry*. 2018;175(2):140-149.
49. Cerimele JM, Chwastiak LA, Chan YF, Harrison DA, Unutzer J. The presentation, recognition and management of bipolar depression in primary care. *J Gen Intern Med*. 2013;28(12):1648-1656.
50. Olfson M, Blanco C, Wall M, et al. National trends in suicide attempts among adults in the United States. *JAMA Psychiatry*. 2017;74(11):1095-1103.
51. National Institute of Mental Health 2017; https://www.nimh.nih.gov/health/topics/suicide-prevention/index.shtml. Accessed Jan 10, 2019.
52. Zalsman G, Hawton K, Wasserman D, et al. Suicide prevention strategies revisited: 10-year systematic review. *Lancet Psychiatry*. 2016;3(7):646-659.
53. Vigo D, Thornicroft G, Atun R. Estimating the true global burden of mental illness. *Lancet Psychiatry*. 2016;3(2):171-178.
54. Oquendo MA, Galfalvy H, Russo S, et al. Prospective study of clinical predictors of suicidal acts after a major depressive episode in patients with major depressive disorder or bipolar disorder. *Am J Psychiatry*. 2004;161(8):1433-1441.
55. Lorant V, de Gelder R, Kapadia D, et al. Socioeconomic inequalities in suicide in Europe: the widening gap. *Br J Psychiatry*. 2018;212(6):356-361.
56. Hogan MF, Grumet JG. Suicide prevention: an emerging priority for health care. *Health Aff (Millwood)*. 2016;35(6):1084-1090.
57. Dube P, Kroenke K, Bair MJ, Theobald D, Williams LS. The p4 screener: evaluation of a brief measure for assessing potential suicide risk in 2 randomized effectiveness trials of primary care and oncology patients. *Prim Care Companion J Clin Psychiatry*. 2010;12(6).
58. Schulberg HC, Lee PW, Bruce ML, et al. Suicidal ideation and risk levels among primary care patients with uncomplicated depression. *Ann Fam Med*. 2005;3(6):523-528.
59. Schulberg HC, Bruce ML, Lee PW, Williams JW Jr, Dietrich AJ. Preventing suicide in primary care patients: the primary care physician's role. *Gen Hosp Psychiatry*. 2004;26(5):337-345.

5

Generalized Anxiety and Related Disorders

INTRODUCTION

Anxiety is a universal, adaptive human experience keeping us alert and safe from danger. It produces our "fight or flight" responses to perceived threats. Anxiety is also a motivating emotion under normal circumstances, driving us to action to achieve goals. When anxiety reaches significant heights, however, it becomes problematic and creates multiple physical symptoms, maladaptive behaviors, and extraordinary human misery—in addition to psychological symptoms of worry or fear.

Anxiety problems may range from mild and annoying physical symptoms that cause little worry to disorders where patients' lives are filled with dread, incapacitating physical symptoms, and avoidant behavior(s) that can reach paralyzing proportions. Anyone who has been acutely frightened or placed in unexpected stressful situations can easily identify the emotional and physical symptoms that accompany the experience of anxiety.

BACKGROUND

Anxiety disorders are the most common psychiatric illnesses overall.[1] Although they may occur at any time in the life cycle, they usually have their onset during adolescence and young adulthood and can become a life-long burden.[2] A recent comprehensive "review of the reviews" of the prevalence of anxiety disorders reveals wide ranges of prevalence, upwards of 25% for "any disorder."[3] The prevalence was particularly high in women, young adults, persons with chronic illnesses, and individuals from Anglo-European cultures.

The neurobiological basis of the anxiety disorders involves "loop networks" within the brain. The fundamental structures recognizing and responding to threat in the environment include the thalamus, amygdala, dorsal anterior cingulate cortex (dACC), hypothalamus, hippocampus, and medial prefrontal cortex (mPFC).[4] The thalamus is the structure that integrates all sensory input, then sending it to the hypothalamus. The amygdala and dACC process threatening stimuli and send it to the hypothalamus which relays it to the basal ganglia and brainstem resulting in rapid, unconscious, and reflexively defensive behaviors such as startle responses and sudden muscular withdrawal. The contextual features of threat are encoded in memory by the hippocampus. The mPFC is then involved in the "top down" regulation of the threat information resulting in an adaptive, conscious response. Several investigative methods have identified specific neural loops producing nuanced differences that correlate with specific anxiety disorders.[4] The major neurotransmitter pathways involved in anxiety are the GABA, noradrenergic, and serotonergic systems that provide the basis for pharmacologic treatment strategies.[5]

DIAGNOSTIC AND TREATMENT ISSUES COMMON TO ALL ANXIETY DISORDERS

The anxiety disorders in DSM-5 have many overlapping symptoms and features in common.[6] They have, however, important distinguishing features critical to effective differential diagnosis. Likewise, anxiety treatments overlap with depression and among the various anxiety disorders themselves. This makes treatment easier because the doses and regimens are similar in the various disorders, although often *starting lower and increasing more slowly with the anxiety disorders.*

Primary care providers must also consider all the patients who struggle with symptoms of anxiety including those whose anxiety does not reach the DSM-5 threshold for a diagnosis. Patients with significant but "subthreshold" anxiety still suffer and their ongoing stress responses complicate all facets of their lives and especially underlying medical problems.

Common Diagnostic Issues. Anxiety is a leading cause of physical symptoms in primary care. To begin, most patients with anxiety disorders have prominent physical symptoms, as reviewed in Chapters 1 and 2. To complicate your diagnostic approach, however, there are many medical conditions associated with anxiety; see Table 5-1. *In general, anxiety manifested*

by physical symptoms in younger people is most likely due to an anxiety disorder itself, while in patients over 50 years of age, it is more likely that anxiety symptoms complicate an underlying medical condition. For example, certain rare or uncommon medical conditions directly cause anxiety; for example, pheochromocytoma, carcinoid, and hyperthyroidism. More commonly, however, chronic medical conditions cause anxiety because of their debilitating and disabling effects. As well, prescribed and over-the-counter medication use and recreational substance use cause anxiety and are additional differential diagnostic considerations; see Table 5-2.

Physical symptoms commonly associated with anxiety disorders include shortness of breath, sleep disturbance (especially initial insomnia—taking more than 30 minutes to get to sleep), muscular tension, headache, restlessness, and gastrointestinal upset. For physical and psychological anxiety symptoms, an easy and helpful strategy to guide the diagnostic workup and intervention is the **A-B-C Model.**[7]

ALARM--------BELIEFS--------COPING

This initial strategy helps to engage patients in how they first became aware of and experienced their anxiety, how they cognitively interpreted it, and the actions they took to cope with it. The following is an example of some of the typical anxiety and physical

TABLE 5-1. Medical Conditions Associated With Anxiety and Their Evaluation

1. **Cardiovascular disorders:** Dysrhythmias, coronary artery disease, congestive failure *Physical examination and ECG*
2. **Endocrine disorders:** Hyperthyroidism, Cushing's disease, Addison's disease, pheochromocytoma, carcinoid *Physical examination, TSH, basic biochemical profile, serum electrolytes* (rarely, studies for cortisol and catecholamine abnormalities)
3. **Gastrointestinal disorders:** GERD, inflammatory bowel disease, appendicitis, pancreatitis *Physical examination, CBC* (with indications: amylase, lipase, abdominal CT)
4. **Hematologic disorders:** Anemias *Physical examination, CBC, stools for occult blood*
5. **Neurologic disorders:** Encephalopathy, seizure, vestibular dysfunction *Physical, neurologic, and mental status examinations* (with indications: EEG, LP, MRI)
6. **Respiratory disorders:** Asthma, COPD, pulmonary embolism *Physical examination, chest x-ray* (with indications: ABG, chest CT, PFT)
7. **Substance abuse/dependency:** *Urine and serum toxicology screens*

TABLE 5-2. Common Drugs and Substances Associated With Anxiety

1. **Anticholinergic:** Benztropine, diphenhydramine, meperidine, oxybutynin
2. **Dopaminergic:** Amantadine, bromocriptine, levodopa, carbidopa, metoclopramide
3. **Stimulants:** Caffeine, nicotine, cocaine, methamphetamines, MDMA, phencyclidine
4. **Herbal preparations:** Any preparations containing ephedra
5. **OTC medications:** Medications with phenylephrine, phenylpropanolamine, or pseudoephedrine
6. **Substances of abuse:** Amphetamines, cannabis, cocaine, MDMA (ecstasy), phencyclidine (PCP), sedative withdrawal (barbiturate, benzodiazepine, alcohol, opioid)
7. **Others:** Aminophylline/theophylline, anabolic steroids, corticosteroids, indomethacin, thyroid

symptoms of pretreatment panic disorder. The patient is a 21-year-old female college student.

> **A**LARM: Initial feelings of uneasiness followed by anxiety and its escalation: "I'm getting really nervous; now my heart is pounding; my chest feels tight, I can't catch my breath; I'm sweating; my lips are tingling. This has never happened to me before. Am I dying?"
> **B**ELIEF: "I'm having a heart attack." Or, "I can't control this, I must be going crazy."
> **C**OPING: "Call 911, I have to get to an emergency room."

Now we see the same patient in the initial phase of a successful intervention:

> **A**LARM: "Here we go again, the emergency room doctor and my primary care doctor said this might happen again before my medication started to work fully."
> **B**ELIEF: "I'm having another panic attack. This will be unpleasant but not dangerous to me."
> **C**OPING: "I will sit down, start my mindfulness and breathing control exercises and manage this."

This strategy also assists in structuring the history, planning an efficient and cost-effective diagnostic workup, and making the best differential diagnosis. Because the interrelationship between anxiety and physical symptoms can be multifactorial, a familiarity with the underlying medical conditions frequently associated with anxiety is important. Typically, workups need not lead to invasive tests and thereby risk iatrogenic complications, especially in young people. (See Table 5-1, where we suggest initial screening testing if the history and physical examination is inconclusive.) Further, summarized in Table 5-2, anxiety can be an adverse effect of commonly prescribed classes of medications, substances of abuse, and both over-the-counter medicines and nutritional supplements; for example, caffeine is a common cause as is excessive thyroid medication. Diligent history-taking in this component of the workup is critical. Treatment may be as simple as dosage adjustment, discontinuation, or switch to another indicated medication.

Common Treatment Issues. The Mental Health Care Model (MHCM) discussed in Chapter 3 provides guidance for diagnosing and managing anxiety disorders.

■ *Patient-centered interactions* are essential. The most important general treatment strategy for all anxiety disorders is establishing a trusting relationship with the primary care provider. Empathy (using NURS skills) is important because many patients with anxiety disorders have been subject to criticism, referred to in pejorative terms, and ridiculed by others. Empathic connection facilitates cooperation with and adherence to instructions made for general self-help measures like a healthy diet, exercise, relaxation techniques, and principles of sleep hygiene. Pharmacologic treatments often do not work immediately while a number of possible untoward/adverse effects may occur early on. The trusting relationship helps patients to have realistic expectations in the trajectory of their recovery and to persist with dosage increases/adjustments of their medications. The clinician-patient relationship is also essential when making a referral to a mental health professional (psychiatrist, psychologist, medical social worker, other counselors), especially if the patient indicates resistance to this suggestion. When making the mental health referral it is critical to reinforce that this will be just one component of their overall primary care. See Chapter 11 for referral principles.

■ *Education:* It is important to always ascertain the patient's understanding of the problem in order to correct any misunderstandings (eg, selective serotonin reuptake inhibitors [SSRIs] don't work for anxiety, benzodiazepines are the best treatment). Once assured that they have a clear and accurate understanding of the problem, you can indicate that very effective treatments exist and that you will prescribe the most appropriate one for them.

■ *Commitment and goals:* Always determine the degree of commitment a patient has, as well as their goals, particularly in describing treatment, looking for any resistances that you may need to address further. It is important to initially establish long-range goals (eg, getting back to work, feeling more comfortable socially), frequently revisiting them at later visits.

■ *Treatment plan:* The remainder of this chapter addresses general and specific treatments as they apply to the various anxiety disorders.

General Self-Help Measures. To review some features of the MHCM especially helpful in anxiety, mindfulness-based therapy is a self-help intervention that involves recognition of one's emotional state followed by "in-the-moment" focused awareness. The mindful awareness achieved is a form of meditation that promotes relaxation and stress reduction. Mindfulness therapies are customized to each individual patient's circumstances.[8] While you are evaluating the patient's progress with pharmacological treatment, be sure to also review clinical progress with self-help efforts. In Chapter 3, see Table 3-4 for a simple meditation procedure.

Patients experiencing significant anxiety require special attention to improvement in their general health, especially a healthy diet and their level of physical fitness. A graded physical exercise program that includes both aerobic and resistance training is effective in both reducing anxiety symptoms and improving overall physical fitness.[9] Exercise programs must be carefully negotiated and tailored to each patient's current health status. Learning to practice Yoga, either by joining a class or individually by following an introductory DVD, assists with neuromuscular anxiety relaxation and reducing anxiety states.[10]

Psychotherapy in all its forms and iterations decreases anxiety symptoms in most anxiety disorders. Although outside the scope of the clinician, it is important to have a sense of what occurs. Cognitive behavioral therapy (CBT) has been foremost and especially successful for long-term remission.[11] (Insight-oriented psychotherapy is a more extensive and deeply reaching process.) Clinicians can refer their patients to mental health professionals trained in this technique. Although most psychiatrists now focus almost exclusively on pharmacological treatment, a psychologist and/or skilled social worker can conduct CBT (or other therapy) and become part of the treatment team. As the clinician, you remain involved with the patient's overall care, often prescribing medications in parallel, as we outline later for each disorder. Patients generally find CBT very useful as they learn new coping strategies and experience symptom reduction. Avoidant behavior is a common consequence of all anxiety disorders and mental health professionals generally address it using exposure techniques. The general principle is "Confronting what makes you anxious makes it better, avoiding what makes you anxious makes it worse." The usual technique is gradual reexposure. For your patients who refuse referral,

encourage them to create their own independent trial of graded confrontation.

With this general backdrop of diagnosis and treatment of anxiety disorders, we now address the specific disorders, including pharmacotherapy for each. A recent meta-analysis indicates that both psychotherapy and medications for anxiety disorders are not only effective but also that they have enduring impact after treatment.[12]

GENERALIZED ANXIETY DISORDER

Generalized anxiety disorder (GAD) is a chronic illness characterized by waxing, especially in times of increased psychosocial stress, and waning as stressors decline.[13] Patients with GAD often have chronically high levels of stress hormones that aggravate and complicate all other coexisting medical conditions.[14] The disorder has a lifetime prevalence of 5.7% and involves near global worry about a wide range of features in the person's life.[1] These include issues that family members and clinicians recognize as mundane in the overall scheme of things, such as having difficulty choosing what to wear or fretting over whether a comment, a gift or a gesture was well received. GAD has even been described in lay terminology as "the worry sickness." Patients themselves often recognize that their worry is excessive and that it interferes with their overall happiness and ability to function in productive ways in interpersonal, social, and work settings.

Patients with GAD generally do not present early in the course of their illness. They typically present after making repeated attempts to cope but failing to bring their emotional and physical symptoms under control. Patients will describe feeling physically and emotionally "drained," which also leads to further feelings of depression and demoralization as their worries expand and their social and occupational functioning suffers. Not surprising is that *anxiety and depression often coexist*. In the physical examination, patients' heart rates are frequently elevated in the mild range, and the symptom that adds greatly to their misery is muscle tension. Patients frequently describe feeling "tied up in knots." Typically, the examination of the muscles in their neck, shoulders, and back reveal areas of localized tension. If long-standing, these areas of chronic muscle spasm may have a hard and "ropey" feel and are tender to palpation. Finally, patients with GAD appear both fatigued and distressed. The fatigue they feel is often

TABLE 5-3. DSM-5 Diagnostic Criteria for Generalized Anxiety Disorder (GAD)

A. Excessive anxiety and worry (apprehensive expectation), occurring more days than not for a least 6 months, about a number of events and activities (such as work or school performance).
B. The individual finds it difficult to control the worry.
C. The anxiety and worry are associated with 3 (or more) of the following 6 symptoms (with at least some symptoms having been present for more days than not for the past 6 mo).
   Note: Only 1 item is required in children.
   1. Restless or feeling keyed up or on edge
   2. Being easily fatigued
   3. Difficulty concentrating or mind going blank
   4. Irritability
   5. Muscle tension
   6. Sleep disturbance (difficulty falling or staying asleep or restless, unsatisfying sleep)
D. The anxiety, worry, or physical symptoms cause clinically significant distress or impairment in social, occupational, or other important areas of functioning.
E. The disturbance is not attributable to the physiological effects of a substance (eg, a drug of abuse, a medication) or another medical condition (eg, hyperthyroidism).
F. The disturbance is not better explained by another mental disorder (eg, anxiety or worry about having panic attacks in panic disorder, negative evaluation in social anxiety disorder [social phobia], contamination or other obsessions in obsessive-compulsive disorder, separation from attachment figures in separation anxiety disorder, reminders of traumatic events in posttraumatic stress disorder, gaining weight in anorexia nervosa, physical complaints in somatic symptom disorder, perceived appearance flaws in the body in body dysmorphic disorder, having a serious illness in illness anxiety disorder, or delusional beliefs in schizophrenia or delusional disorder).

from the combination of both their psychomotor restlessness and built-up sleep deprivation from insomnia. DSM-5 criteria are listed in Table 5-3.[6]

Contemporary primary care practices are busy and efficiency is very important. Since complaints of anxiety and depression are so common, it is helpful to utilize screening tools the patients may complete prior to seeing you. For anxiety, one of the best and most efficient screening instruments is the Generalized Anxiety Disorder Questionnaire-7 (GAD-7), summarized in Table 5-4.[15] It consists of 7 symptom complexes that are consistent with the DSM-5 criteria with the patients rating how frequently they experience each feature and the extent of the difficulty. The clinician can review the areas checked. This facilitates a more efficient evaluation of the patient's history as well as focusing on specific symptom-relief when developing the treatment plan. A score of 10 or more is the recommended cutoff that warrants further evaluation. As well, the GAD-7 should be administered at each follow-up visit to monitor the effectiveness of the treatment plan.

Because patients so commonly complain of both anxious and depressive symptoms together, we recommend that both the PHQ-9 (see Chapter 4) and the GAD-7 be a component of routine patient screening, especially when a mental disorder is a possibility. Both screening instruments are available in the public domain and are easily accessed online—or may be copied from this book.

After initial review of the GAD-7, the patient-centered interview begins by starting with open-ended questions. The term "describe" is always a useful start when beginning the patient's history; for example, "Describe the kinds of worries that bother you." More helpful specific questions include "Would you or others describe you as a nervous person?" A developmental question is also useful: "Would your parents or relatives you grew up with describe you as a 'worrier' or perhaps a 'worry-wart'?" The clinician should then inquire about the specific areas checked in the GAD-7.

Treatment. We now address the details of pharmacological treatment, the mainstay for the clinician managing all anxiety disorders, especially GAD. First-line pharmacologic treatment for GAD is summarized in Table 5-5 and includes the very same SSRI and SNRI antidepressant medications you read about in Chapter 4.[16] Note, however, that the *starting doses are one-half those used for depression.* These newer agents are efficacious and, since treatment will be long term for full recovery/remission, they have the least risk for side effects. Although tolerance also can sometimes be a problem with the newer agents,[17]

TABLE 5-4. Screening for Generalized Anxiety Disorder—The GAD-7 Scale

GAD-7

Over the *last 2 weeks*, how often have you been bothered by the following problems?

	Not at all (0)	Several days (1)	More than half the days (2)	Nearly every day (3)
Feeling nervous, anxious, or on edge	❏	❏	❏	❏
Not being able to stop or control worrying	❏	❏	❏	❏
Worrying too much about different things	❏	❏	❏	❏
Trouble relaxing	❏	❏	❏	❏
Being so restless that it is hard to sit still	❏	❏	❏	❏
Becoming easily annoyed or irritable	❏	❏	❏	❏
Feeling afraid as if something awful might happen	❏	❏	❏	❏
Add the score from each column				
Add column scores =			**Total Score = _____.**	

the severity and extent of the tolerance and habituation often seen with benzodiazepines does not occur. The general strategies include a starting dose with gradual upward titration guided by experience of adverse effect and the trajectory of improvement. The following SSRIs and serotonin–norepinephrine reuptake inhibitors (SNRIs) have FDA approval for the treatment of GAD.

Other SSRIs also effective and used as "off-label" treatment for GAD are citalopram, fluoxetine, and sertraline.

Generally, the same trial-times and therapeutic doses for treating depressive disorders apply in the treatment of anxiety disorders, as described for depression in Chapter 4. Because these medications may initially worsen anxiety (due to their stimulating qualities); however, we recommend starting at half the depression doses; the same reduction applies to those over 60 years old where the therapeutic dose is also reduced by one-half.

These new antidepressant medications are "first-line" because of their milder adverse-effect profiles but patients must still be cautioned to be alert and report adverse experiences. Venlafaxine has been demonstrated to elevate blood pressure as an adverse effect.[18] Since other medications are equally effective in the treatment of GAD, venlafaxine should be avoided in patients with hypertension.

Common adverse-effects were reviewed in Chapter 4; to summarize, they include

1. **Duloxetine** (SNRI) Starting dose: 20 mg qd. Titrate up to 30-60 mg/d
2. **Escitalopram** (SSRI) Starting dose: 5 mg qd. Titrate up to 10-20 mg/d
3. **Paroxetine** (SSRI) Starting dose: 10 mg qd. Titrate up to 20-40 mg/d
4. **Venlafaxine** (SNRI) Starting dose: 37.5 mg qd. Titrate up to 75-225 mg/d

TABLE 5-5. Using Antidepressants for Anxiety Disorders

		ANTIDEPRESSANT MEDICATIONS		ANTIDEPRESSANT SIDE EFFECTS						
CLASS	INITIAL DOSE[a] (mg/d)	THERAP DOSE (mg/d)	HALF-LIFE	SEDATION	WEIGHT GAIN	SEXUAL	CARDIAC	ANTICHO-LINERGIC	SEIZURES	DRUG INTERACTION[b]
SSRI										
Sertraline (Zoloft)	25	100-200	Medium	+/−	+	++	−	+	−	2D6 inhibitor +/− At high doses only
Fluoxetine (Prozac)	10	20-60	Long	−	+/−	++	−	+	−	2D6 inhibitor 4+ Incr. flecainide and β-blocker level
Citalopram (Celexa)	10	20-60	Short	+/−	+	++	QTc increased	−	−	Incr. flecainide level
Escitalopram (Lexapro)	5	10-20	Short	−	+	++	QTc increased	−	−	Incr. flecainide level
Paroxetine (Paxil)	10	20-40	Short	+	++	+++	−	+	−	2D6 inhibitor 4+ Incr. flecainide and β-blocker level

(Continued)

TABLE 5-5. Using Antidepressants for Anxiety Disorders (*Continued*)

CLASS	ANTIDEPRESSANT MEDICATIONS			ANTIDEPRESSANT SIDE EFFECTS						
	INITIAL DOSE[a] (mg/d)	THERAP DOSE (mg/d)	HALF-LIFE	SEDATION	WEIGHT GAIN	SEXUAL	CARDIAC	ANTICHO-LINERGIC	SEIZURES	DRUG INTERACTION[b]
SNRI										
Venlafaxine XR (Effexor XR)	37.5	75-225	Short	–	+/–	+++	Increased BP and heart rate	–	–	Decr. indinavir level
Duloxetine (Cymbalta)	20	30-60	Short	–	+/–	+++	+/–	–	–	2D6 inhibitor 1+

2D6 = P450 2D6 pathway[33-35], BP = blood pressure; QTc = corrected QT interval on an electrocardiogram where abnormal with increased risk for arrhythmias is >470 in women and >450 in men—especially risky when >500; SNRI = serotonin-norepinephrine reuptake inhibitor; SSRI = selective serotonin reuptake inhibitor.

[a]For patients with *anxiety disorders*, this represents **one-half the starting dose for depression**. For patients *older than 60 years*, the **therapeutic dose is reduced by one-half in the table above.**

[b]The following antidepressants should be avoided or used with great caution for the conditions listed because they often interact to increase the levels of medications commonly used for the condition[33-35]:

1. All SSRI/SNRI: (a) on anticoagulation, (b) using centrally acting appetite suppressants; eg, sibutramine, migraine taking 5HT agonists. *Use a tricyclic in these situations.*

2. Paroxetine: constipation, ADHD

3. Venlafaxine: risk for arrhythmia, hypertension, on anticoagulation

4. Duloxetine: difficult to control hypertension, on anticoagulation

5. Fluoxetine: ADHD on stimulants

Also, be aware of need for dosage reductions in patients with comorbid liver and renal disease.

1. *Initial/early activation:* Some patients experience an early significant increase in their anxiety that commonly results in nonadherence/noncooperation. This is usually dose-dependent and diminishes with reassurance, time, and patience—the therapeutic relationship is paramount in conveying this as one reduces the dose. Short-term use of a benzodiazepine (described later), for no more than 2 to 4 weeks, may be necessary to assist patients through this phase of treatment.

2. *Sedation:* Sedation is occasionally a problem, in which case the dosage is reduced or a less sedating antidepressant is used.

3. *Weight increase:* Many of the SSRIs are associated with weight gain, which can compound the patient's anxiety. Switching to (or starting with) an SNRI like duloxetine usually suffices.

4. *Cardiac effects:* Aggravation of hypertension and enhancement of arrhythmias can occur with SNRIs like venlafaxine, so where this is a concern, one begins with an SSRI.

5. *Sexual side effects:* Most common are delayed ejaculation and orgasm. These are also dose-dependent—but do not improve over time. Use of medications for erectile dysfunction like sildenafil, tadalafil, and vardenafil is indicated in these circumstances. Both depressive and anxiety disorders themselves diminish libido and impair satisfying sexual function. Restoring sexual functioning is an important component of successful treatment.[19]

6. *Gastrointestinal discomfort:* The most common patient complaints are nausea and frequent loose stools/diarrhea, while others may develop constipation. These are also dose-dependent but decrease over time.

7. *Discontinuation syndrome:* Once on an SSRI or SNRI for 4 to 6 weeks, they should not be stopped abruptly. When they are, the patient may develop a withdrawal syndrome characterized by acute anxiety and depression, headaches, nausea, vomiting, diarrhea, vertigo, insomnia, paresthesias, tremors, and ataxia. Albeit distressing to patient and clinician alike, this withdrawal phase passes in a few days with supportive measures and re-administering a short-acting antidepressant.

8. *Serotonin syndrome:* This side effect occurs from excessive doses of serotonin-containing antidepressants, usually when given together or sequentially without an adequate washout period (see Table 5-6 for a summary and see Table 5-7 for switching antidepressants).

Length of treatment in GAD is generally long term, typically 1 year before gradual taper and discontinuation of the SSRI/SNRI is begun. If symptoms of anxiety recur, it is a simple matter of titration back up to the prior effective dose. Unfortunately,

---

TABLE 5-6. Serotonin Syndrome

Serotonin syndrome is life-threatening and occurs from very high serotonin levels. Fortunately, it is not common, but most likely to occur when multiple SSRIs and SNRIs are used together (or combined with an MAO inhibitor). This sometimes also occurs when an adequate washout of a prior antidepressant is not observed before beginning a different one, especially when a long acting agent like fluoxetine has not been adequately washed out; see Table 5-7 for the protocols for switching antidepressants. In addition to suicidal overdose, also causing serotonin syndrome there are other possible causative agents: some over-the-counter medications (dextromethorphan); some illegal ones (LSD, ecstasy, cocaine, amphetamines); herbal supplements (St John wort, ginseng, nutmeg); and certain medications (opioids, triptans, carbamazepine, ritonavir, linezolid, metoclopramide, droperidol, ondansetron, lithium, bupropion, tricyclic antidepressants).

Very distressing symptoms first occur.
- *Gastrointestinal:* Nausea and vomiting; diarrhea
- *Cardiovascular:* Tachycardia and hypertension
- *Neurological:* Hyperreflexia, myoclonus, ataxia, muscle twitching, muscular incoordination, muscle rigidity, mydriasis, headache, confusion
- *Autonomic instability:* Hyperthermia, tachycardia, hypertension, profuse sweating, shivering, piloerection

Life-threatening findings can follow if not treated.
- Hyperthermia
- Loss of consciousness
- Seizures
- Arrhythmias

Treatment is removal of the offending drug, which may suffice for minor symptoms, and symptomatic support including benzodiazepines. As well, cyproheptadine may help by blocking serotonin.

TABLE 5-7. Switching Antidepressant Medications in Anxiety[a]

SWITCHING FROM	SWITCHING TO	
Tricyclic	SSRI or SNRI	Taper over 5-7 d; start new drug 2-3 d later
SSRI	SNRI	Taper over 2-5 d, then start SNRI; use lower dose if switch from fluoxetine; longer taper, up to 2 wk, if high doses of fluoxetine were used; monitor serotonin syndrome (see Table 5-6)
SSRI	Different SSRI	Taper over 2-5 d, then start SNRI; use lower dose if switch from fluoxetine; longer taper, up to 2 wk, if high doses of fluoxetine were used; monitor serotonin syndrome (see Table 5-6)
SNRI	SSRI	Taper over 2-5 d; then start SSRI
SNRI	Different SNRI	Taper over 2-5 d; then start new

SNRI = serotonin-norepinephrine reuptake inhibitor; SSRI = selective serotonin reuptake inhibitor.

[a]The material in this table is the same as one in Chapter 4 for switching antidepressants in depression.

data for remission rates from the pharmacologic treatment of anxiety disorders are not available, in contrast to data for the depressive disorders. It is reasonable however to expect an acceptable response after 2 trials. If after 6 to 8 weeks of treatment with an SSRI there is no symptom improvement, it is reasonable to try an SNRI as a second trial, also pushing the dose to maximum recommended levels. See Table 5-7 for the protocols for changing these medications. GAD is a chronic and recurring illness, therefore, long-term treatment

with an SSRI or SNRI is common. As mentioned in Chapter 4, we recommend that you never use MAO inhibitors because of their severe side-effect profile; while they can be used, leave that to psychiatry. Recall, also, do not combine SNRIs and SSRIs at the same time—it risks provoking the serotonin syndrome (Table 5-6).

Second-line pharmacologic treatment of GAD includes the benzodiazepines and buspirone. The major advantage of the benzodiazepines is their rapid onset of action, but the risks for oversedation, impairment of learning/memory, and long-term dependence/abuse are considerable. Their use can typically be avoided in GAD since the symptoms are long-standing. Counseling and self-help recommendations usually suffice as antidepressant medications to take effect. Patients whose symptoms warrant expeditious relief can be started on a benzodiazepine concomitantly with antidepressant medication. As the antidepressant medication takes effect, the benzodiazepine can be gradually tapered and discontinued over no more than 2 to 4 weeks.

Benzodiazepines most useful are

1. Alprazolam (Xanax)—starting dose: 0.25 mg bid-tid—maximum dose: 4 mg/d in divided doses
2. Clonazepam (Klonopin)—starting dose: 0.5 mg q12h—maximum dose: 4 mg/d in divided doses
3. Lorazepam (Ativan)—starting dose: 0.5 mg bid-tid—maximum dose: 10 mg/d in divided doses

Each of these medications has FDA approval for the management of anxiety. Alprazolam and lorazepam have rapid onset and short half-lives. Clonazepam has a longer onset and duration of action which is a distinct advantage when it is time to initiate taper and discontinuation. See the more extensive discussion of tapering benzodiazepines in Chapter 6.

Buspirone (BuSpar) has FDA approval for treatment of GAD and the advantage over benzodiazepines of lower potential for abuse, and it can be used for long term. The disadvantages of buspirone are its lower efficacy than other agents and delayed onset of action. The starting dose is 5 mg tid with a maximum dose of 10 to 15 mg bid.

Older-generation tricyclic and tetracyclic antidepressant medications also are effective in the treatment of anxiety disorders but, due to their higher adverse-effect profiles, they are now considered "fallback" choices.

Calcium channel blockers and anticonvulsants (gabapentin and pregabalin) have also been used in the treatment of GAD. They block physical symptoms of anxiety but do not affect cognitive or emotional symptoms.[20] Generally, we would consider these agents only in refractory cases where clinicians should strongly consider referral to psychiatry for medication consultation; you might try them in patients who refuse or cannot otherwise see a psychiatrist.

With a comprehensive treatment including self-help strategies, first-line medications, and periodic follow-up, clinicians also should expect significant improvement in their GAD patients within 3 months. If patients are not responding the clinician should consider complicating factors, for example, nonadherence/cooperation, substance use/abuse, and misdiagnosis. At this point, clinician's should also consider psychiatric consultation for medication recommendations.

Psychotherapy and Complementary Treatments. Psychotherapy for GAD involves CBT along with training the patient in reflective mindfulness and other relaxation techniques as described earlier in this chapter. Because muscle tension causes significant discomfort, referral to practitioners trained and skilled in massage or musculoskeletal manipulation can also provide welcome relief.

PANIC DISORDER

Panic disorder is common with a lifetime prevalence of 4.7%.[1] Most often, it occurs in adolescence and young adulthood and more often in females, declining with advancing age. Discrete time-limited attacks of acutely heightened anxiety, "panic attacks" may occur in any of the anxiety disorders, but panic disorder itself is a distinct diagnosis. Panic disorder is potentially one of the most devastating of the anxiety disorders because of severe acute and chronic emotional distress as well as physical, interpersonal, social, and occupational dysfunction. The heralding event is a panic attack that is unexpected and not cued or "triggered" by some threat in the patient's environment. Patients describe the occurrence as sudden and coming "out of the blue." The emotional and physical symptoms are often misinterpreted by the patient, especially the first panic attack. Emotional

responses are typically the fear of "going crazy" because the attack cannot be brought under control by "will-power." Among many physical symptoms, the prominent cardiorespiratory symptoms typically engender fear of "fainting" or "having a heart attack." Panic disorder involves periodic recurrences of panic attacks and can lead to serious disability and increasing avoidant behavior to the point where patients fear to leave their homes (agoraphobia). We often see patients with first occurrences of panic disorder in emergency departments or with urgent requests for care in the office. Early diagnosis and rapid treatment to attenuate subsequent panic attacks is the very essence of effective preventive mental health care in the primary care setting.

In the patient-centered interview, it is helpful to ask the patient to describe the attack with a time frame from their first inclination that something was awry, to peak symptoms, to complete resolution. The "A-B-C" model is especially useful here to provide the patient an open-ended opportunity to describe the fear involved, the constellation of physical symptoms, their interpretation of the event, and their coping strategy(ies). Subsequent physical examination and screening laboratory studies usually are enough to reassure patients that their physical symptoms are due to the anxiety disorder itself and they are not at risk of dying or losing their ability to test reality. Shown in Table 5-8, DSM-5 lists the many physical symptoms, such as chest pain and vertigo, that accompany fear during a panic attack; the criteria for a diagnosis of panic disorder is for the patient to experience at least 4 of these. The remaining diagnostic criteria include a specific time frame of 1 month and exclusionary diagnoses which may be causing the symptom complex.[21]

For screening purposes, we present 2 instruments useful in a primary-care practice. Table 5-9 summarizes the panic disorder screener (PADIS), which is a very efficient screening instrument.[22] It includes a list of 4 items corresponding to DSM-5 symptoms and allows the patient to rate the frequency of the number of attacks and the frequency of their worry or anticipation of having another attack in the past month. As well as specific symptoms, it also allows patients to rate the frequency of times they have engaged in avoidant behavior out of their fear of having another panic attack.

TABLE 5-8. DSM-5 Diagnostic Criteria for Panic Disorder

A. Recurrent unexpected panic attacks. A panic attack is an abrupt surge of intense fear or intense discomfort that reaches a peak within minutes, and during which time 4 (or more) of the following symptoms occur:
   Note: The abrupt surge can occur from a calm state or an anxious state.
   1. Palpitations, pounding heart, or accelerated heart rate
   2. Sweating
   3. Trembling or shaking
   4. Sensations of shortness of breath or smothering
   5. Feelings of choking
   6. Chest pain or discomfort
   7. Nausea or abdominal distress
   8. Feeling dizzy, unsteady, light-headed, or faint
   9. Chills or heat sensations
   10. Paresthesias (numbness or tingling sensations)
   11. Derealization (feelings of unreality) or depersonalization (being detached from one-self)
   12. Fear of losing control or "going crazy"
   13. Fear of dying
   Note: Culture-specific symptoms (eg, tinnitus, neck soreness, headache, uncontrollable screaming, or crying) may be seen. Such symptoms should not count as 1 of the 4 required symptoms.
B. At least 1 of the attacks has been followed by 1 month (or more) of 1 or both of the following:
   1. Persistent concern or worry about additional panic attacks or their consequences (eg, losing control, having a heart attack, or "going crazy")
   2. A significant maladaptive change in behavior related to the attacks (eg, behaviors designed to avoid having panic attacks, such as avoidance of exercise or unfamiliar situations)
C. The disturbance is not attributable to the physiological effects of a substance (eg, a drug of abuse, a medication) or another medical condition (eg, hyperthyroidism, cardiopulmonary disorders).
D. The disturbance is not better explained by another mental disorder (eg, the panic attacks do not occur only in response to feared social situations, as in specific anxiety disorder; in response to circumscribed phobic objects or situations, as in specific phobia; in response to obsessions, as in obsessive-compulsive disorder; in response to reminders of traumatic events, as in posttraumatic stress disorder; or in response to separation from attachment figures, as in separation anxiety disorder).

Source: Reprinted with permission from the *Diagnostic and Statistical Manual of Mental Disorders,* Fifth Edition, (Copyright ©2013). American Psychiatric Association. All Rights Reserved.

Another useful screening instrument, seen in Table 5-10, is the PHQ-Panic that asks 15 questions about possible symptoms where patients may simply circle "Yes" or "No" corresponding with their experiences. Scoring is simple, allowing the clinician to rate the panic symptoms into "low," "moderate," and "high" panic symptoms.[23] The PADIS has a 77% sensitivity and 84% specificity[22] and the PHQ-Panic has a 57% sensitivity and 91% specificity.[23] Regardless of which of these instruments is used, use them serially as a measure of the efficacy of the tailored treatment plan.

We screen for medical disorders in panic disorder just as in the workup for GAD. The most important medical disorders to consider are cardiovascular,

especially coronary artery disease. Mitral valve prolapse (MVP) specifically has been associated with but not considered to have a causal effect on panic disorder. It is postulated that the persistent increase in heart rate and elevated blood pressure over time "balloons" a weakened mitral valve.[24] Differential diagnosis includes GAD, posttraumatic stress disorder (PTSD), and phobic disorders. Patients with GAD can have paroxysms of heightened anxiety that produce panic attacks similar to the attacks in panic disorder. Helping to differentiate GAD patients with panic attacks from those with true panic disorder, the latter have inter-panic anticipatory anxiety symptoms. Social anxiety and specific phobias are associated with

TABLE 5-9. Panic Disorder Screener (PADIS)

A sudden feeling of anxiety, fear, discomfort, or uneasiness may indicate a panic episode. A panic episode occurs unexpectedly, peaks within 10 min, and includes 4 or more of the following sensations at the same time.

(1) Skipping, racing, or pounding heart; (2) sweating or clammy hands; (3) trembling or shaking; (4) shortness of breath of difficulty breathing; (5) choking feeling or lump in your throat; (6) chest pain or discomfort; (7) nausea or stomach problems; (8) feeling dizzy, unsteady, light-headed, or faint; (9) feeling strange, unreal, detached, or unfamiliar; (10) fear that you are losing control or going crazy; (11) fear that you are dying; (12) feeling of numbness or tingling; (13) hot flushes or chills

Based on this description, about how many panic episodes have you experienced in the past month?

      None_____ One_____ 2-5_____ 6-10_____ 11 or more_____

Note: Respondents who respond "None" to the 1st item, skip all remaining items and score 0.

In the past month, how often have you been worried about having another panic attack?

      Never_____ Occasionally_____ Often_____ All the time_____

In the past month, how often have you been worried about the consequences of having another panic episode?

      Never_____ Occasionally_____ Often_____ All the time_____

In the past month, how often did you avoid places, situations or activities because you were afraid of having or triggering a panic attack? (For example, avoiding physical exertion or avoiding stressful activities.)

      Never_____ Occasionally_____ Often_____ All the time_____

The 1st item is rated on a 5-point Likert scale scored 0-4, while remaining items are rated on a 4-point Likert scale score 0-3. Severity scores are obtained by summing responses to all items, with scores ranging from 0 to13.

Using a cutoff score of 4 or higher, to indicate criteria for panic disorder, the PADIS had a 77% sensitivity and 84% specificity: higher sensitivity but lower specificity compared to the PHQ-Panic Scale.

Source: Adapted from Batterham et al.[22]

specific cues and/or situations that precipitate a panic attack. Careful interviewing, as outlined in Chapter 7, uncovers the distinguishing features of each.

Treatment. Clinicians can effectively counsel patients by educating them about panic disorder and, providing the panic attacks and inter-panic anxiety are not aggravating another medical condition, reassure them that, albeit distressing, the attacks are not dangerous. The goal is to "cognitively re-structure" thoughts (beliefs) about the attack from, "I am having a heart attack or maybe I am dying" to "Here we go again, I am going to be very uncomfortable for a while," as described earlier in the "A-B-C Model." Patients must be counseled against "yet one more" trip to the emergency department. Rather, clinician's should emphasize multimodal interventions with strategies to manage attacks, including conscious control of breathing and mindful, progressive relaxation.[25]

Pharmacologic treatment is effective and targeted toward halting or attenuating subsequent panic attacks as quickly as possible to prevent development of avoidant behavior. Benzodiazepines are used to bring prompt relief, and we start antidepressant medications at the same time to provide long-term control. Patients must be informed that benzodiazepine treatment will be time-limited, titrated to a dose that controls the attacks while giving the antidepressant medications adequate time to take effect (typically by 6-8 weeks). The clinician then tapers and discontinues the benzodiazepines gradually over 1 to 2 weeks.

Benzodiazepines with FDA approval for panic disorder include alprazolam and clonazepam. SSRIs (fluoxetine, paroxetine, and sertraline) have FDA approval as well as the SNRI (venlafaxine). Dosage instructions are similar to those for the treatment of GAD. See Table 5-5. Frequently patients become concerned about recurrence of the panic attacks when

TABLE 5-10. PHQ-Panic Screener		
General		
a. In the last 4 weeks, have you had an anxiety attack—suddenly feeling fear or panic? *(If "a" above is checked "No," do not present subsequent PHQ Panic Question. If "Yes," continue with Questions).*	Yes	No
b. Has this ever happened before?	Yes	No
c. Do some of these attacks come suddenly out of the blue, ie, in situations where you don't expect to be nervous or uncomfortable?	Yes	No
d. Do you think these attacks bother you a lot or are you worried about having another attack?	Yes	No
Think About Your Last Bad Anxiety Attack		
a. Were you short of breath?	Yes	No
b. Did your heart race, pound, or skip?	Yes	No
c. Did you have chest pain or pressure?	Yes	No
d. Did you sweat?	Yes	No
e. Did you feel as if you were choking?	Yes	No
f. Did you have hot flashes or chills?	Yes	No
g. Did you have nausea or an upset stomach, or feeling that you were going to have diarrhea?	Yes	No
h. Did you feel dizzy, unsteady, or faint?	Yes	No
i. Did you have tingling or numbness in parts of your body?	Yes	No
j. Did you tremble or shake?	Yes	No
k. Were you afraid of dying?	Yes	No
Low panic symptoms = The 1st question is answered "No" **or** the criteria for moderate or high are not met.		
Moderate panic symptoms = The 1st question is answered "Yes" **and** any other of the 1st 4 questions is answered "Yes" **and** 3 of the subsequent questions (a-k) are answered "Yes."		
High panic symptoms = All of the 1st 4 questions are answered "Yes" **and** 4 or more of the subsequent questions (a-k) are answered "Yes."		

Source: Data from Spitzer et al.[23]

anticipating and during benzodiazepine taper. Reassurance by the clinician is usually sufficient to allay these concerns.

Psychotherapy: Patients who continue to struggle with anticipatory anxiety and/or avoidant behavior benefit greatly from referral to mental health professionals skilled in relaxation training (including breathing-control exercises), CBT, and progressive desensitization. The immersion therapy noted earlier is the mainstay of treatment, but we do not recommend that the clinician engage in this without specific training. Multimodal therapies reduce overall stress and promote better general health and fitness.[26]

POSTTRAUMATIC STRESS DISORDER

The lifetime prevalence for PTSD is 6.8%.[1] PTSD is a common and disabling condition that follows a triggering event(s) of significant trauma. War experiences historically have been most extensively researched, especially the emotional and physical sequelae of combat often referred to in the past as "soldier's heart," "shell shock," or "combat fatigue." More recently, PTSD has been recognized as arising from any common traumatic event such as motor vehicle accidents, physical and sexual assault, and other accidents causing serious injury. Sensitizing circumstances now also include experiences of witnessing traumatic events and/or empathic responses in relatives and people who are emotionally connected with victims. Development of PTSD has "dose-related" features (severity of harm and perceived threat of harm) and "frequency of exposure" features. People who have repeated exposures to traumatic events as occurs in law enforcement, firefighters, first responders, and health care personnel who work in emergency medical settings can also develop PTSD.[27] Those most at risk are people who have a prior history of emotional problems, especially by 6 years of age, early developmental hardship or abuse, and female gender. High levels of social support prior to the traumatic event have a protective effect.

Early intervention following the trauma often can prevent the long-term sequelae resulting in life-long disability. Generally, the longer PTSD remains unrecognized and untreated, the more severe and expansive the harmful fallout becomes. Early recognition and intervention(s) are critically important and represent another example of effective preventive mental health care in primary care settings.[28]

DSM-5 Diagnostic Criteria: PTSD and Acute Stress Disorder. Criteria for acute stress disorder (ASD) is the same as for PTSD except patients have symptoms persisting beyond 3 days but not beyond 1 month—compared to 1 month or more for PTSD. The PTSD diagnostic criteria have been expanded to 3½ pages in DSM-5.[6] Rather than present all the new criteria, salient diagnostic features are (1) involuntary, intrusive memories of the event; (2) distressing and recurring dreams/nightmares of the event; and (3) sudden dissociative episodes of reexperiencing the trauma. Dissociative episodes, hallmarks of PTSD, range from brief upsetting intrusions into consciousness, to loss of awareness of surroundings. Episodes often are described as "it was like it was happening all over again." "It was like being right back there." Untreated, patients suffer serious emotional consequences of sadness, fear, guilt, shame, and horror and these become chronic, abiding feelings in their lives, sometimes alternating with periods of emotional blunting where patients describe: "I don't feel anything anymore, I just feel numb." Cognitive distortions eventually develop involving skewed beliefs about themselves, others, and the world; for example, "I'm a bad person," "You can't trust anyone," "Face it, the world is a dangerous place and will never change," "No one can understand how I feel and no one can help me." Such thoughts and feelings lead to increasingly avoidant behavior similar to the progressively constrictive behaviors of patients with panic disorder. Patients become more detached socially, isolating themselves even from concerned loved ones and withdrawing from activities they formerly enjoyed. Hygiene and general personal care

may deteriorate and the self-neglect can progress to more active risky behavior. Patients develop heightened emotional arousal that takes the form of irritability, exaggerated startle, and hypervigilance. The behavioral term, "stimulus generalization," describes the hypervigilance for any circumstance encountered, even remotely, that resembles their sensitizing event, for example, sudden loud noises, shouting, weeping, blood, and even olfactory stimuli—anything that reminds them of the traumatic experience. Substance abuse is common as an attempt at relief from the downward spiral of misery, and this further complicates treatment and recovery. Occupational functioning deteriorates often resulting in increasing dependence and/or homelessness.

PTSD has many overlapping features with depressive disorders and other anxiety disorders, which also often are comorbid (co-occurring) disorders, as described earlier in this and the previous chapter, thus complicating differential diagnosis; that is, there is more than 1 diagnosis. Fortunately, interventions also have overlapping features.

Diagnosis and treatment may be aided by the use of screening instruments. Described in Table 5-11, the PTSD Checklist for DSM-5 (PCL-5) is a new instrument still under study, but it can provide some guidance. It provides both an opportunity for patients to describe the sensitizing event in a more "open-ended" fashion as well as rating a list of 20 symptom-related criteria on a point scale from "Not at all" = 0 to "Extremely" = 4 points; a score of 33 or more is proposed as screening positive for PTSD, pending further research. The symptom check-list and point score features in Table 5-11 are very helpful also in monitoring the progress of multimodal comprehensive interventions.[29]

Treatment. General considerations for primary care treatment of PTSD are consistent with the nature of any other chronic progressive illness: prevention is paramount and the longer the illness goes undiagnosed and untreated, the worse it gets—and the more difficult it becomes to stabilize and reverse.[30]

Clinicians have a critically important role in both the prevention and treatment of PTSD. Prevention involves early diagnosis and debriefing, which can provide supportive reassurance and comforting validation for the emotional reactions that follow the event. Heightened autonomic responses may be

TABLE 5-11(A). PTSD Checklist for DSM-5 (PCL-5)

Instructions: This questionnaire asks about problems you may have had after a very stressful experience involving actual or threatened death, serious injury, or sexual violence. It could be something that happened to you directly, something you witnessed, or something you learned happened to a close family member or close friend. Some examples are a serious accident; fire; disaster such as a hurricane, tornado, or earthquake; physical or sexual attack or abuse; war; homicide; or suicide.

First, please answer of few questions about your worst event, which for this questionnaire means the event that currently bothers you the most. This could be one of the examples above or some other very stressful experience. Also, it could be a single event (eg, a car crash) or multiple similar events (eg, multiple stressful events in a war-zone or repeated sexual abuse).

Briefly identify the worst event (if you feel comfortable doing so):_____

How long ago did it happen?_____ (please estimate if you are not sure)

Did it involve actual or threatened death, serious injury, or sexual violence? Yes_____ No_____

How did you experience it?

_____ it happened to me directly

_____ I witnessed it

_____ I learned about it happening to a close family member or close friend

_____ I was repeatedly exposed to details about it as part of my job (eg, paramedic, police, military, or other first responder)

_____ Other, please describe_____

If the event involved the death of a close family member or close friend, was it due to some kind of accident or violence, or was it due to natural causes?

_____ Accident or violence

_____ Natural causes

_____ Not applicable (the event did not involve the death of a close family member or close friend)

Second, keeping this in mind, read each of the problems on the next page and then circle 1 of the numbers to the right to indicate how much you have been bothered by that problem **in the past month**.

attenuated with medications, generally β-blockers. Early referral to mental health professionals experienced in the treatment of PTSD and/or programs especially designed for PTSD care are usually necessary.[31]

Clinicians also have a role in the care of their patients who have developed full-blown PTSD. Again, the supportive and empathic relationship is important in correcting what, by this point, often is damaged trust. Clinician's may provide "first-line" medication management concomitant with the patient's treatment by the mental health professional for counseling.

Psychotherapy involves general techniques as previously described in the treatment of other anxiety disorders. These include providing a safe forum to process the traumatizing experience and subsequent struggles to cope, encouragement toward improvement in self-care, techniques for reflection and relaxation, and graded exposure for avoidant behaviors. Many PTSD treatment programs include psychotherapy and group counseling, which may include patients who have experienced the same or similar traumatic events.

Pharmacologic Treatment

1. β-Blockers are being used with increasing frequency to attenuate the distressing autonomic symptoms experienced post trauma and can be started in the emergency department. Propranolol is most commonly used in divided doses up to 40 mg/d.[32] From Table 5-5, if you are using β-blockers (for any purpose), avoid paroxetine, fluoxetine, and, perhaps, duloxetine because they can dangerously elevate the drugs levels by their inhibition of the P450 2D6 pathway.[33-35]

TABLE 5-11(B). PTSD Checklist					
In the past month how much have you been bothered by:					
	Not at all (0)	**A little bit (1)**	**Moderately (2)**	**Quite a bit (3)**	**Extremely (4)**
1. Repeated disturbing and unwanted memories of the stressful experience?	❏	❏	❏	❏	❏
2. Repeated disturbing dreams of the stressful experience?	❏	❏	❏	❏	❏
3. Suddenly feeling or acting as if the stressful experience were actually happening again (as if you were actually back there and reliving it)?	❏	❏	❏	❏	❏
4. Feeling very upset when something reminded you of the stressful experience?	❏	❏	❏	❏	❏
5. Having strong physical reactions when something reminded you of the stressful experience (eg, heart pounding, trouble breathing, sweating)?	❏	❏	❏	❏	❏
6. Avoiding memories, thoughts, or feelings related to the stressful experience?	❏	❏	❏	❏	❏
7. Avoiding external reminders of the stressful experience (eg, people, places conversations, activities, objects, or situations)?	❏	❏	❏	❏	❏
8. Trouble remembering important parts of the stressful experience?	❏	❏	❏	❏	❏
9. Having strong negative beliefs about yourself, other people, or the world (eg, having thoughts such as I am bad, there is something seriously wrong with me, no one can be trusted, the world is completely dangerous)?	❏	❏	❏	❏	❏
10. Blaming yourself or someone else for the stressful experience or what happened after it?	❏	❏	❏	❏	❏
11. Having strong negative feelings such as fear, horror, anger, guilt, or shame?	❏	❏	❏	❏	❏

(Continued)

TABLE 5-11(B).   PTSD Checklist (*Continued*)

12. Loss of interest in activities that you use to enjoy?	❑	❑	❑	❑	❑
13. Feeling distant or cutoff from other people?	❑	❑	❑	❑	❑
14. Trouble experiencing positive feelings (eg, being unable to feel happiness or having loving feelings for people close to you?)	❑	❑	❑	❑	❑
15. Irritable behavior, angry outbursts, or acting aggressively?	❑	❑	❑	❑	❑
16. Taking too many risks or doing things that could cause you harm?	❑	❑	❑	❑	❑
17. Being "superalert" or watchful or on guard?	❑	❑	❑	❑	❑
18. Feeling jumpy or easily startled?	❑	❑	❑	❑	❑
19. Having difficulty concentrating?	❑	❑	❑	❑	❑
20. Trouble falling or staying asleep?	❑	❑	❑	❑	❑

Preliminary validation work suggests a cut-point score of 33 to be reasonable until further psychometric work is available.

Source: U.S. Veterans Administration.[29]

2. Prazosin, an α-blocker, is effective to attenuate nightmares in patients with PTSD. The starting dose is usually 1 mg at bedtime with gradual titration to 4 mg. Higher doses may be necessary but merit caution.

3. *Antidepressants:* The SSRIs (fluoxetine, paroxetine, and sertraline) and the SNRI (venlafaxine) are most commonly used for PTSD. Their starting doses and titration strategies are the same as in the treatment for GAD and panic disorder.

4. *Benzodiazepines:* The short-onset-of-action medications alprazolam and lorazepam are indicated for acute control of crisis situations but have limited indications otherwise. Avoid chronic use. For longer, but still limited periods of time, clonazepam represents a safer choice because of its slower onset of action and longer half-life. It is still wisest to use it in conjunction with the above antidepressant medications with gradual taper and discontinuation as the antidepressant shows therapeutic effect.

Benzodiazepines have a higher risk of dependence and abuse and are contraindicated if the patient has a history of or shows problems with self-medication or substance abuse.

SOCIAL ANXIETY DISORDER AND PHOBIAS

Social anxiety and phobias are easily conceptualized as encountering situations or things that would make most people anxious or fearful. Examples of common situations that provoke anxiety include being asked to address a group on short notice (especially if unprepared), climbing a tall ladder, arriving at a social function to find you know no one present except the host, a spider suddenly descending in front of your face, or suddenly encountering a coiled snake during a leisurely hike. Social anxiety disorders can begin at a very young age and include also problems like separation anxiety disorder. This is a common cause in young people of school refusal and social isolation.[36]

When one has an actual disorder, it involves disabling fear greatly out of proportion to the event(s) and interferes with social and occupational functioning. Social anxiety and phobic disorders generally come to the attention of clinicians when fear causes major dysfunction. Attention may also come from spouses/relatives rather than the patient because many times the patients themselves are embarrassed or self-conscious about their fears. Patients themselves usually are aware their anxiety is out of proportion to the thing or event and generally have developed coping strategies, which are more or less successful but, nonetheless, prevent them from experiencing life to the fullest.

Social phobia involves circumstances where the patient feels subject to the scrutiny and critical assessment by others. Patients have intense anxiety when anticipating job interviews, interviews for advancement, or entrance interviews for college or professional school. Fear of humiliation, embarrassment, and failure is very common. The most common social phobia is the fear of public speaking and resultant overcautious avoidance of employment, educational, or social circumstances requiring this. It is a common reason in employment situations to decline offers or opportunities for advancement. If public speaking becomes a new requirement in their advancement, it may result in anxiety sufficiently severe to prompt resignation.

Treatment by the clinician generally involves validation, reassurance, and treatment with propranolol to attenuate the autonomic symptoms of anticipatory anxiety. Use the propranolol in low doses to be taken 30 to 60 minutes prior to the speaking engagement or other social event; as before, use antidepressants other than fluoxetine and paroxetine because they can elevate levels of β-blockers. This facilitates a successful experience and aids in promoting anxiety symptom extinction. If not effective, referral to a mental health care professional for behavioral desensitization often is quite helpful.

Specific phobias (eg, of heights or of animals) are best referred to mental health professionals for treatment with desensitization procedures. Specific phobias respond remarkably well to treatment with relaxation techniques followed by extinction procedures involving graded exposure. Patients with lifelong fears are very commonly surprised and pleased

with the expeditious results. Many comment they only wish they had come for treatment earlier.

OBSESSIVE COMPULSIVE DISORDER

The lifetime prevalence of obsessive compulsive disorder (OCD) is 1.6%.[1] The disorder typically has clear biological components as evidenced by higher concordance in monozygotic twins, responsiveness to medications mediating serotonergic neural systems, and the association with Tourette syndrome (repetitive motor and verbally expressive tics).

Obsessive and compulsive features, like normal levels of anxiety, may be appropriate, adaptive, and necessary. This is especially true in the qualities and characteristics required to become a successful professional or to succeed in any occupation or endeavor where diligence, ability to delay gratification, attention to detail, order, cleanliness, and/or scrupulous adherence to high standards are required. One clear example is the extensive preparation required to become a surgeon, where cleanliness, attention to preparation, step-by-step procedural detail, and high standards are highly valued and required.

Both OCD and obsessive-compulsive personality disorder are exaggerations of these normal situations, both resulting in social and occupational dysfunction. The major distinguishing feature between OCD and the personality disorder is the presence or absence of anxiety. People with the personality disorder often do not feel anxious about their thoughts or behaviors. Moreover, they may even feel a sense of superiority over those who are less clean, organized, or scrupulous than themselves. In OCD, people recognize their thoughts and behaviors are out of proportion to the circumstances and experience even extreme anxiety about them. Generally, they are troubled by their obsessional thoughts and develop compulsive behaviors or rituals to cope with the anxiety, only then to have the thoughts, rising anxiety, and ritualistic behavior repeat.

Obsessions in OCD take the form of intrusive thoughts that distress patients greatly and which they cannot easily suppress. Compulsions appear as ritualistic patterns of behavior that serve to control the level of anxiety. As the obsessions mount, patients are driven to repeat the behaviors that they themselves recognize as irrational. Rituals can intervene and take the form of repetitious mental activities and tasks such as counting, performing calculations, or repetitive silent prayer. Common obsessive themes include cleanliness, contamination, orderliness, symmetry, sex, aggression, and religious faith. The rituals are usually consistent with the obsessive themes and include hand washing, house cleaning, disinfecting, arranging and rearranging things, genuflecting, and repeated checking. Anxiety repeatedly rises to intolerable levels and the compulsions function to relieve it. If stopped from performing the rituals, anxiety levels rise even further. Like phobias, patients many times are embarrassed by their behaviors and come to the attention of clinicians when symptoms interfere with social and occupational functioning. Attention may also come from concerned relatives and loved ones who recognize the patient's misery and dysfunction. The symptoms at times, however, can result in wider family conflict and dysfunction.

Variants of OCD such as trichotillomania also come to the attention of clinician's by the presence of persistent skin irritation/lesions caused by compulsive picking, scratching, and hair pulling. The clinician may notice these and comment upon them when the patient comes in for a visit for another medical problem. Body dysmorphic disorder is a serious and frequently disabling condition seen in primary care in patients who express obsessive dissatisfaction with their appearance and persistently request referral for cosmetic surgery. These obsessions frequently involve facial features or body contour. Many times these issues come to the attention of the clinician only after the patient has already self-referred for repeated cosmetic procedures.

OCD is another psychiatric disorder where clinicians often need to refer to mental health professionals skilled in CBT (or other psychotherapeutic approaches) with the clinician providing pharmacologic management.[37] First-line medications with FDA approval for treatment of OCD include the SSRI's fluoxetine, paroxetine, and sertraline. Dosage strategies are similar to the treatment of anxiety disorders but generally require a longer time for symptom remission and require maximum approved dosages. Other SSRIs and SNRIs not having FDA approval may also be effective. At times it may be necessary to "push the dose" to higher "off-label" proportions. In these cases, psychiatric consultation and added attention to monitoring for adverse-effects may be necessary.

Second-line medications include the SSRI fluvoxamine and the older tricyclic antidepressant: clomipramine. These drugs are effective but represent "fallback" choices due to the higher frequency of interference with the metabolism of other medications and harsher adverse-effect profiles.

OVERLAP OF ANXIETY DISORDERS

The diagnosis of any specific anxiety disorder is at times difficult and complex due to the commonality and overlapping nature of their DSM-5 diagnostic features. Diagnosis and subsequent treatment then become a careful assessment of the constellation of symptoms which predominate and cause patients the most emotional pain and dysfunction. Table 5-12 assists in sorting out these complexities.

The clinician may often need the assistance of mental health professionals. For medication complications, referral to a psychiatrist or an advanced practice psychiatric nurse is advisable. More often, for emotional and behavioral complications, especially constricting or avoidant behavior, referral to a psychologist, clinical social worker, or licensed counselor trained in multimodal psychotherapy and especially in cognitive behavioral therapy (CBT) can be helpful. The movement toward "integrative care" includes the location of these professionals inside primary care practice settings, facilitating communication, expeditious referral, and team-oriented care.[38,39] It also further minimizes any perception on the part of the patient that they are being rejected or abandoned.

CONCLUSION

The anxiety disorders can and should be diagnosed early and treated within the primary care setting. Since a number of drugs have FDA approval for the treatment of anxiety disorders, the clinician should become familiar with and skilled in the use of a select few, those with the fewest and least disabling side effects. Medications should be given sufficient time to work (usually 6-8 weeks) before trying a second one. If the patient has a second medication failure, we recommend referral to psychiatry for further medication recommendations. Teamwork with nonpsychiatrist mental health professionals is also

TABLE 5-12. Overlapping Symptoms in Anxiety Disorders

	GAD	PD	PTSD	SAD	OCD
Arousal	+++	++	+++	+	+/−
Avoidant behavior	+	++++	+++	+++	+
Concentration	++++	++	++	+	+
Expected panic	+	+	+	+++	-
Unexpected panic	+	++++	+	−	−
Fatigue/low energy	++++	++	++	+	+/−
Irritable mood	+++	+	+++	+	+/−
Muscle tension	++++	++	++	+	+
Obsessions	+	+	+	++	++++
Sleep disturbance	+++	+	+++	+	++

GAD = generalized anxiety disorder; OCD = obsessive compulsive disorder; PD = panic disorder; PTSD = posttraumatic stress disorder; SAD = social anxiety disorder.

critical in achieving the best outcomes, and expeditious referral is necessary for several of the disorders, often for CBT.

We now turn in Chapter 6 to the third (and final) group of mental disorders the clinician of the future will need to manage: prescription substance misuse and other substance use disorders.

HELPFUL PATIENT INFORMATION SOURCES

1. *The Anxiety and Phobia Workbook*, 6th ed. Edmund Burke, New Harbinger Publications; 2015. Available online as downloadable PDF. It may be tried as an individual patient self-help effort or in combination with psychotherapy.
2. Anxiety and Disorders Association of America: http://www.adaa.org.
3. National Institute of Mental Health: https://www.nimh.nih.gov/health/topics/anxiety-disorders/index.shtml.
4. *Dare: The New Way to End Anxiety and Stop Panic Attacks*. 2015. B. McDonagh, BMD Publishing.
5. National Center for PTSD: https://www.ptsd.va.gov/.

6. Raja S, Orsillo S, *Overcoming Trauma and PTSD: Workbook*. New Harbinger Publications; 2012.

MOBILE APPLICATIONS

1. PTSD Coach: https://www.ptsd.va.gov/public/materials/apps/PTSDCoach.asp.
2. Pacifica: http://www.thinkpacifica.com/. (Mindfulness and CBT strategies)
3. Breath2Relax: http://t2health.dcoe.mil/apps/breathe2relax. (Breath control guide)

REFERENCES

1. Kessler RC, Berglund P, Demler O, Jin R, Merikangas KR, Walters EE. Lifetime prevalence and age-of-onset distributions of DSM-IV disorders in the National Comorbidity Survey Replication. *Arch Gen Psychiatry*. 2005;62:593-602.
2. Kessler RC, Petukhova M, Sampson NA, Zaslavsky AM, Wittchen HU. Twelve-month and lifetime prevalence and lifetime morbid risk of anxiety and mood disorders in the United States. *Int J Methods Psychiatr Res*. 2012;21(3):169-184.
3. Remes O, Brayne C, van der Linde R, Lafortune L. A systematic review of reviews on the prevalence of anxiety

disorders in adult populations. *Brain Behav.* 2016;6(7): e00497.

4. Duval ER, Javanbakht A, Liberzon I. Neural circuits in anxiety and stress disorders: a focused review. *Ther Clin Risk Manag.* 2015;11:115-126.

5. Dresler T, Guhn A, Tupak SV, et al. Revise the revised? New dimensions of the neuroanatomical hypothesis of panic disorder. *J Neural Transm (Vienna).* 2013;120(1): 3-29.

6. American Psychiatric Association. *Diagnostic and Statistical Manual of Mental Disorders.* 5th ed. Washington, DC: American Psychiatric Association; 2013.

7. Bystritsky A, Khalsa SS, Cameron ME, Schiffman J. Current diagnosis and treatment of anxiety disorders. *P T.* 2013;38(1):30-57.

8. Khoury B, Lecomte T, Fortin G, et al. Mindfulness-based therapy: a comprehensive meta-analysis. *Clin Psychol Rev.* 2013;33(6):763-771.

9. Jayakody K, Gunadasa S, Hosker C. Exercise for anxiety disorders: systematic review. *Br J Sports Med.* 2014;48(3): 187-196.

10. Chugh-Gupta N, Baldassarre FG, Vrkljan BH. A systematic review of yoga for state anxiety: considerations for occupational therapy. *Can J Occup Ther.* 2013;80(3): 150-170.

11. Hofmann SG, Smits JA. Cognitive-behavioral therapy for adult anxiety disorders: a meta-analysis of randomized placebo-controlled trials. *J Clin Psychiatry.* 2008;69(4): 621-632.

12. Bandelow B, Sagebiel A, Belz M, Gorlich Y, Michaelis S, Wedekind D. Enduring effects of psychological treatments for anxiety disorders: meta-analysis of follow-up studies. *Br J Psychiatry.* 2018;212(6):333-338.

13. Bandelow B, Michaelis S. Epidemiology of anxiety disorders in the 21st century. *Dialogues Clin Neurosci.* 2015;17(3):327-335.

14. Rodrigues SM, LeDoux JE, Sapolsky RM. The influence of stress hormones on fear circuitry. *Annu Rev Neurosci.* 2009;32:289-313.

15. Spitzer RL, Kroenke K, Williams JB, Lowe B. A brief measure for assessing generalized anxiety disorder: the GAD-7. *Arch Intern Med.* 2006;166(10):1092-1097.

16. Bandelow B, Michaelis S, Wedekind D. Treatment of anxiety disorders. *Dialogues Clin Neurosci.* 2017;19(2):93-107.

17. Katz G. Tachyphylaxis/tolerance to antidepressants in treatment of dysthymia: results of a retrospective naturalistic chart review study. *Psychiatry Clin Neurosci.* 2011;65(5):499-504.

18. Thase ME. Effects of venlafaxine on blood pressure: a meta-analysis of original data from 3744 depressed patients. *J Clin Psychiatry.* 1998;59(10):502-508.

19. Arafa M, Shamloul R. A randomized study examining the effect of 3 SSRI on premature ejaculation using a validated questionnaire. *Ther Clin Risk Manag.* 2007;3(4): 527-531.

20. Farach FJ, Pruitt LD, Jun JJ, Jerud AB, Zoellner LA, Roy-Byrne PP. Pharmacological treatment of anxiety disorders: current treatments and future directions. *J Anxiety Disord.* 2012;26(8):833-843.

21. Bandelow B. Comparison of the DSM-5 and ICD-10: panic and other anxiety disorders. *CNS Spectr.* 2017;22(5): 404-406.

22. Batterham PJ, Mackinnon AJ, Christensen H. The panic disorder screener (PADIS): development of an accurate and brief population screening tool. *Psychiatry Res.* 2015;228(1):72-76.

23. Spitzer RL, Kroenke K, Williams JB. Validation and utility of a self-report version of PRIME-MD: the PHQ primary care study. Primary Care Evaluation of Mental Disorders. Patient Health Questionnaire. *JAMA.* 1999;282(18):1737-1744.

24. Filho AS, Maciel BC, Martin-Santos R, Romano MM, Crippa JA. Does the association between mitral valve prolapse and panic disorder really exist? *Prim Care Companion J Clin Psychiatry.* 2008;10(1):38-47.

25. Kim S, Roth WT, Wollburg E. Effects of therapeutic relationship, expectancy, and credibility in breathing therapies for anxiety. *Bull Menninger Clin.* 2015;79(2):116-130.

26. Plag J, Gaudlitz K, Schumacher S, et al. Effect of combined cognitive-behavioural therapy and endurance training on cortisol and salivary alpha-amylase in panic disorder. *J Psychiatr Res.* 2014;58:12-19.

27. Skogstad M, Skorstad ML, Lie A, Conradi H, Heri T, Weisaeth L. Work-related post-traumatic stress disorder. *Occup Med (Lond).* 2017;63:175-182.

28. Sareen J. Posttraumatic stress disorder in adults: impact, comorbidity, risk factors, and treatment. *Can J Psychiatry.* 2014;59(9):460-467.

29. Veterans Administration 2017; https://www.ptsd.va.gov/ professional/assessment/adult-sr/ptsd-checklist.asp. Accessed December 14, 2017.

30. Qi W, Gevonden M, Shalev A. Prevention of posttraumatic stress disorder after trauma: current evidence and future directions. *Curr Psychiatry Rep.* 2016;18(2):20.

31. Burbiel JC. Primary prevention of posttraumatic stress disorder: drugs and implications. *Mil Med Res.* 2015;2:24.

32. Steenen SA, van Wijk AJ, van der Heijden GJ, van Westrhenen R, de Lange J, de Jongh A. Propranolol for the treatment of anxiety disorders: systematic review and meta-analysis. *J Psychopharmacol.* 2016;30(2): 128-139.

33. Ayano G. Psychotropic medications metabolized by cytochromes P450 (CYP) 2D6 enzyme and relevant drug interactions. *Clin Pharmacol Biopharm*. 2016;5:4.

34. British Psychological Society. Appendix 16. Table of drug interactions. In: National Collaborating Centre for Mental Health (UK). *NICE Clinical Guidelines* No. 91. Depression in Adults with a Chronic Physical Health Problem. Leicester (UK): The British Psychological Society; 2010.

35. Spina E, Santoro V, D'Arrigo C. Clinically relevant pharmacokinetic drug interactions with second-generation antidepressants: an update. *Clin Ther*. 2008;30(7):1206-1227.

36. Mohatt J, Bennett SM, Walkup JT. Treatment of separation, generalized, and social anxiety disorders in youths. *Am J Psychiatry*. 2014;171(7):741-748.

37. Hirschtritt ME, Bloch MH, Mathews CA. Obsessive-compulsive disorder: advances in diagnosis and treatment. *JAMA*. 2017;317(13):1358-1367.

38. Huffman JC, Niazi SK, Rundell JR, Sharpe M, Katon WJ. Essential articles on collaborative care models for the treatment of psychiatric disorders in medical settings: a publication by the academy of psychosomatic medicine research and evidence-based practice committee. *Psychosomatics*. 2014;55(2):109-122.

39. Kroenke K, Unutzer J. Closing the false divide: sustainable approaches to integrating mental health services into primary care. *J Gen Intern Med*. 2017;32(4):404-410.

Misuse of Prescription Substances and Other Substances

6

INTRODUCTION

In this chapter, we address substance use, the final topic for which future clinicians will need considerable mastery in handling mental health problems in medical settings. We'll focus mainly on prescription-based disorders where the prescribing clinician has great control. Physicians unfortunately received little clinical training in chronic pain or in using opioids when in medical school or in most residencies, just one among many factors contributing to the current opioid crisis.

The Mental Health Care Model (MHCM) from Chapter 3 provides the overarching structure for managing prescription substance problems, including chronic pain. In this chapter, we'll address the pharmacologic and related nonpharmacologic management of patients with problematic substance use. Let's start with the opioid crisis, the worst of the prescription drug problems.

PRESCRIPTION OPIOID MISUSE

Background

Considerable research shows *there is little, if any, clinically significant benefit for opioid use in chronic noncancer pain.*[1-4] The Centers for Disease Control and Prevention (CDC) has recently underscored this fact, including that opioids should be prescribed for acute pain only and for no more than 3 to 7 days.[1] For the unfortunate millions of people already addicted to or otherwise dependent on chronic opioid use, the CDC advises that the safe dose is no more than 50 morphine milligram equivalents (MME) per day, and that the maximum acceptable dose is 90 MME each day; more on how to calculate MME shortly. Unfortunately, we have seen people taking as much as 2200 MME and commonly see them taking 200 to 400 MME. These are lethal amounts for someone not accustomed to this high dose. For example, if a teenager steals them from an addicted parent and takes the same dose written on the bottle for their parent, it could be lethal.

You will, we believe, be encouraged to learn that there are effective ways to manage these patients. Informed by a rich body of research from psychiatry, multidisciplinary pain management, and primary care,[5-15] the authors' research group identified an evidence-based model for medical physicians and other clinicians, the MHCM, which you've already learned in Chapter 3. It is designed to guide clinicians in conducting mental health care in medical settings. This model includes treating chronic pain and co-occurring mental disorders, reducing and discontinuing opioids while replacing them with something effective, and handling patients demanding more narcotics.[13,14,16-20] In addition to demonstrating that it is a very effective model to care for patients, we also have shown it is easily learned.[16,21]

Misuse

Many opioid prescriptions are "misused," which we define as use for *nonprescribed* reasons such as for recreation, to satisfy an addiction, to self-treat one's pain, to give to someone else, or to sell.[22] Importantly, there is no agreed-upon definition of misuse, abuse, or addiction,[23,24] and we have chosen to use this as the most straightforward way to understand misuse. Here's what makes the misuse problem harder for clinicians: it's difficult to determine who is misusing opioids. Certainly, the majority who use opioids do not misuse them, but each year in America more than 11 million will.[25,26] All told, at some point in their lives, 52 million adults have used prescription drugs for nonmedical reasons.[27] Especially worrisome, about one-half of teenagers believe that prescription drugs are safer than street drugs, preferring them recreationally. Compounding this problem, over half of prescription drug users get them free from a friend or relative.[27] Both facts have serious implications for deaths from suicidal overdoses and accidental overdoses when using the drug recreationally.

Diagnosing Misuse

Let's first look at some clinical clues suggestive of opioid misuse. These clues can raise your suspicion and help direct your questioning and subsequent investigation to arrive at a more definitive misuse diagnosis.

Interviewing the Patient Wanting an Opioid Prescription. For patients using opioids for chronic pain and often associated symptoms of depression, anxiety, and insomnia, the greater the number of the patient behaviors in Table 6-1, the more likely the patient is misusing the prescribed opioid.[22,28] These aberrant, often drug-seeking behaviors represent the impact of opioids on the patient's personal and professional life. Certainly, they are not diagnostic, and patients may occasionally lose a prescription or have it stolen. Rather, it is the repetitive pattern that is the clue to potential issues.

In addition to detecting misuse, in taking a careful history, you'll learn of important *contraindications to any opioid use*: prior history overdoses, especially on opioids, any substance use disorder (prescription, alcohol, illicit), or an untreated mental disorder.

While one is always patient-centered, obtaining substance-related information often requires the more specific, closed-ended questioning characteristic of clinician-centered inquiry.[29] As well, important information about opioid use often comes from relatives or others familiar with the patient because they are concerned about the patient's medication use.[29] Knowing that these interactions can be a stressful, often guarded discussion for the patient, assure them that you ask

TABLE 6-1. Clinical Clues to Possible Prescription Opioid Misuse

1. Noncoordinated prescribers from multiple practice settings
2. Multiple patient requests for visits without appointment
3. Multiple patient requests for early medication
4. Multiple patient reports of lost/stolen medication
5. Increased dose without approval
6. Using opioid for nonpain symptoms, such as insomnia or anxiety
7. Using alcohol for pain
8. Missing appointments because of pain
9. Hoarding opioids
10. Sedated from opioids
11. Intoxicated from opioids
12. Complaints about the patient's misuse from other providers/emergency room/family
13. Patient reluctance to reduce medication in face of no benefit
14. Patient reluctance to participate in other methods to control pain
15. Violation of terms in medication contract
16. Involved in complication of using opioids, work injury, traffic accident

these questions of everyone where opioids are being prescribed or requested—and that the information obtained is part of providing the best care possible. In particular, you need to determine the following information about possible risk factors[30]:

1. Use of opioids: first use; doses; duration; present use; time of most recent use; side effects and complications; problems with work, school, relationships, or the law; any accidental or deliberate overdosing
2. Other substances used now and in the past with similar details obtained, particularly alcohol and illicit drugs
3. Mental disorders and the details of these
4. Family history of drug or alcohol abuse or mental health problems
5. Specific medical/surgical problems sometimes associated with opioid misuse: hepatitis B and C, HIV, frequent accidents and trauma, and frequent skin infections
6. Nicotine dependency
7. Pain that is unexplained, occurs after a motor vehicle accident, or occurs in more than 3 body areas

Systematic Screening for Opioid Misuse. Careful as you may be in your history, we still need systematic drug screening for misuse in all patients *prior to* beginning opioids (or prior to the next refill if already on them). To identify aberrant, misuse behaviors, we recommend the Opioid Risk Tool (ORT) in Table 6-2.[31] The revised Screener and Opioid Assessment for Patients with Pain (SOAPP-R)[30,32] is much longer, but has good psychometrics and a higher rate of identifying patients who eventually evince misuse.

Observing aberrant behaviors, however, also is insufficient and may underestimate misuse.[30] There are 2 necessary items of information you will need in all patients on or beginning on opioids: (1) the patient's pattern of filling prescriptions from your state's prescription drug monitoring program (PDMP); and (2) a urine drug screen. They are key elements in making a diagnosis of misuse and are reflected in the first 2 items in Table 6-3.

Prescription Drug Monitoring Program. PDMPs are statewide electronic databases that collect data on controlled substances dispensed in that state. Data are available to individuals, such as clinicians or

TABLE 6-2. The Opioid Risk Tool		
This tool should be administered to patients upon an initial visit prior to beginning or renewing opioid therapy for pain management. **Mark each box that applies**	**Female**	**Male**
Family history of substance abuse		
Alcohol	1	3
Illegal drugs	2	3
Prescription drugs	4	4
Personal history of substance abuse		
Alcohol	3	3
Illegal drugs	4	4
Prescription drugs	5	5
Age between 16 and 45 years	1	1
History of preadolescent sexual abuse	3	0
Psychological disease		
ADD, OCD, bipolar disorder, schizophrenia	2	2
Depression	1	1
Scoring totals		

ADD = attention deficit disorder; OCD = obsessive compulsive disorder.

Scoring: A score of 3 or lower indicates low risk for future opioid abuse, a score of 4 to 7 indicates moderate risk for opioid abuse, and a score of 8 or higher indicates a high risk for opioid abuse.

Questionnaire developed by Lynn R. Webster, MD to assess risk of opioid addiction.

Webster LR, Webster R. Predicting aberrant behaviors in opioid-treated patients: preliminary validation of the opioid risk too. *Pain Med.* 2005;6(6):432.

TABLE 6-3. Evidence of Prescription Substance Misuse[a]

1. Prescription drug monitoring program indicates substances obtained from providers/pharmacies not part of the contract—or not filling prescriptions for prescribed substances in the contract
2. Urine toxicology positive for any nonprescribed addicting substance—or negative for prescribed opioids
3. Tolerance
4. Withdrawal
5. Selling/stealing medications
6. Buying prescription drugs from nonmedical sources
7. Prescription forgery
8. Injection of oral preparations

[a]Substances include opioids, benzodiazepines, and stimulants.

pharmacists, authorized to receive the information from the state agency administering the program. The intent is to provide a means of monitoring controlled substance use by both physicians and patients, to prevent and deter drug abuse and diversion, to identify patients with addiction problems, to inform public health initiatives, and to educate people about drug abuse. Although each system is state based, there are some that communicate with other states. All states and the District of Columbia have operating PDMPs. Although practices vary considerably, it has been demonstrated that mandatory checking of the PDMP before prescribing an opioid has reduced overdose deaths.[33] Current PDMP contact information can be obtained from the Alliance of States with Prescription Monitoring Programs (www.nascsa.org/rxMonitoring.htm).[34]

Often required by state regulations, it is imperative to check the PDMP *before* prescribing opioids to your patient, particularly for any new patient requesting them. When pharmacists dispense controlled substances, they enter these data into the PDMP, increasingly doing so immediately so that data are current; unfortunately, some states still allow delays ranging up to a month, which reduces their value, but they still should be used.[33,35] Most reports from the PDMP provide the time and date of all controlled substance prescriptions filled (and when it was written), the prescriber, the location, and the number of pills and dose actually filled.

From the PDMP you determine what prescriptions a patient has received, when, and from whom. For example, if you had a contract to be the only prescriber and for the patient to use only one pharmacy and the only controlled substance you prescribed was 3 tablets (10 mg) per day for 30 days of oxycodone, you should find this prescription to be the only entry into the PDMP for that period. In general, there are several possibilities from a PDMP report:

1. As in the example above, the opioid(s) prescribed is the only one listed in the PDMP and it is in the amount prescribed over the correct duration—this suggests adherence and no misuse.
2. If the opioid(s) prescribed is not present—this suggests diversion or other misuse, but the patient's inability to obtain the medication must be reviewed with the patient; for example, pharmacy did not have it, patient could not pay for it.
3. If opioids (or other substances) not prescribed in your contract appear in the PDMP—this means there are additional prescribers (they would be listed if from your state) and strongly suggests misuse—again, this requires discussion with the patient for some alternative explanation; for example, went to the emergency department because of a fractured arm or the dentist prescribed opioids following a tooth extraction.

Urine Drug Testing (UDT). You can see that the PDMP is imperfect, so (also imperfect) laboratory testing of the urine for drugs is needed in all patients. In fact, from 30% to 50% of all patients on chronic opioids have abnormal UDTs.[30] The idea is similar to that of the PDMP: ensuring that what is prescribed is present and that there are no nonprescribed controlled substances present and no illicit drugs. But there are pitfalls in interpretation of UDTs.

Urine drug testing is often conducted in 2 phases: (1) screening immunoassay and (2) confirmatory chromatography/mass spectrometry. All guidelines recommend that a positive test on the former be confirmed by the latter to exclude the very common false positives.[30,36-41] Some believe that only the confirmatory test should be done in most instances because of the low sensitivity (high false negative rates) and low specificity (high false positive rates) of the immunoassay.[30,41]

Screening immunoassay: The attributes of the immunoassay are that it is immediately available (point of care or laboratory testing), detects drugs used in the preceding 5 to 7 days, and is inexpensive using test cups or test strips. Its immediate availability is sometimes important, say, in new patient requesting opioids where the PDMP from another state is not available—and you need to know if the drug reported is indeed present. Unfortunately, however, the immunoassay has so many false positives and false negatives that confirmatory testing is required in the opinion of most, unanimously when screens are positive for a substance of interest.[30,36-40] As well, however, the high false negative rate also means that negative screens would benefit from confirmatory testing.

Confirmatory mass spectrometry testing: These tests are done in the laboratory only (no point of care option), are more expensive, detect substances used in the preceding 1 to 2 days, and may take several days to obtain a report. But confirmatory testing has much greater sensitivity and specificity, is able to differentiate among drugs of the same class, is able to measure semisynthetic and synthetic opioids (such as hydromorphone, fentanyl, and oxycodone), and has the ability to check for drug metabolites that sometimes are the key evidence of use.[41] Many believe confirmatory testing should be obtained once or twice yearly in all patients on chronic opioids.[30] The objection to confirmatory testing by mass spectrometry has been cost, but recent evaluations propose that immunoassay is not more cost-effective and should be discarded. The main issue of cost is whether the laboratory invests in the mass spectrometry equipment or sends specimens out for analysis.[41]

There are many important issues in UDT to attend to

1. You must know your laboratory, what its routine panel contains, how to order specific drugs that match your needs, what algorithms are used, and what cutoff values are used.[41] The latter are particularly important because cutoffs are often set too high, resulting in false negatives.[36] A standardized set of cutoffs recently was reported that identifies controlled substances and illicit substances in 97.5% of patients; see Table 6-5 *in the reference* for cutoffs.[37]

2. Likely already obtained during the history, it is critical to know the patient's recent drug history, including the specific times when they last took each medication during the preceding week; this history should include alcohol and marijuana use, which often must be measured via urine testing due to under-reporting or failure to disclose use.

3. One must be very systematic in how the urine is collected to preclude dilution or adulteration, whether deliberate or inadvertent.[30,36,38] Urine should be collected in the clinic or laboratory, preferably early in the morning and evaluated within 3 to 4 minutes of collection if immunoassay is done. If possible, use a dedicated toilet facility with no running water and add a blue color to the water in the toilet. Table 6-4 reviews the characteristics of normal and adulterated urine samples. If the urine is not completely normal, a repeat urine is obtained under direct supervision. The effect of a diluted urine is to decrease the concentration of the drug being measured, while adulteration can destroy the drug.[36,37]

If the urine appears normal, it can be evaluated by immunoassay and/or sent to the lab for confirmatory testing (often collected at the lab). The result

TABLE 6-4. Evaluating a Urine Specimen for Adulteration			
URINE TEST	**NORMAL**	**ABNORMAL**	**LIKELY ADULTERATION OR DILUTION**
Temperature	90-100°F	<90°F	Cold substance, like tap water, added
pH	4.5-8.0	<3.0 or >11.0	Adulteration
Specific gravity	1.002 and 1.030	<1.001	<1.001 is not human urine
Creatinine, random	>20 mg/dL	<20 mg/dL	<20 suggests dilution <5 is not human urine
Appearance	Variations of yellow	Nonyellow	Small bubbles suggest soap

TABLE 6-5. Interpreting Unexpected UDT Results

FINDING	MISUSE	ALTERNATIVE	OPTIONS
Prescribed drug absent	Diversion	Patient could not afford Drug stolen or lost Over use and ran out early Rapid metabolizer	Consult with patient
Nonprescribed drug present	Other prescriber Used others' drug for recreation or self-medication	Legitimate other prescriber, such as emergency room or dentist for acute problem	Consult with patient Refer to addiction specialist
Illicit drug present	Illicit drug use		Consult with patient Refer to addiction specialist
Low specific gravity and creatinine	Deception	Renal tubular abnormality Over-hydration	Consult with patient and review medical issues Refer to addiction specialist
Very high concentration of drug prescribed	Additional drug taken	Metabolic variability	Consult with patient Refer to addiction specialist
Low concentration of unexpected drug	Remote use		Consult with patient Follow-up to ensure clears

should be known before prescribing any opioids. If an immunoassay result is positive for opioids, confirmatory testing is obligatory to exclude false positives. If the result is negative and there is high suspicion of some substance use, confirmatory testing also should be ordered.

Although quantification of results is reported, it cannot be used to judge the actual doses taken by patients.[30] Table 6-5 reviews some possible unexpected results from UDT. It is essential in all cases to discuss them with the patient, always using the patient-centered skills central to the MHCM.

Risk Profile

With information from the history and your screening with the ORT and UDT, we construct a risk profile. This includes the dose and type of opioid medication, polypharmacy (especially opioids and benzodiazepines), history of mental or substance use disorder, and other data. The profile guides in determining the frequency of visits and refills and how often to obtain UDTs. Table 6-6 outlines the features of high-, moderate-, and low-risk patients.[30,38]

We recommend initially monitoring everyone after 1 month (sometimes sooner if high risk) until we are clear on stability of the risk stratification.[30] Then continue to monitor high-risk patients at monthly intervals (including UDT) until stable, including getting the opioid dose to 90 MME or lower. When this is achieved, see them at 2 and then 3 month intervals as long as stable, hopefully moving high-risk patients into the moderate- and lower-risk groups. Moderate risk groups are followed every 4 months and low-risk groups every 6 months. We will return to the details of management soon.

Other items in Table 6-3 also provide evidence of potential misuse. **Tolerance** means that there is less effect from the same amount of drug and/or that increased doses are needed to achieve the desired effect.[42] And opioids may affect body systems differently, for example, motor coordination, respiratory depression, and sedation. Laboratory testing often is needed to make the diagnosis, observing high drug levels with little evidence of effect. **Withdrawal** is the development of symptoms when the substance is stopped—and relief of symptoms when resuming it.[42]

TABLE 6-6. Risk Stratification

RISK GROUP	MME DOSE	ORT	UDT	TAKING FENTANYL OR METHADONE	ON BENZODIAZEPINES[a]	USING MARIJUANA	MENTAL DISORDER[b]	SUBSTANCE USE DISORDER[b]
High	>90	>7	Unexpected	+	+	+	+	+
Moderate	40-90	4-7	Expected or minor issues	−	−	−	−	−
Low	<40	<4	Expected	−	−	−	−	−

MME = morphine milligram equivalent; ORT = opioid risk tool; UDT = urine drug testing.

[a]Also includes zolipidem, carisoprodol, and muscle relaxants.

[b]Mental and substance use disorders are a contraindication to opioids unless they are under expert ongoing treatment for those problems and the opioid treatment is integrated with the treatment plan; otherwise these patients should be referred to specialty care.

The presence of any one risk factor for the high-risk group is sufficient to qualify for this group; the more high-risk factors present, the greater the risk.

The remaining items in Table 6-3 are infrequent and often come to your attention from legal sources or from concerned relatives.

Prescribing Opioids

It is important to reiterate that there are few, if any, data suggesting clinically significant, long-term benefit from using opioids in chronic pain, and that they are causing great harm from overdose deaths, suicidal deaths, misuse, diversion,[1-4] and the severe side effects outlined in Table 6-7.[3,43-47] Before addressing actual treatment with opioids, there are 2 key tasks: calculating MMEs and how to ascertain the patient's response to opioids if you use them.

Calculating Morphine Milligram Equivalents. Most adverse effects relate directly to the opioid dose.[38] The intent in calculating MME is to provide a common denominator for estimating opioid risk. From a widely varying literature and relying mostly on a report from the Centers for Disease Control and Prevention (CDC), we have guidelines for "safe" doses and "dangerous" doses.[1]

We calculate doses in MMEs from research showing the relative potency on a milligram basis of all different opioids. This means that the dose of each opioid preparation is converted to the equivalent amount of morphine as a common reference point. Some prescription monitoring programs will provide you with this information, but it is important for you to be comfortable with the calculation yourself for quick,

bedside assessment. With an agent like hydrocodone, for example, its potency on a milligram basis is the same as morphine. But many opioids are more potent on a milligram basis, and they need to be converted by a multiplier to MME. For example, oxycodone is

TABLE 6-7. Adverse Effects from Using Opioids

1. Respiratory depression—this is important in overdoses, especially in patients with compromised lung function; even in small opioid doses, severe pulmonary disease patients often present with respiratory failure
2. Sedation and confusion—this leads to accidents at work and while driving as well as to falls
3. Pregnant or nursing mothers taking opioids risk having infants dependent on opioids
4. Depression—this is a common comorbid condition with opioid use, and the opioids make it worse
5. Insomnia—also part of depression made worse
6. Opioid hyperalgesia is a paradoxical response to opioids where pain actually increases
7. Constipation—this is so common and severe, it now is recognized as narcotic bowel syndrome
8. Decreased libido with decreased testosterone levels
9. Osteopenia
10. Hypotension
11. Impaired immunologic responsivity
12. Common side effects: itching, nausea/vomiting, fatigue, difficulty with urination

TABLE 6-8. Table for Calculating Morphine Milligram Equivalents (MME)

OPIOID (mg/d EXCEPT FENTANYL)	MULTIPLY TO GET MME
Morphine	1×
Hydrocodone (Vicodin, Norco)	1×
Oxycodone (Oxycontin)	2× (1.5× from CDC)
Fentanyl transdermal (in µg/h)	3× (2.4× from CDC)
Oxymorphone (Opana)	3×
Hydromorphone (Dilaudid)	4×
Methadone	
1-20 mg/d	4×
21-40 mg/d	8×
41-60 mg/d	10×
61-80 mg/d	12×
Codeine (Tylenol 3 or 4)	0.15×
Tramadol (Ultram)	0.1

nearly twice as potent as morphine, meaning 20 mg are equal to 40 MME. Similarly, hydromorphone is 4 times as potent, so we multiply by 4 to get MME. Adapted from the CDC, we developed Table 6-8 to assist you in calculating MME.

With a variable literature and to keep the calculations conservative and simple, we slightly modified the CDC recommendations: for oxycontin, use a multiplier of 2× rather than the 1.5; for fentanyl, use a multiplier of 3 rather than 2.4. In doing this, the clinician does not need to go to a calculator or website to determine the MME. Instead, they simply memorize the whole-number multipliers to calculate on the spot the MME a patient is taking:

1 × hydrocodone dose in mg = MME
2 × oxycodone dose in mg = MME
3 × fentanyl dose in µg/h = MME
4 × hydromorphone dose in mg = MME

Here's an example:

A patient was taking 10 mg of oxycodone 4 times daily, a total of 40 mg each day. Multiply this by 2 (from

the table) and this is 80 MME. He also used fentanyl skin patches with a dose of 25 µg/h; multiply this by 3 and this is 75 MME. Combining 80 and 75 MME, he is taking a total of 155 MME daily, a dangerous level.

A safe dose is defined as 50 MME or less, and borderline safe doses are up to 90 MME.[1] Beyond that, the risk of death and other complications increases in direct proportion to MME doses. Noted earlier, we have seen (tolerant) patients taking as many as 2200 MME and often see them taking in the range of 200 to 400 MME. Here are a couple sobering figures. In a patient taking a low dose of opioids, the later development of the DSM-5 Opioid Use Disorder[42] is 15 times more likely than someone not on opioids; for those on high doses (> 120 MME), the risk is 122 times greater.[38] Further, a person taking >100 MME per day is 9 times more likely to overdose than a patient taking < 20 MME. One overdose in 7 is fatal.[38] The MME is an important number to know as you are prescribing opioids, and it's also important for patients to know when you are working with them to reduce their dose level.

Monitoring Pain Responses to Treatment. If you prescribe opioids, their impact should be monitored, just as you would, for example, monitor blood sugars and glycohemoglobins in patients taking insulin. While the old standard of having patients rate their pain on a 1 to 10 scale can be used, it provides no sense of the functional impact of a patient's pain—just the subjective severity. For example, a level 2 severity might be associated with the inability to work, but we would not know that and assume the patient was doing well. Alternatively, we might hear of a pain rating score of 8 and wonder about increasing the dose without learning whether the patient's enjoyment in life and general activity were satisfactory or improved.

The Pain Intensity, Enjoyment of Life, and Interference with General Activity (PEG) Tool in Table 6-9 takes little additional time and informs you of the impact of pain on enjoyment of life and on general activity.[38,48] We learn about the impact of pain as well as its subjective severity.

Because you will see patients using harmful doses of opioids, the PEG allows you to determine if, from the patient's perspective, there is any benefit—defined as a 30% reduction in the overall score from the time the opioid was initiated or the dose increased. This method defines the minimal clinically significant improvement we can expect if, indeed, the opioids

TABLE 6-9. Measuring Pain Intensity, Enjoyment of Life, and Interference with General Activity (PEG) Tool

PEG Tool

1. What number best describes your **pain on average** in the past week?

0	1	2	3	4	5	6	7	8	9	10

| No pain | | | | | | | Pain as bad as you can imagine | | | |

2. What number best describes how, during the past week, pain has interfered with your **enjoyment of life?**

0	1	2	3	4	5	6	7	8	9	10

| Does not interfere | | | | | | | Completely interferes | | | |

3. What number best describes how, during the past week, pain has interfered with your **general activity?**

0	1	2	3	4	5	6	7	8	9	10

| Does not interfere | | | | | | | Completely interferes | | | |

SCORING:

There is no cutoff. Rather, the higher the score, the more severe the pain, lack of enjoyment, and interference with general activity. If the patient is responding to treatment, there should be a 30% reduction in the score, recalling that failure to respond to opioid treatment does not mean an increase in dose is indicated; rather, it means the opioid is not working and should be tapered and discontinued.

actually worked. *Failure to achieve this minimal level of improvement does not mean that the dose needs to be increased but, rather, that the opioid is not working and needs to be tapered and discontinued.*

Opioids as Treatment

We have indicated that opioids have little, if any, value in chronic noncancer pain[1,38] *but, nonetheless, they are often used.* You will encounter many patients already taking opioids, and the material here provides guidelines for evaluating and treating them. We begin by outlining where opioids should not be prescribed without advice from a mental health and/or addiction consultant. We then describe in detail how to use them, which includes how to taper and discontinue them.

Never Prescribe Opioids

1. *Opioid use disorder:* Almost always associated with misuse, this is a severe disorder resulting from opioid use, one constituting a DSM-5 diagnosis, as outlined in Table 6-10.[42]
2. Comorbid mental and nonopioid substance use disorders unless they are under effective treatment for this problem and opioid treatment is integrated into the care plan. These DSM-5 disorders are presented elsewhere in this book.[42]

3. History of a suicidal attempt, especially with opioids. Unfortunately, we know that opioids continue to be prescribed to many following a nonfatal opioid overdose, in which case fatal drug-associated

TABLE 6-10. Opioid Use Disorder

Two of the following occur within a 12-month period and lead to clinically significant impairment or distress.

1. Opioids taken in larger amount or over a longer period than intended
2. Persistent desire or unsuccessful efforts to cut down or otherwise control opioid use
3. Much time spent obtaining the opioid, using the opioid, or recovering from its use
4. Craving and strong desire or urge to use opioids
5. Failure to fulfil major role obligations at work, home, or school
6. Continued use despite recurrent social or interpersonal problems from opioids
7. Social, occupational, or recreational activites given up or reduced because of opioid use
8. Recurrent use in situations where it is physically hazardous
9. Continued use despite knowledge of having recurrent problems caused by the opioid
10. Tolerance
11. Withdrawal

outcomes 1 year later are 132 times higher than in the general population. These patients need careful follow-up and care, not more opioids.[49]

4. History of nonsuicidal overdose, especially with opioids.

5. Not currently taking them. There are 2 groups of patients:

   a. Never have had opioids for chronic pain
   b. Have had opioids for chronic pain in the past but have been off for a week or more when you first see them

An exception to these recommendations, implemented only in consultation with a mental health and/or an addiction specialist, is for a patient who has tried all other treatment described later in this chapter and by the MHCM (Chapter 3) and obtained incomplete relief. This would particularly apply to a patient who has responded in the past to safe doses of opioids but is not now taking this. The nonopioid treatment outlined shortly is always tried first and continued if you add an opioid. Thus, one would never begin opioids until after exhausting all other means of treatment.

Opioids in Acute Pain. The CDC has indicated that opioids in acute pain should be used for no more than 3 to 7 days.[1] Further, they advise that you rely on nonsteroidal analgesic drugs and use opioids only when these are incompletely effective, that is, opioids are a secondary choice, not the first treatment provided to an acute pain patient. This practice targets clinicians (including dentists) who prescribe opioids routinely for any pain problem, especially when they provide a 1-month supply with refills. Encouragingly, a recent emergency department study demonstrated that treatment of severe, acute extremity pain with 400 mg of ibuprofen combined with 1000 mg of acetaminophen was as effective as three different opioid-acetaminophen combinations in relieving pain.[50] If opioids are used in the acute setting, the state's PDMP is first queried to determine if they already are taking them or have been in the past.

Acute treatment is straightforward if the patient has never used opioids regularly and has a clear-cut new acute pain problem, such as an ankle fracture or sprain, acute low back strain, acute appendicitis, or recent dental surgery. We strongly recommend that acute pain patients requesting refills after the initial 3-7-day prescription is gone be evaluated instead of filling the prescription by phone even though the latter may be easier.

This is especially the case in patients with acute back pain where the natural course of resolution often lasts more than 1 week. In general, if a patient is not back to full activity within 2 to 4 weeks, they require careful evaluation to be certain of the diagnosis and of the appropriate, nonopioid treatment needed; for example, physical therapy and osteopathic manipulative therapy.

There is a good reason that we devote so much time to the management of acute pain. You can prevent chronic pain. One study found that more than 50% of patients on opioids for 90 or more days remained on them for years, and that the factors most associated with continuation were intermittent prior exposures, doses of 120 MME per day or greater, and indications of misuse.[51] As well, you will not be surprised to learn, there is little, if any, clinically significant benefit from opioids for chronic low back pain where misuse is found in 24%.[52] Be similarly wary in patients with what may have begun as an acute migraine headache or other acute problems that frequently recur. Properly treated, acute problems will improve over the short term. When patients are not improving on narcotics, it means the opioid is not effective, not that the dose is increased or the drug refilled.

But it's not all this easy! There is a large group of patients who repeatedly present with acute problems, such as low back pain, abdominal pain, chest pain, or headache, yet there is no objective evidence of currently active disease even though the patient may have had, for example, a myocardial infarction in the past. Many of these patients also take opioids chronically and request increased doses for the acute flare, often repeatedly hospitalized where they typically receive very liberal opioid dosing, sometimes intravenously. If the patient is not on opioids regularly and the investigative work-up shows no objective disease explanation for the pain, whether in the office or in the emergency department, treatment is symptomatic and narcotics are used for no more than 3 to 7 days at less than 50 MME. For patients already taking narcotics, the opioid is not increased but is continued at the present dose, and the patient is entered into the treatment regimen that follows later in this chapter. For patients hospitalized who have received large doses of narcotics, often intravenously, they are quickly tapered over 1 to 2 days to the dose they took prior to admission and entered into the treatment regimen below. Similar principles apply in patients undergoing surgery, tapering the narcotic before discharge, if possible, or rapidly when they return home. If already on an opioid, the same or a slightly increased dose can be used to address the acute surgical needs, and the patient is then tapered back to their usual home dose. Recent data indicate an increased use of chronic opioids after perioperative exposure, and that switching from intravenous to oral or subcutaneous routes of administration works just as well in the perioperative period and reduces total opioid exposure.[53]

Opioids in Chronic Pain. For the patients *already on chronic opioids*, we have therapeutic options leading to 3 possible outcomes:

1. Taper and discontinue the opioid.
2. Taper the opioid to the lowest possible dose that is in the semi-safe range of less than 90 MME, aiming at less than 50 MME.
3. Prescribing opioids to someone who cannot achieve 1 of the first 2 outcomes. In unstable patients, this undesired option often requires consultation for comanagement with a mental health and/or addiction specialist—if they are available—and very careful follow-up.

Tapering Opioids. The obvious issue in chronic opioid use is tapering opioids, and we now discuss how to do that.[44,45,54] Tapering is integrated with the MHCM, in particular the need for a respectful, patient-centered approach. As well, recall the use of nonaddicting medications, such as antidepressants and nonsteroidal anti-inflammatory drugs (NSAIDs), in negotiating the treatment plan. For now, though, we'll specify exactly how to taper and, perhaps, discontinue narcotics.

Rapid taper in patients with misuse: This approach assumes you have checked and there is evidence on the PDMP that the patient has received the drug as prescribed and on the UDT that they have actually taken the medication (rather than diverted it), for example, misusing by taking more than prescribed and/or getting opioids from another source. This can be safely done when the patient needs to quickly come off the drug because of misuse.

We recommend tapering over about 7 days, at approximately 30% of the preceding day's dose each day; see Table 6-11 for an example. This rate is sufficient to avoid most physiological withdrawal symptoms. Withdrawal symptoms sometimes occur though and can be treated as presented in Table 6-12, keeping the doses lower and observing closely for side effects in those over 65 years old.[38] While rapid tapering can usually be performed on an outpatient basis, when patients have abruptly stopped their opioid and developed psychosis or stress cardiomyopathy, they require urgent inpatient management.[44]

Slow taper and discontinuation: Slow tapering likely will be your most common approach in trying to help those on long-term opioids who are

---

TABLE 6-11. Example of Rapid Reduction of an Opioid

1. Assume the patient has been on 100 mg of oxycontin in divided doses per day. Checking Table 6-7 and seeing that the multiplier to obtain MME for oxycontin is 2×, this means the patient was on 200 MME per day.
2. We want to reduce by approximately 30% of each preceding day's MME although more rapid and slower regimens may be used, not shorter than 3 days or longer than 10.

DAY	30% MME REDUCTION FROM PRECEDING DAY'S DOSE	NEW MME DOSE FOR THIS DAY	TOTAL OXYCONTIN DOSE (DOSES DIVIDED DURING DAY)
1	30% of 200 MME (baseline) = 60	(200 − 60 =) 140	7 tablets (10 mg)
2	30% of 140 MME (day 1) = ~40	(140 − 40 =) 100	5 tablets (10 mg)
3	30% of 100 MME (day 2) = 30	(100 − 30 =) 70	3 tablets (10 mg) + 1 tablet (5 mg)
4	30% of 70 MME (day 3) = ~20	(70 − 20 =) 50	2 tablets (10 mg) + 1 tablet (5 mg)
5	30% of 50 MME (day 4) = 15	(50 − 15 =) 35	3 tablets (5 mg) + 1 tablet (2.5 mg)
6	30% of 35 MME (day 5) = ~10	(35 − 10 =) 25	2 tablets (5 mg) + 1 tablet (2.5 mg)
7	30% of 25 MME (day 6) = ~10	(25 − 10 =) 15	3 tablets (2.5 mg) – **THEN, STOP THE DRUG**

TABLE 6-12. Treating Opioid Withdrawal
1. Sweats, tremors, anxiety, restlessness, or hypertension—0.1 mg clonidine 3 times daily
2. Insomnia—diphenhydramine (25 mg) or hydroxyzine (25 mg) at bedtime for insomnia
3. Anxiety or restlessness—diphenhydramine (25 mg) or hydroxyzine (25 mg) 3 times daily
4. Fever or pain—NSAID or acetaminophen
5. Nausea and vomiting—promethazine (25 mg) or metoclopramide (10 mg) every 6 h
6. Diarrhea—loperamide, 4 mg initially and then 2 mg with each loose stool, up to 16 mg daily
7. Muscle spasm—methocarbamol (1000 mg) as needed every 6 h
8. Dyspepsia—symptomatic measures

Use reduced doses and observe closely for side effects in those over 65 years old.

not misusing. Slow tapering considers the impact of psychological dependence, and its success depends on both effective opioid management, as we've described, and a strong clinician-patient relationship. Recall that tapering is just one part of a treatment approach that also uses, for example, medications for depression and insomnia to address these 2 commonly associated problems.

Dosage decreases must be negotiated using shared decision making rather than being prescribed unilaterally. It is helpful in negotiating with patients to emphasize that you do not stop medications "cold turkey" as many fear. Indicate, rather, that they will be slowly tapered at a pace the patient sets and, then, only after starting adequate doses of what you can frame as a "better pain medication," which refers to antidepressant and other measures in the MHCM. The slow pace of reduction is for psychological withdrawal, not physiological, and addresses the patient's long dependence on the medications. At the outset of treatment, we also tell patients that if this tapering program is not effective in reducing them to less than 90 MME, consultation with a pain/addiction specialist is indicated and inpatient detoxification may be necessary.

Procedure: You first establish from the history what their starting total dose in the taper should be. You ask how much of the opioid they think they would need on a typical worst day, explaining to them that they will be taking the same dose each day throughout tapering

so that it is important that they begin with enough. For example, a patient may occasionally take only 4 per day, but is usually in the range of 7 to 8 per day. You and the patient then agree to begin the taper at the high end with, say, 8 tablets per day of the oxycodone.

Next, great detail then goes into the specific scheduling of exactly what time of day each of the 8 tablets will be taken. Ask your patient how they would like to distribute the 8 tablets during the day, eliciting when the pain is usually at its worst and its best helps focus this discussion. Here's an example: 2 upon arising (when getting the household going), 1 mid-morning (with shopping), 1 at noon (when needing to do some heavy housework), 2 at 4:00 PM (when the kids get home from school), 1 at supper, and 1 at 10:00 PM just before going to bed.

It is essential the patient understand that they will always adhere to the schedule you are negotiating. This means making clear that they never take the opioid at a different time or take more or less at the same times. If the patient expresses concern about what to do if the pain is not controlled, you indicate that the tablet distribution can be renegotiated at the next visit.

This all occurs at the first visit and there is no effort yet to reduce the dose, which may even be a bit higher than their previous dose. In this example, you would provide them with 56 tablets to be taken as above during the following week. Having already agreed to taper, you also ask them to begin thinking about which 1 of the 8 tablets could be removed at the next visit (in 1 week). You can encourage this by indicating that, by then, some of the other medications will have begun to work. Recall from the depression chapter, the use of trazodone or mirtazapine to help with sleep.

At the follow-up visit in 1 week, in addition to other issues we'll discuss with the MHCM, you ask how the pain is going and which of the tablets they decided to remove. They might say that the mid-morning dose would be best, so they now are down to 7 tablets in the otherwise same distribution—unless the patient wishes to renegotiate parts of it. You then write the new prescription for 49 tablets and ask the patient to be thinking about which one to remove in 1 week at the next visit.

At follow-up visits, we verify the patient's specific time of use, and one ascertains that they are taking the full dose even if having fewer problems and not going beyond it if having greater problems. Reframing tapering to "when" patients take the medications, rather than arguing about "if" they are to take them, helps with the relationship and getting an effective reduction in dose over time. Generally, if there is no misuse, you continue this way, recalling that the PDMP and UDT are obtained according to the risk profile you have formulated. You may be able to increase to 2-week visit intervals as long as stable and later to 3-week intervals.

By 8 to 12 weeks, many will have completely discontinued the medications at rates of a 1 tablet per day reduction every 1 to 3 weeks. During tapering, watch carefully for an increase in pain and depression, especially manifest by lack of enjoyment of life (anhedonia). This withdrawal phenomenon simply means to slow down the pace of tapering, not that they have reached a drug dose beneath which they cannot go.[43] There is absolutely no hurry in tapering. Remember, they have often taken opioids for years and are psychologically dependent on them. In some patients, the beginning of a taper is a very stressful and often unstable time so relying on the provider-patient relationship for support is key. By the slow taper on a time-contingent schedule (non-prn), you are slowly ameliorating the dependence—and other parts of the treatment will be working. The taper occurs as part of the treatment, not the only thing you will be doing.

Naltrexone: Once having stopped the opioid, if you and the patient are concerned about relapse to opioid use, naltrexone can be implemented after the patient has been completely off opioids for 7 days or more (10-14 days for buprenorphine and methadone). Naltrexone is a long-acting opioid antagonist, similar otherwise to the short-acting naloxone, and blocks the effects of opioids if they are used, preventing intoxication and dependence from recurring. However, they can precipitate severe opioid withdrawal if the patient has had opioids in the last 7 to 14 days. A naloxone challenge can be performed if there is any question: up to 0.8 mg of naloxone is administered and the patient is observed for 1 hour for signs of opioid withdrawal; see Table 6-12. Using naltrexone applies also to the patient, described earlier, who has been off opioids when you first see them but who wants help and is considering resuming the narcotic; a naloxone challenge may be advisable to verify abstinence. If abstinent, add naltrexone and treat with the nonopioid plan outlined here rather than resuming the opioid.

Table 6-13 summarizes the use of naltrexone. It is generally well tolerated but side effects can be reduced by beginning with the lower 25 mg dose and then increasing to 50 mg daily. The injectable preparation also can be used with monthly administration. When naltrexone is used, careful follow-up continues to be

TABLE 6-13. Medications for Problematic Opioid and Alcohol Use					
	ACTION	DOSE	SIDE EFFECTS (SERIOUS)	SIDE EFFECTS (OTHER)	PRECAUTIONS
Naltrexone, oral *Depade, ReVia*	Blocks opioid receptors	25 mg/d for 3 d → 50 mg/d; some advise increasing to 100 mg/d after 7 d[81]	Hepatotoxic in high doses	Anorexia, nausea/vomiting, headache, fatigue, anxiety, dizzy, sleepy	Hepatic/renal disease, monitor Do not use when on opioids in prior 7-14 d
Naltrexone, intramuscular *Vivitrol*	Blocks opioid receptors	380 mg per month	Hepatotoxic Suicidal—rare	(Same as oral) Reaction at injection site, muscle/joint aches	(Same as oral) May have bleeding problems
Acamprosate, oral *Campral*	Affects GABA and glutamate	666 mg 3 times daily	Suicidal—rare	Diarrhea, somnolence	Monitor renal function Adjust dose with CrCl 30-50

necessary. The greatest success has been in highly motivated patients, often for legal reasons.

Implementing the tapering procedure: Initially, you negotiate that patients use one pharmacy, pick up medications themselves, and receive prescriptions from their clinicians only at the time of visits. Early on, provide sufficient medications only until the next visit, generally giving one "grace period" in the event the medication is "lost." When stable and there is no evidence of misuse from PDMP and UDT, we recommend refills by phone from Tuesday through Fridays only—to avoid problems with vacations and uninformed on-call clinicians becoming involved in deciding if a refill is needed.

Other medication issues:

1. Because of greater overdose risk, we recommend that you do not use extended release preparations,[38] and that patients taking fentanyl patches or hydromorphone be switched to morphine, hydrocodone, or oxycodone at the same MME level.

2. Methadone and buprenorphine are opioid agonists used in specialty clinics for detoxification. These are considerations by the addiction specialist if you need to refer a refractory patient. Some medical clinicians are receiving training in using these agents and this represents an important step forward in addressing the problem by making these valuable measures more available in medical settings.[55,56] The following link provides information on the required 8-hour training courses: https://www.samhsa.gov/medication-assisted-treatment/training-resources/buprenorphine-physician-training

3. For patients taking more than 50 MME per day, taking simultaneous benzodiazepines at any opioid dose, with a history of overdose on any drug, or a history of any substance use disorder, prescribe injectable naloxone or intranasal spray (Narcan; Adapt Pharma) or an autoinjector (Evzio; Kaleo). Because over one-half of overdoses occur in the home, explain the use to significant others as well as to the patient—instructing them to immediately go the emergency department for definitive care.[25,38,57,58] Naloxone is an important but overlooked adjunct, and the Office of the Surgeon General has declared the opioid crisis to be a public health emergency and that naloxone should become routine treatment in an attempt to reduce the present death rate of 115 persons dying each day of opioid overdoses.[58]

4. You need to be aware that many opioids contain acetaminophen, and that high doses of the opioid may contain more than the 4 g maximum allowable acetaminophen dose; this includes incorporating into your calculations over-the-counter preparations like Tylenol. If liver disease or alcoholism in remission is present, acetaminophen should not be used, relying on NSAIDs such as ibuprofen.

5. Symptomatic medications, such as acetaminophen and NSAIDs (for pain) and stool softeners (for opioid-induced constipation), can be used.

6. Not uncommonly, patients are taking more than 1 opioid and may also be taking 1 or more sedative-hypnotics. Negotiate with the patient whether they wish to taper these concomitantly or sequentially.

7. Gabapentinoids (pregabalin-Lyrica; gabapentin-Neurontin) have not been approved for their increasingly widespread use in chronic pain for a good reason: they have no conclusive evidence of effectiveness.[59] FDA approval exists for both drugs only for postherpetic neuralgia; pregabalin is approved also for use in fibromyalgia and the neuropathic pain of diabetes and spinal cord injury; the few rigorous studies conducted in chronic noncancer pain patients have shown no conclusive benefit.[59] As well, gabapentinoids are attended by significant side effects of sedation, dizziness, and cognitive difficulties. They also have been misused and abused for a euphoric effect and withdrawal occurs when stopped.[59] Worrisome also is that both drugs, when combined with opioids, have increased opioid-related deaths compared to using opioids alone.[60] While one might give a brief trial of these medications, without concomitant opioid use and using objective measures of its impact (see PEG Tool in Table 6-9), the MHCM outlined here is a far better and proven effective treatment because, in addition to proven effective pharmacologic measures, it highlights the clinician-patient relationship and the motivational features needed for successful outcomes.

Slow taper without discontinuation: To this point, we have described the ideal situation—a cooperative patient who is able to discontinue opioids altogether. Unfortunately, many are not able to do this because of dependence on the drugs. But these patients can be managed effectively using the same procedures described earlier. The difference here is that patients have much more difficulty reducing the medications.

Procedurally, recalling the goal-setting part of the MHCM, you share your MME goals with the patient. And that, if they are unable to at least reduce to less than 90 MME, you will no longer be able to prescribe for them without first obtaining a mental health and/or addiction consultation—and that this may entail out- or in-patient detoxification, a common recommendation. This contingency can be quite motivating to patients. These patients often have a greater risk stratification and, accordingly, are more likely to misuse. They will be on a more frequent schedule of checking PDMP and UDT.

You determine that a patient is unable to reduce the opioid further by observing and talking with them. You will note that patients in this group tend to have more severe comorbid problems, presenting with physical as well as mental disorders, and that life is more overwhelming for these patients than for those with complete tapers. While all patients evince resistance and complain about tapering, these complaints are more persistent and vociferous—or sometimes hopeless and passive. Some also have irremediable social situations and low self-esteem.

MME levels less than 90: If a patient is well controlled and functioning effectively on levels of less than 90 MME but strongly resisting tapering, it is satisfactory for them to continue this as long as they are fully adherent to the complete MHCM treatment plan.[61] In fact, tapering a stable patient at the upper acceptable MME range, can precipitate craving and drug-seeking behaviors.[43] If the full MHCM plan has not been tried, as is often the case with the many patients on regular doses of 90 MME or less, it should be implemented before deciding to continue prescribing opioids for the patient at this level. If on the full MCHM plan and not misusing, it is satisfactory to prescribe opioids. You, of course, try to get them down to 50 MME or less.

MME levels greater than 90: The psychological dependence in this group is even greater, often with very distressing life situations and many associated comorbid disorders, both physical and mental, and large numbers of pain locations in the body.[62] They also tend to be on higher doses, often in the 200 to 400 MME range. It is quite appropriate to attempt, as described above, to taper these patients in conjunction

with the other parts of the treatment plan. For those who cannot achieve MME levels less than 90, especially those who can't get below 200 MME or who have severe comorbid depression or other mental disorders, referral to mental health and/or addiction specialists is needed; buprenorphine may be effective in these patients, in which case you comanage the patient with the addiction specialist. It is not always this easy, though, because you may not have access to specialty care with the severe shortage of psychiatry and other addiction specialists. In this case, you do not abandon these often very distressed people but, rather, provide maintenance opioid (and other) treatment as long as they are adhering to monitoring and other MHCM treatment. It helps to view this approach as "comfort care" with the caveat that there should be far fewer patients on these high doses than there are today.[62]

Formal pain contract: What we have described to this point has been an oral contract or agreement on how both the clinician and patient agree to interact. While many protocols require written contracts for all patients, we have found a simple oral agreement satisfactory—as long as there is no evidence of misuse and the patient follows the monitoring plan and the treatment plan in the MHCM, including satisfactory tapering and discontinuation. We judge that tapering is satisfactory if a daily 1 pill reduction occurs every 1 to 3 weeks.

However, there are many situations when a written contract is needed: high risk for misuse; history of any substance abuse; comorbid mental disorder; or any significant abrogation of the oral contract.[38] The contract should contain the items in Table 6-14.[38] Numerous sample contract forms are available and must be adapted to each individual's specific practice setting. It is also important to check with your own state regulations, as some states require a specific contract to be used.

When patients misuse: With minor violations of the contract, it is best to be patient but firm. With greater violations of the contract, including nonadherence to other aspects of the treatment plan, you will rapidly taper and discontinue the opioid after full discussion with the patient. Whether you discharge the patient from your care is another issue, one the patient often decides by seeking care elsewhere. A related issue is whether other clinicians in your clinic will accept the patient and, if so, if they will provide opioids.

TABLE 6-14. Content of a Written Contract

1. Clinician's agreement to provide opioid and other medications as negotiated with the patient as long as the patient adheres to the contract.
2. Patient's agreement to provide UDT samples upon request.
3. Patient's acknowledgement that PDMP will be monitored.
4. Patient's agreement to take opioid and other medications as scheduled.
5. Patient's agreement to obtain prescriptions only from the clinician or their surrogate.
6. Patient's agreement to use only one pharmacy (or pharmacy system).
7. Patient's agreement not to abuse alcohol or to use any illicit substances.
8. Patient's agreement that the clinician release the contract's contents to local emergency departments, urgent care facilities, pharmacies, and other practitioners—and for the recipients to report back any violations of the contract.
9. Patient's agreement to safeguard all medications in a secure location, and to report any stolen or lost medications.
10. Patient's agreement that the clinician may notify the proper authorities if there is a reason to believe the patient has engaged in illegal activity.
11. Patient's agreement that violation of the contract may result in rapid tapering or discontinuation of the opioid medications and discharge from care.
12. Patient's agreement that any violations of the contract and the clinician's response to them will be docmented in the patient's electronic health record, including the rationale for changes in the treatment.

Clinic policies should be constructed to address these contingencies.

While many clinicians understandably are concerned about patient satisfaction ratings such as the Hospital Consumer Assessment of Healthcare Providers and Systems or Press Ganey, it is important to recall your greater obligation to cause no harm. Indeed, it is important to remember that being patient-centered does not mean patients must be satisfied. While patient satisfaction often results from being patient-centered in other dimensions of medicine, it may not occur when patients demand treatment that is inappropriate or harmful to them. Indeed, being patient-centered does not equal satisfying patients, it means doing what is best for them.[63] Expanded upon in the MHCM in Chapter 3, this means being firm and respectful, stating what you can and cannot do and not arguing.

THE OTHER PRESCRIPTION SUBSTANCE USE PROBLEM—BENZODIAZEPINES

Physicians are also the sole legal source of another misused and abused class of addicting medication: benzodiazepines, such as diazepam, alprazolam, and lorazepam. Even though nearly 9000 people died from benzodiazepine overdoses in 2015, three-fourths of them also involved opioids, and this factor may account for the considerably lesser attention this problem has received.[64] Patients using both opioids and benzodiazepines often have especially severe comorbid mental disorders such as PTSD. From 1996 to 2013, there was a 67% increase in usage, from 8.1 million U.S. citizens to 13.5 million; as well, rates of co-prescribing with opioids nearly doubled from 2001 to 2013.[64] The problem has been greatest among the elderly.[65-68] For example, in 2014, 7% of adults aged 21 to 64 years and 32% of adults older than 64 years had received benzodiazepines (or one of the Z-drugs sleep aids such, as zolpidem, which are also dangerous, especially combined with opioids[64]—and the rate was 49% in adults 85 years or older. Worse yet, 59% of older users were chronic users, and 21% who were short-term users who became long-term users by the following year.[68]

Further worrisome, among all patients, prescriptions for benzodiazepines have been given to especially vulnerable groups of (often elderly) patients with depression, substance abuse, osteoporosis, chronic obstructive pulmonary disease, alcohol abuse, sleep apnea, and asthma.[69] That this is a high-risk group is underscored by increased numbers of outpatient and emergency room visits as well as hospitalizations. One can only speculate that the benzodiazepines may actually be responsible for the severity of some problems;

for example, respiratory suppression in patients with sleep apnea or obstructive lung disease, depression in the elderly. Equally worrisome, the *indications* for using benzodiazepines are things they actually may *cause* when used chronically: depression, insomnia, and anxiety.[67,68] In one study, 42% of depressed patients were receiving benzodiazepines.[68]

Indications for Use

For their main purported indication, insomnia and anxiety, benzodiazepine impact does not exceed placebo after about 2 weeks.[65] The reason for this effect is development of tolerance and, in turn, withdrawal symptoms from what has become an insufficient dose.[70] This, unfortunately, may lead to increasing the dose. Most agree that there is nothing other than a short-term (2-4 weeks) indication for using benzodiazepines.[70,71] We have reviewed the pharmacology and specific uses of benzodiazepines in Chapter 5—mainly used for brief periods to manage acute anxiety in panic disorder and during the initial period when starting antidepressants for anxiety and/or depression. We do not address in this book the more useful role of benzodiazepines for the inpatient management of alcohol detoxification or seizure disorders; or their use for severe muscle spasms in neurologic disorders.

Long-term use should not be undertaken without a psychiatry referral for medication consultation and/or consultation for nonpharmacologic treatment from psychiatry or other mental health professionals. Most also agree that benzodiazepines should not be used at all in the elderly, in those on opioids, or in those with a history of substance use disorders of any type. Long-term use is fraught with the complications described next.

Complications of Benzodiazepine Use

The complications of taking benzodiazepines are well known and very common: dependence and addiction, depression, increased anxiety and insomnia, overdoses, injuries/falls/fractures, confusion and worsening of organic mental syndromes, traffic accidents, and respiratory suppression in patients with compromised pulmonary function.[64,65,71,72] Intoxication with benzodiazepines resembles that of alcohol intoxication with slurred speech, ataxia, and poor physical coordination.[72]

In contrast to opioids, *withdrawal* symptoms are common, can be troublesome, and can be very serious and life-threatening, particularly when benzodiazepines have been given at high doses and/or in conjunction with opioids. Withdrawal syndromes have symptoms that may span a wide range: insomnia, agitation and irritability, anxiety and panic attacks, tremor, difficulty in concentration, dry heaves and nausea, weight loss, palpitations, headache, muscular pain and stiffness, and a host of perceptual changes.[70,72,73]

More serious and life-threatening are the delirium, psychosis, and seizures that can attend withdrawal, a risk that also can occur when the competitive antagonist *flumazenil* is administered in emergency rooms for overdoses.[72] Importantly, withdrawal seizures may occur without any preceding symptoms of withdrawal, and delirium may occur in the elderly with only mental status changes, without the autonomic hyperactivity that usually attends withdrawal.[72]

The usual *"rebound" anxiety* with insomnia occurs 1 to 4 days after stopping the drug, depending on the half-life of the drug, and lasts 2 to 3 days, while the *full-blown withdrawal* syndrome lasts 10 to 14 days. Later, upon discontinuation, the original anxiety symptoms may then return.[70,73] Physical and psychological dependence is very common, even at low doses. At 4 to 6 months of use, about one-half will experience withdrawal, so that the drug must be tapered slowly.[70-72] This means that withdrawal and rebound anxiety often attend discontinuation or dosage reduction. This, in turn, inclines patients to resume the drug, making cessation difficult.[71] Benzodiazepines should never be stopped abruptly, regardless of the dose or duration of use—unless taking them for only a few days or taking the very short-acting triazolam (Halcion).[70,72]

Tapering and Discontinuing Benzodiazepines

Tapering can be more difficult than with opioids because of withdrawal symptoms. You can taper on an outpatient basis as long as the patient and family are informed and motivated, and there are no complicating substance use problems or medical disorders. Families need to be informed that delirium and seizures may occur and how to respond if they do—and provided with the withdrawal symptoms to watch for that might warn of more serious symptoms.[72] This

TABLE 6-15. Benzodiazepines and Their Withdrawal Equivalents for Outpatient Management

	THERAPEUTIC DOSE (mg/d)	HALF-LIFE (h) (ACTIVE METABOLITE)	EQUIVALENT DOSES (mg) FOR WITHDRAWAL USE[a]
Long-Acting Benzodiazepines			
Diazepam (Valium)	4-40	20-100 (36-200)	**10**
Chlordiazepoxide (Librium)	15-100	5-30 (36-200)	25
Clonazepam (Klonopin)	0.5-4.0	18-50	2
Short-Acting Benzodiazepines			
Alprazolam (Xanax)	0.75-6.0	6-12	**1**
Lorazepam (Ativan)	1-16	10-20	2
Triazolam (Halcion)	0.125-0.50	2	0.25
Oxazepam (Serax)	10-120	4-15	10
Temazepam (Restoril)	15-30	8-22	15

[a]Based on equivalence of each to 30 mg phenobarbital. These are the amounts of the drug that 30 mg of phenobarbital will substitute for. Thus, the listed doses for each benzodiazepine are equivalent. These are not therapeutic equivalencies.

danger is particularly the case around times of dosage reductions. Frequent reevaluations are essential for often more complex and longer tapers than with opioids.

Tapering should be conducted using *long-acting* (Table 6-15) benzodiazepines, such as diazepam or chlordiazepoxide. Clonazepam has also been used but has a shorter half-life, is more potent and, practically, has fewer options in tablet size.[70] We recommend a slow taper over a few months, even over a year for high baseline doses. As with opioids, there is no hurry.[70] For patients taking *short-acting* benzodiazepines, it is best to slowly switch them to a long-acting agent before tapering because the more constant blood level decreases withdrawal symptoms. Equivalent doses for converting short-acting to long-acting agents, for

the purpose of withdrawal, are given in Table 6-15[72]; the doses differ in some instances from the equivalent therapeutic doses found elsewhere.[70] Table 6-16 describes a gradual, stepwise switching from alprazolam to diazepam, tapering, and discontinuation over more than 6 months. This suggestion, however, is simply an example. If significant withdrawal occurs at any point, the schedule can stop for a few weeks but you do not return to a higher dose. Also, be sensitive to the patient's interests and beliefs in deciding on exact times of changes.

For patients on high doses (nontherapeutic) of benzodiazepines, withdrawal should be conducted in the hospital setting. Because seizures usually occur within 24 to 48 hours of reducing the dose, even on therapeutic doses, hospitalization also may be needed initially

TABLE 6-16. Sample Reduction Schedule to Switch From Alprazolam (3 mg/d) to Equivalent Dose of Diazepam (30 mg/d) and Then Taper[a]

	BREAKFAST	LUNCH	SUPPER	DAILY DIAZEPAM EQUIVALENT
Baseline	Alprazolam 1 mg	Alprazolam 1 mg	Alprazolam 1 mg	30 mg
1 week later	Alprazolam 1 mg	Alprazolam 1 mg	Alprazolam 0.5 mg Diazepam 5 mg	30 mg
1 week later	Alprazolam 0.5 mg Diazepam 5 mg	Alprazolam 1 mg	Alprazolam 0.5 mg Diazepam 5 mg	30 mg
1 week later	Alprazolam 0.5 mg Diazepam 5 mg	Alprazolam 0.5 mg Diazepam 2.5 mg	Alprazolam 0.5 mg Diazepam 5 mg	27.5 mg
2 weeks later	Alprazolam 0.5 mg Diazepam 5 mg	Alprazolam 0.5 mg Diazepam 2.5 mg	Alprazolam 0.25 mg Diazepam 5 mg	25 mg
2 weeks later	Alprazolam 0.5 mg Diazepam 5 mg	Alprazolam 0.5 mg Diazepam 2.5 mg	Alprazolam stopped Diazepam 5 mg	22.5 mg
2 weeks later	Alprazolam 0.25 mg Diazepam 5 mg	Alprazolam 0.5 mg Diazepam 2.5 mg	Diazepam 5 mg	20 mg
2 weeks later	Alprazolam 0.25 mg Diazepam 5 mg	Alprazolam 0.25 mg Diazepam 2.5 mg	Diazepam 5 mg	17.5 mg
2 weeks later	Alprazolam stopped Diazepam 5 mg	Alprazolam 0.25 mg Diazepam 2.5 mg	Diazepam 5 mg	15 mg
2 weeks later	Alprazolam stopped Diazepam 5 mg	Alprazolam stopped Diazepam 2.5 mg	Diazepam 5 mg	12.5 mg
2 weeks later	Diazepam 5 mg	Diazepam stopped	Diazepam 5 mg	10 mg[b]

[a]See Table 6-15 where 1 mg of alprazolam is equal to 10 mg diazepam for withdrawal purposes.

[b]From this point on, taper by 1.0 mg diazepam every 2 weeks; when down to 1.0 mg/d, stop after the next 2 weeks; 2 mg tablets of diazepam are scored and can be broken in half.

if home circumstances are not supportive, especially in the elderly, or if there are comorbid substance use or significant medical disorders.[72]

It is important to recognize the extreme stress that withdrawal can cause in patients and ensure that they have adequate support, especially helping them to avoid either relapsing or using alternative substances like alcohol. Like any addiction, relapses occur but do not bode poorly. One simply resumes the effort. It has been useful also for insomnia to use trazodone during benzodiazepine withdrawal.[70,71] And it is important to treat comorbid depression if present.[71]

Benzodiazepine withdrawal is far more cumbersome and difficult than opioid withdrawal, and you often will want to consult a psychiatrist or an addiction specialist. To best avoid the problem, avoid long-term benzodiazepines.

ALCOHOL USE

At this point, we move from prescribed agents, where we have considerable control over outcomes (we control prescribing), to alcohol use where we have far less control. Nevertheless, we can be effective with this far more common problem using the following recommendations. Let's begin with a look at the magnitude of the problem.

- In 2016, 44.7 million adults (18 years or older), 18.3% of the U.S. population, had *some type of mental disorder* (mostly the depressive and anxiety disorders you've already heard about in earlier chapters); 10.4 million had what is called *serious mental illness*, which means it is extremely disabling and often found in the psychotic and personality disorders you'll learn about in Chapters 9 and 10, respectively.[74]

- In 2016, 20.1 million Americans, 12 years or older, had *some type of substance use disorder* of some type, broken down as follows:
  - 15.1 million had an *alcohol* use disorder
  - 7.4 million had an *illicit drug* use disorder
    - 4.0 million had a *marijuana* use disorder
    - 2.1 million had an *opioid* use disorder
      - 1.8 million had a *prescription pain reliever* use disorder
      - 0.6 million had a *heroin* use disorder[74]

- You've already learned about the problem of comorbid disorders, so how often do mental and substance use disorders occur together? In 2016, 8.2 million adults, 18 or more years old, had both some type of mental disorder and some type of substance use disorder; 2.6 million adults had a comorbid serious mental illness and a substance use disorder.[74]

These data tell us that substance use disorders are important by dint of sheer numbers, magnified by their extreme adverse impact on morbidity and mortality.

Definitions of Potentially Harmful Use

The unit of alcohol consumption is 1 drink of the following size and content: 1.5 oz of hard liquor, 12 oz of beer, or 5 oz of table wine. *Acceptable*, "moderate" drinking is defined as 2 drinks per day for men and 1 per day for women; of note, however, is that recent studies are showing there is no safe or acceptable level from a health standpoint.[75] *At-risk* drinking is defined as more than 14 drinks per week (or > 3 on one occasion) for men and more than 7 drinks a week (or > 1 on one occasion) for women or anyone over 65 years of age. *Binge* drinking is defined as 5 or more drinks on one occasion in the preceding month for men and 4 or more in the last month for women. *Heavy* alcohol use is more than 4 bingeing episodes in the preceding month.[74,76]

In 2016, for people older than 12 years, 136.7 million Americans *used alcohol*, including 65.3 million with *binge drinking* and 16.3 million with *heavy alcohol use*. Among those between 12 and 20 years of age, 4.5 million reported binge drinking and 1.2 million were heavy alcohol users—in the past month. About 40% of young adults from 18 to 25 years of age were binge users, and 10% were heavy alcohol users.[74] We can conclude that alcohol use is a huge problem beginning early in our young people in the United States, where about 30% of adults drink in amounts that increase their risk for physical, mental, and social problems.[76]

Accordingly, although often difficult to elicit, it will be important to identify problem drinkers.

Diagnosis

Interviewing the Patient. Information on potentially stress-laden discussion material, such as substance use, may not arise during the patient-centered component of the interview. It is essential to understand that eliciting data about alcohol use requires specific and repeated clinician-centered inquiry.[29] In all patients, ask about specific amounts and patterns so that you can identify the above drinking levels: acceptable, at risk, bingeing, and heavy. You ask something like, "Do you drink alcohol, beer, wine, or hard liquor?" Then ask how much and if alcohol has ever been a problem in the patient's life with, for example, divorce, loss of a job, or with the legal system.[29] Patients may minimize their use of alcohol, likely more to delude themselves than not wanting to tell you. In these sometimes fraught-with-tension discussions, remain respectful and nonjudgmental, recalling the centrality of the clinician-patient relationship to success with mental and substance use disorders. In patients using large amounts of alcohol, determine if they have tried to stop drinking and the results of this effort, and if they are interested in getting help.[29,76] Surprising perhaps, they are often interested in help, but you need to ask to find out. If not interested, ask if they see a problem with their drinking. Recalling that mental and substance use problems may be comorbid, you determine these key facts as well. Although some prefer to use

TABLE 6-17. CAGE Questionnaire[77]
1. Have you ever felt you should cut down on your drinking?
2. Have people annoyed you by criticizing your drinking?
3. Have you ever felt bad or guilty about your drinking?
4. Have you ever had a drink first thing in the morning to steady your nerves or to get rid of a hangover (eye opener)?

Scoring: Item responses on the CAGE are scored 0 or 1, with a higher score an indication of alcohol problems. A total score of 2 or greater is considered clinically significant.

the following questions initially, they ordinarily fit best integrated with the above. The specific screening questions, the CAGE questions, follow here and in Table 6-17[77]:

"Have you ever:

- Felt the need to **C**ut down on your drinking?
- Felt **A**nnoyed by criticism of your drinking?
- Had **G**uilty feelings about your drinking?
- Taken a morning **E**ye opener?"

An affirmative answer to 2 or more makes problematic alcohol use likely.

Screening. With any suspicion of a possible alcohol problem, patients should complete the Alcohol Use Disorders Identification Test (AUDIT).[76] Table 6-18 has both English and Spanish (Table 6-18[2]) versions. As noted in Table 6-18(3), a cut point of 8 for men and 4 for women has greater sensitivity and will allow you to find more patients with problematic use.

Classification. You now classify the patient's drinking habits.[74,76]

- *Acceptable drinking:* Two drinks per day for men and 1 per day for women
- *At-risk drinking:* More than 14 drinks per week (or > 3 on one occasion) for men and more than 7 drinks a week (or > 1 on one occasion) for women or anyone over 65 years of age
- *Binge drinking:* Five or more drinks on one occasion in the preceding month for men and 4 or more in the last month for women

- *Heavy drinking:* More than 4 bingeing episodes in the preceding month.

Is There Associated Abuse or Dependence? You must now determine whether there has been clinically significant impairment or distress and if there are features of an alcohol use disorder.[42,76]

- If, in the last 12 months, the patient's drinking has repeatedly caused or contributed to *any one of the following*, the patient has **alcohol abuse**:
  1. Risk of bodily harm from driving, operating machinery, or swimming
  2. Relationship problems with family or friends
  3. Failure to perform their role at home, work, or school
  4. Contacts with the legal system, arrests or otherwise

- If, in the last 12 months, the patient has had *3 or more* of the following, the patient has **alcohol dependence:**
  1. Unable to stick to drinking limits
  2. Unable to cut down or stop
  3. Shown tolerance (need to drink more to get same effect)
  4. Shown withdrawal (tremors, sweats, nausea/vomiting, insomnia) when cutting down
  5. Persisted in drinking despite problems (recurrent physical/psychological problems)
  6. Spent much time drinking (or anticipating or recovering from drinking)
  7. Spent less time on activities that had been important or pleasurable

Treatment

Nonpharmacologic Measures. A critical starting point is to negotiate with the patient exactly what they will do (cut down, quit) and when. It is also critical to know the specifics of their drinking habits, the circumstances, the stressors or enforcers, and even the times of day. Jointly, try to determine what prompts them to drink. Then, as part of the plan, have them avoid these triggers to the extent possible; for example, stop bowling with the boys for the first month or going to happy hour after work—whether quitting or cutting down. It also helps to have them commit to keeping track of exactly how much, when, and with whom they drink. Have them set specific goals. For example, if cutting

TABLE 6-18. Screening Instrument: The Alcohol Use Disorders Identification Test (AUDIT)

PATIENT: Because alcohol use can affect your health and can interfere with certain medications and treatments, it is important that we ask some questions about your use of alcohol. Your answers will remain confidential, so please be honest.

Place an X in one box that best describes your answer to each question.

QUESTIONS	0	1	2	3	4	
1. How often do you have a drink containing alcohol?	Never	Monthly or less	2-4 times a month	2-3 times a week	4 or more times a week	
2. How many drinks containing alcohol do you have on a typical day when you are drinking?	1 or 2	3 or 4	5 or 6	7-9	10 or more	
3. How often do you have 5 or more drinks on one occasion?	Never	Less than monthly	Monthly	Weekly	Daily or almost daily	
4. How often during the last year have you found that you were not able to stop drinking once you had started?	Never	Less than monthly	Monthly	Weekly	Daily or almost daily	
5. How often during the last year have you failed to do what was normally expected of you because of drinking?	Never	Less than monthly	Monthly	Weekly	Daily or almost daily	
6. How often during the last year have you needed a first drink in the morning to get yourself going after a heavy drinking session?	Never	Less than monthly	Monthly	Weekly	Daily or almost daily	
7. How often during the last year have you had a feeling of guilt or remorse after drinking?	Never	Less than monthly	Monthly	Weekly	Daily or almost daily	
8. How often during the last year have you been unable to remember what happened the night before because of your drinking?	Never	Less than monthly	Monthly	Weekly	Daily or almost daily	
9. Have you or someone else been injured because of your drinking?	No		Yes, but not in the last year		Yes, during the last year	
10. Has a relative, friend, doctor, or other health care worker been concerned about your drinking or suggested you cut down?	No		Yes, but not in the last year		Yes, during the last year	
					Total	

TABLE 6-18(2). Spanish Version of AUDIT

PACIENTE: Debido a que el uso del alcohol puede afectar su salud e interferir con ciertos medicamentos y tratamientos, es importante que le hagamos algunas preguntas sobre su uso del alcohol. Sus respuestas serán confidenciales, así que sea honesto por favor.

Marque una X en el cuadro que mejor describa su respuesta a cada pregunta.

PREGUNTAS	0	1	2	3	4	
1. ¿Con qué frecuencia consume alguna bebida alcohólica?	Nunca	Una o menos veces al mes	De 2 a 4 veces al mes	De 2 a 3 más veces a la semana	4 o más veces a la semana	
2. ¿Cuantas consumiciones de bebidas alcohólicas suele realizar en un día de consumo normal?	1 o 2	3 o 4	5 o 6	De 7 a 9	10 o más	
3. ¿Con qué frecuencia toma 5 o más bebidas alcohólicas en un solo día?	Nunca	Menos de una vez al mes	Mensualmente	Semanalmente	A diario o casi a diario	
4. ¿Con qué frecuencia en el curso del último año ha sido incapaz de parar de beber una vez había empezado?	Nunca	Menos de una vez al mes	Mensualmente	Semanalmente	A diario o casi a diario	
5. ¿Con qué frecuencia en el curso del último año no pudo hacer lo que se esperaba de usted porque había bebido?	Nunca	Menos de una vez al mes	Mensualmente	Semanalmente	A diario o casi a diario	
6. ¿Con qué frecuencia en el curso del último año ha necesitado beber en ayunas para recuperarse después de haber bebido mucho el día anterior?	Nunca	Menos de una vez al mes	Mensualmente	Semanalmente	A diario o casi a diario	
7. ¿Con qué frecuencia en el curso del último año ha tenido remordimientos o sentimientos de culpa después de haber bebido?	Nunca	Menos de una vez al mes	Mensualmente	Semanalmente	A diario o casi a diario	
8. ¿Con qué frecuencia en el curso del último año no ha podido recordar lo que sucedió la noche anterior porque había estado bebiendo?	Nunca	Menos de una vez al mes	Mensualmente	Semanalmente	A diario o casi a diario	
9. ¿Usted o alguna otra persona ha resultado herido porque usted había bebido?	No		Sí, pero no en el curso del último año		Sí, el último año	
10. ¿Algún familiar, amigo, médico o profesional sanitario ha mostrado preocupación por un consumo de bebidas alcohólicas o le ha sugerido que deje de beber?	No		Sí, pero no en el curso del último año		Sí, el último año	
					Total	

TABLE 6-18(3). Scoring the AUDIT

Record the score for each response in the blank box at the end of each line. Then total these numbers. The maximum possible total is 40.

Total scores of 8 or more for men up to age 60 or 4 or more for women, adolescents, and men over 60 are considered positive screens. For patients with totals near the cut-points, clinicians may wish to examine individual responses to questions and clarify them during the clinical examination.

Note: The AUDIT's sensitivity and specificity for detecting heavy drinking and alcohol use disorders varies across different populations. Lowering the cut-points increases sensitivity (the proportion of "true positive" cases) while increasing the number of false positives. Thus, it may be easier to use a cut-point of 4 for all patients, recognizing that more false positives may be identified among men.

down, exactly how much and when they drink. See if you can get them to commit, for example, to alternating nonalcoholic drinks and to drink alcohol slowly and on a full stomach. It helps to have them carry a list of why they want to cut down (or quit) and for them to agree to review it when they have the craving or urge to drink beyond their commitment. It also helps to talk with someone and this is where AA becomes key. It can also be helpful for the patient to announce their plans to key others and enlist their support and help.

Medications.[76,78,79] The former standby, disulfiram (Antabuse), is seldom used because compliance is poor and because it is contraindicated in patients who have not agreed to completely abstain. On the other hand, oral naltrexone (Depade, ReVia), injectable naltrexone (Vivitrol), and oral acamprosate (Campral) are effective in reducing drinking, avoiding relapse to heavy drinking, and achieving and maintaining abstinence. Patient adherence has been the key.

Outlined in Table 6-13, these medications should be considered in all instances where cessation or reduction in drinking is recommended—or in those who have stopped but continue to have cravings or slips ("falling off the wagon"). Patients who have failed with nonpharmacologic approaches are prime candidates. Ideally, patients will have the goal of abstaining, but it is acceptable to use the medications in those who simply want to reduce their drinking. Injectable naltrexone and acamprosate are approved only for those who abstain prior to treatment. This often means that you will be using oral naltrexone. There has been no evidence that combining any of these medications is helpful, but if one medication has not been effective it is reasonable to try an alternative. With patients who achieve abstinence, the relapse rate is very high in the

first 6 to 12 months, so continuing the medications for at least 3 months and up to 12 months is recommended. Close follow-up after cessation of the medication is essential.

These medications are safe and, themselves, not prone to abuse, and they can be used during other types of treatment. Note, though, that *naltrexone should not be used in a patient on opioids or in opioid withdrawal.* Before starting naltrexone, patients should have been off opioids completely for 7 to 10 days.

Support Groups and Other Resources[76]

- Alcoholics Anonymous (www.aa.org) are groups of volunteers in recovery and have a proven record of success. Virtually all problem drinkers should attend.

- Al-Anon (http://al-anon.org/) is also a successful resource for families and friends concerned about someone's drinking.

- Other mutual help organizations (http://rethinking drinking.niaaa.nih.gov/Help-links/).

- National and local rehabilitation facilities for inpatient and/or outpatient care. These are highly recommended for people with a refractory drinking problem. Call local hospitals to see if they have addiction services available. You also can call the National Drug and Alcohol Treatment Referral Routing Service (1-800-662-HELP) or visit the Substance Abuse Facility Treatment Locator Web site at http://findtreatment.samhsa.gov. These services have done remarkable work with patients everyone else had given up on.

- Referral to psychiatry and other mental health professionals, often working in concert with rehabilitation facilities. These are highly recommended for people with a refractory drinking problem and can be very effective.

- Expect that failures will occur and indicate that they do not bode poorly but, rather, that they are part of the process. The more severe the alcohol problem, the more refractory it is to your efforts; the more you need to encourage the other treatment elements above. This is particularly the case with obtaining specialist help and systematic rehabilitation. As well, with serious comorbid problems, both mental and physical, these often dictate upping the ante to higher levels of care. Unfortunately, many of the more severe alcohol problems have comorbid severe depression, unipolar or bipolar, and these disorders must be addressed as well. Problems of using multiple substances also usually indicate the need for specialty assistance.

- Your effort is identifying the problem, fostering awareness in the patient, being supportive, seeing if you can effect change with the measures we've outlined in this book (including managing comorbid mental disorders), and facilitating specialty care if you are not successful.

In closing, it is important that research shows that alcohol use can be significantly reduced by as much as 9 drinks weekly in users who are not dependent. Brief interventions also reduce blood pressure, levels of gamma-glutamyl transferase (GGT), psychosocial problems, hospital days, cost-savings, and hospital-related admissions for alcohol-related trauma.[76] For alcohol-dependent patients, monthly interventions can lead to significant reduction in or cessation of drinking.[76]

MENTAL HEALTH CARE MODEL

The MHCM in Table 6-19 is reproduced from Chapter 3 in order to reemphasize that the material in the last 3 chapters (depression, anxiety, substance use) fits into this overarching treatment model. It is of particular importance in addressing substance use problems, especially when they are comorbid with depression, anxiety, and/or medical problems. Let's review how the MHCM fits here in patients with these problems, using examples of problematic opioid use and of problematic alcohol use.

Patient-Centered Approach[29]

Probably nowhere is the patient-centered interaction (PCI) more important than with addiction problems. Patients have often been shunned by others and/or are self-recriminating and/or feeling hopeless. The ability to effectively communicate and establish a strong therapeutic relationship is key to having success. You know by now the conduct of the PCI, but it bears emphasis that you must first understand the patient psychologically and emotionally, and then respond empathically to them, usually doing so multiple times over multiple visits. Patients often lack the healthy support you can provide. Patients who succeed in controlling their addiction problem typically report that their success was due to an understanding and trusting relationship they established with their provider. A healthy and empathic relationship does not discount other aspects of treatment, however, but it does foster adherence to the rest of treatment.

But the PCI is only the centerpiece of the MHCM. The remaining parts, derived from motivational interviewing and shared decision making, are also essential to success.[78,80] Let's review the specifics of ECGN (education, commitment, goals, negotiated plan).

Education

Recalling that you first must determine what the patient understands about their problem, we ask patients their understanding is of, for example, their opioid or alcohol use. This will vary considerably from those without a clue to someone who knows everything about it. In the former instance, you clarify both a deficient knowledge base ("...yes, alcohol causes bad liver disease...") and in both instances frequent misunderstandings ("...I know the opioid seems to help but it is actually making you worse" OR "...it makes no difference that your father lived to be 80 and drank every day in his life, you are at great risk...").

Once you are on the same page about an understanding of the problem, you make a succinct diagnosis and recommendation, such as, "...we need to reduce your opioid slowly and stop it over time, and we have a better treatment for your pain..." OR "You have a drinking problem, and you need to stop or at least decrease your drinking, I'm here to help you if you wish," always listening to the patient's response

TABLE 6-19. Mental Health Care Model (MHCM)

Education

1. *ASK* – "What's Your Understanding"
   a. Their problem/diagnosis, why they have it, its outcome
   b. What they want done
2. *TELL*—
   • "I Have Good News"
      a. Clarify misunderstandings and what needs to be done
      b. Ominous conditions not found (from prior work-up)
      c. More testing/consultation not now necessary
         i. You will follow-up for any change
      d. You know diagnosis; addressed in last 3 chapters: depression, anxiety, chronic pain, prescription substance disorder, alcoholism (and comorbid medical problem)—name/explain it
   • "You Need Better Treatment"
      e. Depression (anxiety) makes pain (other symptom) worse → needs medication
         i. Problem is "real" or "not in head" (not a "psych case")
      f. Addicting prescription medications (opioids, benzodiazepines, stimulants) make pain and depression worse → need to slowly taper and discontinue
      g. Need to stop or cut down alcohol use
3. *ASK*—"Please summarize what you've heard"

Commitment

1. ASK—"Are you committed to treatment?"
2. TELL—"You need to be active, I can't do it by myself"
3. ASK—"Please summarize your commitment"

Goals

1. Obtain *long-term goals*

Negotiate Plan

1. *ALL plans are scheduled*—nothing is "as needed"
2. *Medications*—details of the following examples presented in last 3 chapters
   a. *Antidepressant*—for depression or anxiety
   b. *Trazodone*—for sleep
   c. *Naltrexone*—for alcohol withdrawal
3. *Addicting medications* (prescription opioid; benzodiazepine and amphetamine detoxification often require referral)
   a. Determine present dose
   b. Regularize dose schedule—no PRN dosing regimens
   c. Start taper at 1 pill per day each week
   d. Ask them to think about which pill in their dosing schedule they can stop at the next visit
4. *Symptomatic and other medication for medical problem*
5. *Exercise* program—determine present level → prescribe small increase
6. *Social activity*—determine present level → prescribe small increase
7. *Regular follow-up visits*
8. Have *patient summarize* treatment plan
9. *Praise* patient for commitment
10. *Other aspects of treatment* plan (relaxation, diet, PT, OMT)—later
11. Do *not* advise more tests or consultation (other than PT or OMT)

ASK for EMOTIONS and use NURS at each step.

to this statement, learning their feelings about it, and responding empathically using NURS (Naming, Understanding, Respecting, Supporting). Remember, these are loaded situations and you can elicit negative emotions, but responding empathically is how you establish a trusting relationship.

You end this education segment by asking the patient their understanding of what you have discussed.

Commitment

Now you determine the patient's readiness to change[81] by asking directly, "Can you commit to this recommendation?" If they cannot or will not, you explore if they are willing to cut down, "What, then, about cutting down?"

If they refuse both recommendations, don't be offended, argue, or get angry with them. Instead, here is how we recommend you handle what are 2 different problems.

1. For *problematic opioid use*, you indicate that you cannot manage them or prescribe opioids for them if they cannot follow the rest of the treatment program you have outlined for them. Fortunately, most patients are willing to participate.
2. For *problematic alcohol use*, accept their decision and indicate you will not brow-beat them about it, but that you will continue to raise the issue when you see them in the future. Compliment them on being willing to discuss the issue and indicate understanding of their decision. In these so-called precontemplators, you may find that they become more inclined to follow your recommendations in the future, although that is not always the case.[81]

Goals

To facilitate decisions to commit to treatment, you establish their goals as a way to reinforce their decision to participate in your plan, emphasizing some of the positive things in their lives to motivate them. These long-range goals will vary with each person, but often fall into some common categories: better home, work, or school relations and performance; save money; feel better about themselves; avoid/remove legal problems.

Negotiating the Treatment Plan[76]

We have identified these specifics in great detail where discussed in Chapters 4 to 6. At follow-up visits, first see how things have gone and provide support in the face of both failure and success. Reviewing their understanding, commitment, and goals is helpful along with plentiful use of NURS. Review the specifics of what went well and what did not and problem solve around how to avoid the latter. Then, carefully determine what the plans will be before the next return visit. These visits should take no more than 15 to 20 minutes and can incorporate other issues you need to address for comorbid disorders.

CONCLUSION

We have now completed the core curriculum for which we recommend competence for all future medical clinicians: depression, anxiety, prescription substance use, and alcohol use. You have learned diagnoses and treatment. The common denominator of the latter is the MHCM into which fit the various unique pharmacologic and nonpharmacologic aspects of treatment.

In Chapter 7, we look more closely at the interview. We will identify what its structure is, what information you need to gather, and how you go about this.

REFERENCES

1. Centers for Disease Control and Prevention. Prescribing opioids for chronic pain. In: Centers for Disease Control and Prevention, ed. Washington, DC: CDC; 2016.
2. Ballantyne JC. Is lack of evidence the problem? *J Pain*. 2010;11(9):830-832.
3. Ballantyne JC, Shin NS. Efficacy of opioids for chronic pain: a review of the evidence. *Clin J Pain*. 2008;24(6):469-478.
4. Manchikanti L, Helm S II, Fellows B, et al. Opioid epidemic in the United States. *Pain Physician*. 2012;15(3 suppl): ES9-E38.
5. Cutler RB, Fishbain DA, Rosomoff HL, Abdel-Maty E, Khalil TM, Rosomoff RS. Does nonsurgical pain center treatment of chronic pain return patients to work? A review and meta-analysis of the literature. *Spine*. 1994;19:643-652.
6. Kashner TM, Rost K, Cohen B, Anderson MA, Smith GR Jr. Enhancing the health of somatization disorder patients: effectiveness of short-term group therapy. *Psychosomatics*. 1995;36:462-470.

7. Klimes I, Mayou RA, Pearce MJ, Coles L, Fagg JR. Psychological treatment for atypical noncardiac chest pain: a controlled evaluation. *Psychol Med*. 1990;20:605-611.

8. Peters J, Large RG, Elkind G. Follow-up results from a randomised controlled trial evaluating in- and outpatient pain management programmes. *Pain*. 1992;50:41-50.

9. Rost K, Kashner TM, Smith GR Jr. Effectiveness of psychiatric intervention with somatization disorder patients: improved outcomes at reduced costs. *Gen Hosp Psychiatry*. 1994;16:381-387.

10. Sharpe M, Peveler R, Mayou R. The psychological treatment of patients with functional somatic symptoms: a practical guide. *J Psychosom Res*. 1992;36:515-529.

11. Smith GR Jr, Rost K, Kashner TM. A trial of the effect of a standardized psychiatric consultation on health outcomes and costs in somatizing patients. *Arch Gen Psychiatry*. 1995;52:238-243.

12. Warwick HMC, Clark DM, Cobb AM, Salkovskis PM. A controlled trial of cognitive-behavioural treatment of hypchondriasis. *Brit J Psychiatry*. 1996;169:189-195.

13. Smith R, Gardiner J, Luo Z, Schooley S, Lamerato L. Primary care physicians treat somatization. *J Gen Int Med*. 2009;24:829-832.

14. Smith RC, Lyles JS, Gardiner JC, et al. Primary care clinicians treat patients with medically unexplained symptoms—a randomized controlled trial. *J Gen Intern Med*. 2006;21:671-677.

15. Katon W, von Korff M, Lin E, et al. Collaborative management to achieve treatment guidelines: impact on depression in primary care. *JAMA*. 1995;273:1026-1031.

16. Smith R, Laird-Fick H, Dwamena F, et al. Teaching residents mental health care. *Patient Educ Couns*. 2018; 101:2145-2155.

17. Smith R, D'Mello D, Freilich L, Osborn G, Laird-Fick H, Dwamena F. *Essentials of Pschiatry in Primary Care: Behavioral Health in the Medical Setting*. New York, NY: McGraw-Hill, Inc.; 2019.

18. Smith R, Laird-Fick H, D'Mello D, et al. Addressing mental health issues in primary care: an initial curriculum for medical residents. *Patient Educ Couns*. 2014;94:33-42.

19. Dwamena F, Laird-Fick H, Freilich F, et al. Behavioral health problems in medical patients. *J Clin Outcomes Management*. 2014;21:497-505.

20. Smith RC, Lein C, Collins C, et al. Treating patients with medically unexplained symptoms in primary care. *J Gen Intern Med*. 2003;18:478-489.

21. Smith RC, Lyles JS, Mettler J, et al. The effectiveness of intensive training for residents in interviewing. A randomized, controlled study. *Ann Intern Med*. 1998;128:118-126.

22. Smith RC, Frank C, Gardiner JC, Lamerato L, Rost KM. Pilot study of a preliminary criterion standard for prescription opioid misuse. *Am J Addict*. 2010;19(6):523-528.

23. Sullivan M. Clarifying opioid misuse and abuse. *Pain*. 2013;154(11):2239-2240.

24. Smith SM, Dart RC, Katz NP, et al. Classification and definition of misuse, abuse, and related events in clinical trials: ACTTION systematic review and recommendations. *Pain*. 2013;154(11):2287-2296.

25. McCance-Katz E, Houry D, Collins F. Testimony on addressing the opioid crisis in America: prevention, treatment, and recovery before the Senate Subcommittee. Senate Appropriations Subcommittee on Labor, Health and Human Services, Education and Related Agencies. Bethesda, MD: National Institutes of Health; 2017.

26. Han B, Compton WM, Blanco C, Crane E, Lee J, Jones CM. Prescription opioid use, misuse, and use disorders in U.S. adults: 2015 National Survey on Drug Use and Health. *Ann Intern Med*. 2017;167(5):293-301.

27. Talbott Recovery 2015; https://talbottcampus.com/2015-prescription-drug-abuse-statistics/. Accessed August 15, 2017.

28. Fleming MF, Davis J, Passik SD. Reported lifetime aberrant drug-taking behaviors are predictive of current substance use and mental health problems in primary care patients. *Pain Med*. 2008;9(8):1098-1106.

29. Fortin AH VI, Dwamena F, Frankel R, Lepisto B, Smith R. *Smith's Patient-Centered Interviewing—An Evidence-Based Method*. 4th ed. New York, NY: McGraw-Hill, Lange Series; 2018.

30. Owen GT, Burton AW, Schade CM, Passik S. Urine drug testing: current recommendations and best practices. *Pain Physician*. 2012;15(3 suppl):ES119-E133.

31. Webster LR, Webster RM. Predicting aberrant behaviors in opioid-treated patients: preliminary validation of the Opioid Risk Tool. *Pain Med*. 2005;6(6):432-442.

32. Butler SF, Fernandez K, Benoit C, Budman SH, Jamison RN. Validation of the revised screener and opioid assessment for patients with pain (SOAPP-R). *J Pain*. 2008;9(4):360-372.

33. Compton WM, Wargo EM. Prescription drug monitoring programs: promising practices in need of refinement. *Ann Intern Med*. 2018;168(11):826-827.

34. National Association of State Controlled Substances Authorities 2016; http://www.nascsa.org/rxMonitoring. htm. Accessed March 22, 2018.

35. Centers for Disease Control and Prevention 2017; https://www.cdc.gov/drugoverdose/pdmp/states.html. Accessed March 22, 2018.

36. Moeller KE, Kissack JC, Atayee RS, Lee KC. Clinical interpretation of urine drug tests: what clinicians need to know about urine drug screens. *Mayo Clin Proc*. 2017;92(5):774-796.

37. Pesce A, West C, Egan City K, Strickland J. Interpretation of urine drug testing in pain patients. *Pain Med*. 2012;13(7):868-885.

38. Kaiser Foundation Health Plan of Washington. Patients on Chronic Opioid Therapy for Chronic Non-Cancer Pain Safety Guideline. Washington State Agency Medical Directors' Group (AMDG); 2016.

39. Saitman A, Park HD, Fitzgerald RL. False-positive interferences of common urine drug screen immunoassays: a review. *J Anal Toxicol*. 2014;38(7):387-396.

40. Reisfield GM, Salazar E, Bertholf RL. Rational use and interpretation of urine drug testing in chronic opioid therapy. *Ann Clin Lab Sci*. 2007;37(4):301-314.

41. Melanson S, Petrides A. Economics of pain management testing. *J Appl Lab Med*. 2017.

42. American Psychiatric Association. *Diagnostic and Statistical Manual of Mental Disorders*. 5th ed. Washington, DC: American Psychiatric Association; 2013.

43. Ballantyne JC, Sullivan MD, Kolodny A. Opioid dependence vs addiction: a distinction without a difference? *Arch Intern Med*. 2012;172:1342-1343.

44. Berna C, Kulich RJ, Rathmell JP. Tapering long-term opioid therapy in chronic noncancer pain: evidence and recommendations for everyday practice. *Mayo Clin Proc*. 2015;90(6):828-842.

45. Scherrer JF, Salas J, Sullivan MD, et al. Impact of adherence to antidepressants on long-term prescription opioid use cessation. *Br J Psychiatry*. 2018;212(2):103-111.

46. Silverman SM. Opioid induced hyperalgesia: clinical implications for the pain practitioner. *Pain Physician*. 2009;12(3):679-684.

47. Scherrer JF, Salas J, Copeland LA, et al. Prescription opioid duration, dose, and increased risk of depression in 3 large patient populations. *Ann Fam Med*. 2016;14(1):54-62.

48. Krebs EE, Lorenz KA, Bair MJ, et al. Development and initial validation of the PEG, a three-item scale assessing pain intensity and interference. *J Gen Intern Med*. 2009;24(6):733-738.

49. Olfson M, Crystal S, Wall M, Wang S, Liu SM, Blanco C. Causes of death after nonfatal opioid overdose. *JAMA Psychiatry*. 2018;75(8):820-827.

50. Chang AK, Bijur PE, Esses D, Barnaby DP, Baer J. Effect of a single dose of oral opioid and nonopioid analgesics on acute extremity pain in the emergency department: a randomized clinical trial. *JAMA*. 2017;318(17):1661-1667.

51. Martin BC, Fan MY, Edlund MJ, Devries A, Braden JB, Sullivan MD. Long-term chronic opioid therapy discontinuation rates from the TROUP study. *J Gen Intern Med*. 2011;26(12):1450-1457.

52. Martell BA, O'Connor PG, Kerns RD, et al. Systematic review: opioid treatment for chronic back pain: prevalence, efficacy, and association with addiction. *Ann Intern Med*. 2007;146(2):116-127.

53. Ackerman AL, O'Connor PG, Doyle DL, et al. Association of an opioid standard of practice intervention with intravenous opioid exposure in hospitalized patients. *JAMA Intern Med*. 2018;178(6):759-763.

54. Dowell D, Haegerich TM. Changing the conversation about opioid tapering. *Ann Intern Med*. 2017;167(3):208-209.

55. Wakeman SE, Barnett ML. Primary care and the opioid-overdose crisis—buprenorphine myths and realities. *N Engl J Med*. 2018;379(1):1-4.

56. Samet JH, Botticelli M, Bharel M. Methadone in primary care—one small step for congress, one giant leap for addiction treatment. *N Engl J Med*. 2018;379(1):7-8.

57. Rudd RA, Seth P, David F, Scholl L. Increases in drug and opioid-involved overdose deaths—United States, 2010-2015. *MMWR Morb Mortal Wkly Rep*. 2016;65(5051):1445-1452.

58. Adams JM. Increasing naloxone awareness and use: the role of health care practitioners. *JAMA*. 2018;319(20):2073-2074.

59. Goodman CW, Brett AS. Gabapentin and pregabalin for pain—is increased prescribing a cause for concern? *N Engl J Med*. 2017;377(5):411-414.

60. Gomes T, Greaves S, van den Brink W, et al. Pregabalin and the risk for opioid-related death: a nested case-control study. *Ann Intern Med*. 2018;169:732-734.

61. Kroenke K, Cheville A. Management of chronic pain in the aftermath of the opioid backlash. *JAMA*. 2017;317(23):2365-2366.

62. Sullivan MD, Ballantyne JC. What are we treating with long-term opioid therapy? *Arch Intern Med*. 2012;172(5):433-434.

63. Kupfer J, Bond E. Patient satisfaction and patient-centered care—necessary but not equal. *JAMA*. 2012;308:139-140.

64. Lembke A, Papac J, Humphreys K. Our other prescription drug problem. *N Engl J Med*. 2018;378(8):693-695.

65. Moore N, Pariente A, Begaud B. Why are benzodiazepines not yet controlled substances? *JAMA Psychiatry*. 2015;72(2):110-111.

66. Olfson M, King M, Schoenbaum M. Benzodiazepine use in the United States. *JAMA Psychiatry*. 2015;72(2):136-142.

67. Simon GE, Ludman EJ. Outcome of new benzodiazepine prescriptions to older adults in primary care. *Gen Hosp Psychiatry*. 2006;28(5):374-378.

68. Steinman MA, Low M, Balicer RD, Shadmi E. Epidemic use of benzodiazepines among older adults in Israel: epidemiology and leverage points for improvement. *J Gen Intern Med*. 2017;32(8):891-899.

69. Kroll DS, Nieva HR, Barsky AJ, Linder JA. Benzodiazepines are prescribed more frequently to patients already at risk for benzodiazepine-related adverse events in primary care. *J Gen Intern Med*. 2016;31(9):1027-1034.

70. Ashton H. *Benzodiazepines: How They Work and How to Withdraw*. Copyright 1999-2013. Newcastle upon Tyne, UK: Institute of Neuroscience, Newcastle University; 2002.

71. Rickels K, Schweizer E. Anxiolytics: indications, benefits, and risks of short-term and long-term benzodiazepine therapy: current research data. In: Cooper JR, Czechowicz DJ, Molinari SP, Petersen RC, eds. *Impact of Prescription Drug Diversion Control Systems on Medical Practice and Patient Care %7 NIDA Research Monograph 131.* Rockville, MD: National Institute on Drug Abuse; 1993:51-67.

72. Substance Abuse Mental Health Services Administration 2015; https://store.samhsa.gov/shin/content/SMA15-4131/SMA15-4131.pdf. Accessed April 3, 2018.

73. Petursson H. The benzodiazepine withdrawal syndrome. *Addiction.* 1994;89(11):1455-1459.

74. National Survey on Drug Use and Health 2017; https://www.samhsa.gov/data/sites/default/files/NSDUH-FFR1-2016/NSDUH-FFR1-2016.htm#summary. Accessed March 2, 2018.

75. Collaborators GBDA. Alcohol use and burden for 195 countries and territories, 1990-2016: a systematic analysis for the Global Burden of Disease Study 2016. *Lancet.* 2018;392(10152):1015-1035.

76. Department of Health and Human Services 2016; https://pubs.niaaa.nih.gov/publications/practitioner/cliniciansguide2005/guide.pdf. Accessed April 5, 2018.

77. National Institute on Alcohol Abuse and A 2002; https://pubs.niaaa.nih.gov/publications/inscage.htm. Accessed April 5, 2018.

78. Miller W, Rollnick S. *Motivational Interviewing—Helping People Change.* 3rd ed. New York, NY: The Guilford Press; 2013.

79. Kranzler HR, Soyka M. Diagnosis and pharmacotherapy of alcohol use disorder: a review. *JAMA.* 2018;320(8):815-824.

80. Gulbrandsen P, Clayman ML, Beach MC, et al. Shared decision-making as an existential journey: aiming for restored autonomous capacity. *Patient Educ Couns.* 2016;99(9):1505-1510.

81. Prochaska JO, Velicer WF. The transtheoretical model of health behavior change. *Am J Health Promot.* 1997;12:38-48.

7

The Diagnostic Interview

At this point, it's time to consider the diagnostic interview. By now you know the major mental disorders you will need to master in medical settings—depression, anxiety, and prescription and other substance misuse. In the interview, you're looking for criteria that distinguish among these disorders and their subsets. The interview format we now present describes the categories of data needed and how it can be written up for your records.

You learned in Chapter 3 to begin all interviews with the patient-centered interview.[1] To briefly review, one begins any interaction by ensuring the patient's comfort (step 1) and setting an agenda for the visit (step 2). You then proceed to the true patient-centered part of the interaction (steps 3 and 4) to determine open-endedly the patient's physical symptom and personal story. You next elicit any emotion associated with these stories and empathically respond by **N**aming it, expressing **U**nderstanding of it, **R**especting it, and offering **S**upport (**NURS**). See Table 3-1 in Chapter 3.

Following this 3- to 5-minute patient-centered introduction, you transition to develop the details of the chief concern you elicited during agenda setting (step 2). Even in patients with a mental disorder, this step will often involve physical symptoms, and you need to pin down these details as you normally would via the history of present illness (HPI), past medical history (PMH), social history (SH), family history (FH), and review of systems (ROS). For mental disorders, the format is essentially the same.

You may have already uncovered psychological symptoms (of a mental disorder) in your patient-centered interviewing. As you expand the patient's physical and personal stories, you will often identify them. Once you have identified these symptoms, you proceed to the clinician-centered part of the interaction to pin down crucial diagnostic details, as outlined in Chapters 4 to 6. On the other hand, recall that you may not have gotten many psychological symptoms in the patient-centered component, and that you will need to actively inquire about them during clinician-centered inquiry.

So how might you elicit the psychological symptoms? What are some questions you can use to screen for a mental disorder during clinician-centered interviewing? Table 7-1 presents the disorders discussed in Chapters 4 to 6; your clinician-centered questions will focus on differentiating among them. Table 7-2 suggests some specific screening questions for depression, mania/hypomania, and drug/alcohol abuse. Now, you generally do not ask all the questions in Table 7-2 in screening; rather, you should focus on the areas where you have suspicions. These concerns will commonly include depression and/or anxiety because the 2 are the most common disorders and often occur together. When answers to screening questions are positive, you conduct your subsequent history to elicit the differentiating material described in Chapters 4 to 6. Tables 7-3 and 7-4 list some less common mental disorders and present some screening questions for them. We will cover these in more detail later in the book,

TABLE 7-1. Common Mental Disorders: Depression, Anxiety, and Substance Abuse

DEPRESSION	ANXIETY	SUBSTANCE ABUSE
Major depression	Generalized anxiety disorder	Illicit drug abuse
Chronic depression	Panic disorder	Prescription drug abuse Opioids Benzodiazepines Stimulants
Depression variants	Posttraumatic stress disorder	Alcohol abuse
Bipolar disorders I and II	Obsessive-compulsive disorder	
	Social phobia Other phobias	

TABLE 7-2. Screening Questions for Common Mental Disorders

DEPRESSION	MANIA/HYPOMANIA	ANXIETY	SUBSTANCE ABUSE
Depressed mood "Have you felt sad, depressed, blue, or hopeless over the last 2 weeks?"	Elation "Have you felt higher or happier than usual, the opposite of depression, for 4 or more days in a row?" "Have you had excessive amounts of energy or racing thoughts or talking a lot where you didn't need much sleep for 4 or more days in a row?"	"Do you have persistent problems with being nervous or anxious?" "Are there specific situations in which you regularly become anxious?"	"How much alcohol do you drink per day?" "Do you use street drugs?" "What prescribed medications are you taking for pain?"
Anhedonia (lack of joy) "What have you done for fun in the last 2 weeks?" "Have you had decreased interest or energy for pleasurable activities in the last 2 weeks?"	Irritability "Have you ever been so unusually (for you) irritable that you did things you would not ordinarily do, like start arguments or fights over 4 or more days in a row?"		
Insomnia "Does it take you more than 30 minutes to get to sleep or get back to sleep if you waken in the last 2 weeks?" "Have you been sleeping more than usual in the last 2 weeks?"			

TABLE 7-3. Less Common Mental Disorders

PSYCHOSES	ORGANIC	OTHER
Schizophrenia	Various dementias	Attention-deficit/hyperactivity disorder (ADHD)
Schizoaffective disorder	Medications	Eating disorder
Bipolar I (mania)	Chronic disease	Personality disorder
Depressive psychosis	Human immunodeficiency virus (HIV)	Borderline personality disorder
Dementia	Traumatic brain injury	
Organic—delirium		

but know for now that they are less common and often more easily recognized.

DIAGNOSTIC INTERVIEW—NEW PATIENT WITH A MENTAL DISORDER

1. Circumstances of the interview and patient's understanding of it—this may be a patient new to you or one you already know, but in whom you have just identified a mental disorder.
2. Patient-centered HPI
   a. Set stage and agenda (steps 1 and 2 of patient-centered interview).
   b. Use focused, open-ended questions to obtain physical and personal contextual stories. Next, elicit emotion and address using NURS to establish the clinician-patient relationship (steps 3 and 4).
   c. Transition to clinician-centered HPI for details (step 5).
3. Clinician-centered HPI
   a. Chronology and other details of *physical* symptoms, for example chronic pain, dyspnea, weight loss.
   b. Chronology and other details of *psychological* symptoms, for example fearful, depressed.
   - Significant positive and negative symptoms *from onset* (recalling that many disorders begin in childhood or adolescence) and detail the *course since then*. This stage is where you will often make your diagnosis of mental disorder by identifying the key features you have learned from Chapters 4 to 6.
   - In all patients, ask specifically about the following:
     - Precipitants/stressors: Severity
     - Self-harm and suicidal ideation and intent
     - Illicit drug and alcohol use
     - Psychopharmacologic medications: Doses, effectiveness, side effects, problems with medications or reasons for discontinuing
     - Impact of problem on the patient's life and ability to function, highest and lowest functional levels
     - Support system, for example spouse, family, work, Alcoholics Anonymous, church

TABLE 7-4. Screening Questions for Uncommon Mental Disorders

PSYCHOSES	ORGANIC
"Have you heard or seen things that others don't seem to?"	"Do you know where you are?"
"Have you suspected other people were spying on you or following you or want to harm you?"	"Do you know what year it is?"
"Does the radio or television say things meant just for you?"	"What is your telephone number?"

- Comorbid medical illness (and medications/treatment) and link to mental disorder
    - NURS throughout.
4. Past history of mental disorders (included in HPI if relevant)
    - Symptoms, duration, severity, treatment/response.
    - Prior hospitalizations and treatments, for example medications, counseling. Duration of any hospitalization provides clues about how severe the problem was, for example overnight versus 3 weeks.
    - Prior nonhospitalized contacts with mental health professionals, for example community mental health, psychiatry, counseling.
5. Family history
    - Any mental disorder in blood relatives, including first cousins.
    - Specifically ask about bipolar disorder, depression, anxiety, "nervous breakdowns," schizophrenia.

6. Social history
    - Interpersonal relationships (number, availability), living circumstances, housing/homeless; many have histories of troubled, dysfunctional relationships.
    - Developmental history, for example what childhood was like (walking, talking, sibling interactions, progress in education, educational level, social interactions, parental interactions/surrogate parents, interests/goals).
    - Abuse history: Physical, sexual, psychological.
    - Legal problems, for example arrested, jailed.
    - Socioeconomic status: Financial situation, employment, Medicaid, Medicare, and insurance status.
7. Integrate results of questionnaires
    - Patient Health Questionnaire-9 (PHQ-9): Obtained on all patients suspected of a mental disorder (see Table 7-5)

TABLE 7-5. Screening for Patient Health Questionnaire (PHQ-9) Scale

Over *the last 2 weeks*, how often have you been bothered by any of the following problems?

	Not at all (0)	Several days (1)	More than half the days (2)	Nearly every day (3)
1. Little interest or pleasure in doing things	❑	❑	❑	❑
2. Feeling down, depressed, or hopeless	❑	❑	❑	❑
3. Trouble falling or staying asleep, or sleeping too much	❑	❑	❑	❑
4. Feeling tired or having little energy	❑	❑	❑	❑
5. Poor appetite or overeating	❑	❑	❑	❑
6. Feeling bad about yourself—or that you are a failure or have let yourself or your family down	❑	❑	❑	❑
7. Trouble concentrating on things, such as reading the newspaper or watching television	❑	❑	❑	❑
8. Moving or speaking so slowly that other people could have noticed? Or the opposite—being so fidgety or restless that you have been moving around a lot more than usual	❑	❑	❑	❑
9. Thoughts that you would be better off dead or of hurting yourself in some way	❑	❑	❑	❑
Add the score from each column				
Add column scores =			**Total Score =** _____	

TABLE 7-6. Screening for Generalized Anxiety Disorder-7 (The GAD-7) Scale				
Over the _last 2 weeks_, how often have you been bothered by the following problems?				
	Not at all (0)	**Several days (1)**	**More than half the days (2)**	**Nearly every day (3)**
Feeling nervous, anxious or on edge	❏	❏	❏	❏
Not being able to stop or control worrying	❏	❏	❏	❏
Worrying too much about different things	❏	❏	❏	❏
Trouble relaxing	❏	❏	❏	❏
Being so restless that it is hard to sit still	❏	❏	❏	❏
Becoming easily annoyed or irritable	❏	❏	❏	❏
Feeling afraid as if something awful might happen	❏	❏	❏	❏
Add the score from each column				
Add column scores =			**Total Score = _____**	

- Generalized Anxiety Disorder-7 (GAD-7): Obtained on all patients suspected of a mental disorder (see Table 7-6)
- As necessary: Other screeners for substance use, bipolar disorder, attention-deficit/hyperactivity disorder (ADHD), eating disorder
8. Integrate results of existing data
   - Prescription Drug Monitoring Program (PDMP) for controlled medication use. Be aware that in many states including the search results in the medical record is not allowed, but you can and should summarize the report in your documentation.
   - Urine (and blood) drug screens.
9. Physical examination
   - Mental status evaluation (as needed): We recommend screening, but not a full Mini-Mental Status Examination unless one is suspicious of an organic mental syndrome, acute or chronic, or a psychotic disorder.
   - Remainder of physical examination.
10. Assessment
   - Medical diseases: Almost always more than 1, typically 3 to 5 diseases.
   - Mental disorder(s) according to Diagnostic and Statistical Manual of Mental Disorders,

5th ed. (DSM-5)[2]: Often more than 1. Also indicate "subsyndromal" disorders, those that don't quite meet criteria in DSM-5.
11. Institute treatment plan: You now have diagnosed 1 or more mental disorders and are ready to deploy the Mental Health Care Model (MHCM) described in Chapter 3, and you know the disorder-specific medications and other treatments for depression, anxiety, and prescription substance misuse discussed in Chapters 4 to 6.

In the following chapters, we now address some of the less common mental disorders that are nonetheless important in primary care, often because early detection can lead to early referral and treatment.

REFERENCES

1. Fortin AH VI, Dwamena F, Frankel R, Lepisto B, Smith R. _Smith's Patient-Centered Interviewing—An Evidence-Based Method._ 4th ed. New York: McGraw-Hill, Lange Series; 2018.
2. American Psychiatric Association. _Diagnostic and Statistical Manual of Mental Disorders._ 5th ed. Washington, DC: American Psychiatric Association; 2013.

Other Disorders and Issues in Primary Care

In this chapter, we consider some other important mental health issues encountered in medical settings. Recognizing the signs and symptoms of these disorders can prevent misdiagnoses and medication errors, as well as help the patient to get started on an effective course of treatment early on, often by timely referral.

ATTENTION-DEFICIT/HYPERACTIVITY DISORDER

Introduction

Attention-deficit/hyperactivity disorder (ADHD) is a neurodevelopmental disorder characterized by age-inappropriate levels of motor hyperactivity, impulsivity, and inattention.[1] It is a common disorder of childhood and adolescence and persists into adulthood in about 50% of cases.[2] The prevalence of ADHD in Americans aged 18 to 44 years is estimated to be 4.4%.[3] Like prescribed opioids, the stimulant drugs commonly used to treat ADHD have posed a problem of misuse, so it is important to know how to diagnose these patients so that those with true ADHD can receive the effective treatment you have at your disposal. Also, diagnosis is especially important because persistence of childhood ADHD into adulthood and adult-onset ADHD are associated with increased mental health problems and substance abuse, in addition to the diminished economic and physical health outcomes that characterize remitted childhood ADHD.[4]

Diagnosis and Screening

The differential diagnosis of ADHD in adults includes disorders that are also commonly comorbid with ADHD such as mood disorders, anxiety disorders, substance use disorders, learning disabilities, and impulse control disorders.[3,5] Medical disorders that can mimic ADHD include endocrine and metabolic disorders (thyroid disorders), neurologic disorders (including traumatic brain injury), sleep disorders (obstructive sleep apnea), and side effects of medications.[1]

The *Diagnostic and Statistical Manual of Mental Disorders*, 5th ed. (DSM-5) diagnostic criteria for ADHD (Table 8-1), originally developed to diagnose ADHD in children, need slight modifications for use with adults. Adults with ADHD present primarily with deficits in executive functioning such as memory deficits, problems with initiating and shifting tasks, and difficulty with inhibiting or monitoring themselves. This leads to problems with organizing, prioritizing, remaining focused, and following through with tasks and assignments.[5] While these manifestations of inattention are prominent, symptoms of hyperactivity or impulsivity are less or overt in adults.

The objectives of the assessment of an adult for ADHD is to identify symptoms and behaviors consistent with DSM-5 criteria for ADHD, evaluate the patient for any impairment attributable to these symptoms, rule out other psychiatric and other comorbid disorders, and refer doubtful cases for neuropsychological testing, as described shortly. A careful history, including documenting when the symptoms

TABLE 8-1. DSM-5 Criteria for ADHD

A. A persistent pattern of inattention and/or hyperactivity-impulsivity that interferes with functioning or development, as characterized by (1) and/or (2):

1. **Inattention:** Six (or more) of the following symptoms have persisted for at least 6 months to a degree that is inconsistent with developmental level and that negatively impacts directly on social and academic/occupational activities: **Note:** The symptoms are not solely a manifestation of oppositional behavior, defiance, hostility, or failure to understand tasks or instructions. For older adolescents and adults (age 17 or older), at least five symptoms are required.
   a. Often fails to give close attention to details or makes careless mistakes in schoolwork, at work, or during other activities (e.g., overlooks or misses details, work is inaccurate).
   b. Often has difficulty sustaining attention in tasks or play activities (e.g., has difficulty remaining focused during lectures, conversations, or lengthy reading).
   c. Often does not seem to listen when spoken to directly (e.g., mind seems elsewhere, even in the absence of any obvious distraction).
   d. Often does not follow through on instructions and fails to finish schoolwork, chores, or duties in the workplace (e.g., starts tasks but quickly loses focus and is easily sidetracked).
   e. Often has difficulty organizing tasks and activities (e.g., difficulty managing sequential tasks; difficulty keeping materials and belongings in order; messy, disorganized work; has poor time management; fails to meet deadlines).
   f. Often avoids, dislikes, or is reluctant to engage in tasks that require sustained mental effort (e.g., schoolwork or homework; for older adolescents and adults, preparing reports, completing forms, reviewing lengthy papers).
   g. Often loses things necessary for tasks or activities (e.g., school materials, pencils, books, tools, wallets, keys, paperwork, eyeglasses, mobile telephones).
   h. Is often easily distracted by extraneous stimuli (for older adolescents and adults may include unrelated thoughts).
   i. Is often forgetful in daily activities (e.g., doing chores, running errands; for older adolescents and adults, returning calls, paying bills, keeping appointments).

2. **Hyperactivity and impulsivity:** Six (or more) of the following symptoms have persisted for at least 6 months to a degree that is inconsistent with developmental level and that negatively impacts directly on social and academic/occupational activities: **Note:** The symptoms are not solely a manifestation of oppositional behavior, defiance, hostility, or a failure to understand tasks or instructions. For older adolescents and adults (age 17 and older), at least five symptoms are required.
   a. Often fidgets with or taps hands or feet or squirms in seat.
   b. Often leaves seat in situations when remaining seated is expected (e.g., leaves his or her place in the classroom, in the office or other workplace, or in other situations that require remaining in place).
   c. Often runs about or climbs in situations where it is inappropriate. (**Note:** In adolescents or adults, may be limited to feeling restless.)
   d. Often unable to play or engage in leisure activities quietly.
   e. Is often "on the go," acting as if "driven by a motor" (e.g., is unable to be or uncomfortable being still for extended time, as in restaurants, meetings; may be experienced by others as being restless or difficult to keep up with).
   f. Often talks excessively.
   g. Often blurts out an answer before a question has been completed (e.g., completes people's sentences; cannot wait for turn in conversation).
   h. Often has difficulty waiting his or her turn (e.g., while waiting in line).
   i. Often interrupts or intrudes on others (e.g., butts into conversations, games, or activities; may start using other people's things without asking or receiving permission; for adolescents and adults, may intrude into or take over what others are doing).

B. Several inattentive or hyperactive-impulsive symptoms were present prior to age 12 years.

C. Several inattentive or hyperactive-impulsive symptoms are present in two or more settings (e.g., at home, school, or work; with friends or relatives; in other activities).

(Continued)

TABLE 8-1. DSM-5 Criteria for ADHD (*Continued*)

D. There is clear evidence that the symptoms interfere with, or reduce the quality of, social, academic, or occupational functioning.

E. The symptoms do not occur exclusively during the course of schizophrenia or another psychotic disorder and are not better explained by another mental disorder (e.g., mood disorder, anxiety disorder, dissociative disorder, personality disorder, substance intoxication, or withdrawal).

ADHD = attention deficit/hyperactivity disorder; DSM-5 = *Diagnostic and Statistical Manual of Mental Disorders*, 5th edition. Reprinted with permission from the *Diagnostic and Statistical Manual of Mental Disorders*, Fifth Edition, (Copyright ©2013). American Psychiatric Association. All Rights Reserved.

started, will often help to exclude ADHD.[5] There should almost always be a history of onset by age 12 to entertain a diagnosis of ADHD.[5] What often is called adult-onset ADHD usually is due to a comorbid mental health disorder rather than ADHD.[6] A new adult ADHD questionnaire has a high sensitivity and specificity for DSM-5 ADHD.[7] It may be a useful tool in primary care for screening and evaluating treatment efficacy.

Approach to Diagnosis and Referral

If the patient has a history compatible with ADHD and if they have been treated previously, we request records from their prior physician, including medication use and doses. If this material indicates a prior history of ADHD and a response to stimulants, we continue the medications and follow the treatment plan that follows.

If this past information is not forthcoming or if the patient does not have a clear childhood history of ADHD, we recommend referral to a mental health professional skilled in ADHD diagnosis and neuropsychological testing. Neuropsychologic assessment consists of a series of tests that evaluate intellectual abilities, academic achievement, memory, language skills, visual-motor coordination, attention, reasoning abilities, executive functioning skills, and emotional dysfunction. Most testing also will evaluate possible other psychological problems that might contribute to the problem, such as learning disabilities. Such a referral can also help weed out those seeking to simulate ADHD, perhaps having reviewed the symptom criteria for it, for financial gain and other misuse.

If testing indicates a likely diagnosis of ADHD, we follow the treatment plan given next. If there is a history of substance use, we do not prescribe stimulants but offer the patient referral for addiction counseling.

Use of the Prescription Drug Monitoring Program and urine drug screening is needed, as outlined in Chapter 6.[8]

Treatment

Adults with ADHD usually do not receive treatment for ADHD. This is unfortunate because untreated persons with ADHD compared with unaffected controls experience higher rates of academic failure, low occupational status, increased risk of substance use disorders (tobacco, alcohol, or drugs), accidents and delinquency, and have fewer social relationships or friends.[9] Even with treatment, unfortunately, patients may not get to the level of non-ADHD patients.[10]

An approach that combines appropriate pharmacotherapy with the Mental Health Care Model (MHCM) described in Chapter 3 works best with these patients. Patients especially benefit from education about ADHD and comorbid disorders, as well as cognitive behavioral therapy, coaching and family therapy, and medications for ADHD and any comorbid disorders.[9] Referral to a mental health professional can be helpful.

We strongly recommend treatment of comorbid disorders before making a diagnosis of ADHD. Many believe a diagnosis of ADHD cannot be made until after this occurs. In addition, an approved nonstimulant medication such as bupropion should be used first with the patient's understanding that they may take 1 to 2 weeks to exhibit an effect. Also, the serotonin noradrenaline reuptake inhibitor (SNRI) atomoxetine is approved for use in ADHD. See Table 8-2. The nonstimulant medications, however, have lower effect sizes in ADHD than the stimulants.

Stimulants (amphetamine/dextroamphetamine and lisdexamfetamine; methylphenidate) are *absolutely contraindicated* with a history of substance abuse; their nontherapeutic effects such as euphoria may place the patient at added risk of abuse. They are *relatively*

TABLE 8-2. Stimulant and Nonstimulant Medications

STIMULANT	STARTING DOSE	USUAL DOSE	MAXIMUM DOSE
(Amphetamine/dextroamphetamine)	2.5-5 mg bid	10-20 mg/day	40-60 mg/day
Adderall XR (amphetamine/dextroamphetamine)	20 mg in AM	20-40 mg/day	40-60 mg/day
Vyvanse (lisdexamfetamine)	30 mg/day	50-60 mg/day	70 mg/day
Ritalin (methylphenidate)	5 mg bid	10 mg bid	60 mg/day
Ritalin LA (methylphenidate)	20 mg/day	40 mg/day	60 mg/day
Ritalin SR (methylphenidate)	20 mg/day	40 mg/day	60 mg/day
NONSTIMULANT			
Strattera (atomoxetine)	40 mg/day	80-100 mg/day	100 mg/day
Wellbutrin SR (bupropion)	100 mg/day	100-150 mg bid	200 mg bid
Wellbutrin XL (bupropion)	150 mg/day	300 mg/day	450 mg/day

Common side effects for all stimulants: headache, abdominal pain, decreased appetite, insomnia.
Uncommon side effects for all stimulants: tics, agitation, anxiety, increased pulse rate and blood pressure.
Common side effects for atomoxetine: headache, decreased appetite, insomnia, nausea, dry mouth, fatigue.
Common side effects for bupropion: headache, decreased appetite, insomnia, dry mouth.

contraindicated in patients with structural heart disease, hyperthyroidism, hypertension, anxiety, and glaucoma. In patients with contraindications, bupropion or atomoxetine can be used. Stimulants are generally quite safe, however, and can have a major impact on ADHD. See Table 8-2 for dosing. One caveat: contrary to popular perception, they should not be used diagnostically because neither a response nor lack of response has diagnostic value. While the different drug classes of stimulants are of equal effect in ADHD, failure to respond to one does not necessarily mean the other will also be ineffective, so switching drugs is recommended with an initial poor response. We recommend using the extended release forms from the outset and for maintenance. Unfortunately, many primary

care physicians have historically been reluctant to prescribe stimulants, in part, because they are controlled substances that have the potential for abuse.[11]

Amphetamine side effects stem from sympathetic overstimulation and can lead to agitation and delirium accompanied by hypertension, tachycardia, hyperthermia, sweating, paranoia, and dilated pupils. Symptoms can progress to violent behavior and seizures. Death usually stems from hyperthermia, arrhythmias, and cerebral hemorrhage. In contrast to alcohol or opioid withdrawal where we expect symptoms opposite those of intoxication, the symptoms of stimulant withdrawal can often at least partly mimic intoxication, for example, agitation, hyperarousal, and sleeplessness. See Table 8-3. While there is little evidence that tapering the

	WITHDRAWAL (DAYS TO SEVERAL WEEKS, DEPENDING ON STIMULANT)
TABLE 8-3. Symptoms and Signs of Stimulant Intoxication and Withdrawal	
INTOXICATION	
Overly confident	*Initial 1-2 day "crash" with excessive sleeping, irritability, nausea, and headache precedes the withdrawal manifestations that follow:*
Agitation, irritable, hypervigilant	Agitation
Physical overactivity	Lethargic, exhausted
Insomnia, anxiety	Insomnia, anxiety
Poor appetite	Increased appetite
Excited, talkative	Craving drug
Tachycardia, hypertension, palpitations	Depression, dysphoria, poor concentration, anhedonia
Hyperthermia, sweating, dilated pupils, dry mouth, clenched jaw	
Psychosis, seizures	

drugs is of value or that other medications are helpful during withdrawal, because of the potentially serious nature and difficulty of withdrawal, we recommend referral of addicted patients or those showing signs of intoxication or withdrawal be referred to addiction specialists for supervised withdrawal.[12]

END-OF-LIFE ISSUES

Introduction

In 2016, over 2.7 million people died in the United States. These deaths came in many different ways and under a variety of circumstances. Lunney et al[13] have identified 4 trajectories of dying: (1) *Sudden death* is progression from normal function to death with little warning and often with little interaction with the health care system; (2) *terminal illness* is death after a distinct phase of terminal illness (sufferers may function relatively well for a prolonged period and then suffer a sudden decline, eg, cancer); (3) people with *organ failure* experience gradual decline with acute exacerbations (eg, congestive heart failure; chronic obstructive pulmonary disease), each episode of which can potentially result in death; and (4) *frailty* often occurs in people with long-term diseases (eg, dementia and stroke) that show a slow and gradual decline. The

main sources of health care expenditures in the first 3 groups are physicians and ambulatory care, inpatient care, and long-term care and skilled nursing facilities, respectively. Sources of costs in the last category are highly variable, but use of nursing homes or other long-term care is higher than with other groups.[14]

The wide variability of the end-of-life (EOL) experience, coupled with current advances in medicine, has complicated the process of dying for many people. Clinicians, patients, and their families often are faced with an overwhelming number of options and decisions. Nevertheless, most people identify effective pain and symptom management, communication with their physicians, adequate preparation for death, and/or the opportunity to achieve a sense of completion as their most important value(s) at the end of their lives.[15]

Diagnosis and Screening

Despite national efforts to improve EOL care, troubling symptoms like dyspnea, severe fatigue, incontinence, anorexia, and frequent vomiting have remained prevalent, while pain, depression, and delirium have become more common. Debilitating symptoms increase notably beginning in the last 5 months prior to death and may be a prospective marker for the EOL

TABLE 8-4. Edmonton Symptom Assessment System: (Revised Version) (ESAS-R)													
Please circle the number that best describes how you feel *now*:													
No Pain	0	1	2	3	4	5	6	7	8	9	10	Worst Possible Pain	
No Tiredness (*Tiredness = lack of energy*)	0	1	2	3	4	5	6	7	8	9	10	Worst Possible Tiredness	
No Drowsiness (*Drowsiness = feeling sleepy*)	0	1	2	3	4	5	6	7	8	9	10	Worst Possible Drowsiness	
No Nausea	0	1	2	3	4	5	6	7	8	9	10	Worst Possible Nausea	
No Lack of Appetite	0	1	2	3	4	5	6	7	8	9	10	Worst Possible Lack of Appetite	
No Shortness of Breath	0	1	2	3	4	5	6	7	8	9	10	Worst Possible Shortness of Breath	
No Depression (*Depression = feeling sad*)	0	1	2	3	4	5	6	7	8	9	10	Worst Possible Depression	
No Anxiety (*Anxiety = feeling nervous*)	0	1	2	3	4	5	6	7	8	9	10	Worst Possible Anxiety	
Best Well-being (*wellbeing = how you feel overall*)	0	1	2	3	4	5	6	7	8	9	10	Worst Possible Well-being	
No _____ Other Problem (*eg, constipation*)	0	1	2	3	4	5	6	7	8	9	10	Worst Possible _____	

Scoring: There is no cutoff, but scores are compared from one time to the next, seeing improvement or deterioration. In the referenced study, many of the various baseline scores were in range of 5-6 before chemotherapy, falling to range of 1-2 at the completion of chemotherapy.[17]

period in patients with chronic conditions who appear relatively healthy.[16]

Primary care providers can screen for symptoms and monitor effects of treatment in appropriate patients, using simple tools like the revised Edmonton Symptom Assessment System in Table 8-4.[17] Referral to palliative care at an earlier stage of an advanced disease or life-threatening illness may reduce the symptom burden of patients and better prepare them for the last stages of life.[18,19]

Comorbid Conditions

Common comorbid conditions at the EOL include hypertension, arthritis, myocardial infarction, diabetes mellitus, lung disease, cancer, congestive heart failure, stroke, advanced dementia, and hip fracture.[16] Delirium occurs in 28% to 83% of patients near the

EOL and can significantly complicate EOL care if not managed properly.[20] Management of pain and other comorbidities complicates the diagnosis and treatment of delirium at the EOL. Untreated delirium frightens many patients, robs them of valuable time, and curtails opportunities to make final choices and plans. It may also lead to premature separation from family members who then suffer and express regret. Therefore, it is paramount for providers to recognize and treat delirium at the EOL.[20]

Treatment

Treatment at the EOL includes managing symptoms (eg, pain, dyspnea, nausea/vomiting, and fatigue); establishing goals of care that are in keeping with the patient's values and preferences; consistent and sustained communication between patients and all those involved in their care; psychosocial, spiritual, and practical support both to patients and their families; and coordination across sites of care.[18,19]

Primary care providers generally feel more comfortable treating pain than other symptoms such as dyspnea and depression.[21] Open conversations between health care professionals and patients as the EOL approaches are the first step in ensuring that well-planned care is delivered.[22] The effective use of NURS (Naming, Understanding, Respecting, Supporting) and other aspects of the MHCM are paramount.

Primary care providers may be especially suited in helping individuals establish goals of care and determine treatment preferences.[21] However, some providers perceive many barriers to providing emotional support.[23] While studies of interventions to improve EOL communications have yielded mixed results,[24,25] training that simultaneously targets physicians and patients/caregivers may be most effective.[25] Decision aides may also help patients, surrogates, and physicians (especially in cases of terminal illness, organ failure, or frailty) to navigate complex EOL decision making. These tools may be especially useful for decisions where prognostic data are known (eg, with major interventions, procedures, and treatments).[26]

Patients sometimes request help in speeding up the dying process, and laws increasingly allow this in some states. One option is physician-assisted death, but many physicians are uncomfortable accepting this role. Another option is for patients to voluntarily stop eating and drinking (VSED). While some patients might do this on their own, it is almost always more comfortable and effective for the patient to have their physician's participation for ongoing management. Viewed by many as the most humane way to assist death, VSED is perhaps a more palatable option for responding to patient's requests to assist in dying.[27]

NEUROCOGNITIVE DISORDERS

Introduction

The term *dementia*, now referred to as neurocognitive disorders (including Alzheimer's dementia and delirium), comprises a heterogeneous group of conditions characterized by loss of previous levels of cognition, executive function, and memory that results in impairment in role functioning and independence.

It is a growing problem in the United States, which affects 3% to 11% of persons older than 65 years and 25% to 47% of those older than 80 years.[28] Recent data indicate that cardiovascular dysregulation and cognitive decline are associated and preceded by depressive symptoms.[29] See Table 8-5 for a review of the criteria.

Delirium is a state of confusion that develops over a period of hours to days and is not explained by a pre-existing, established, or evolving dementia. It is a common life-threatening, often preventable syndrome, but research demonstrates persistent under-recognition in 60% of adults 65 years and older; it accounts for over $164 billon in health care expenditures.[30] See Table 8-5.

Diagnosis and Screening

Neurocognitive Disorders/Dementia. The diagnosis of neurocognitive disorders often is delayed because of its insidious and variable nature. The Alzheimer's Association has offered the following key warning signs that may be useful to primary care physicians in making a timely diagnosis (https://www.alz.org/10-signs-symptoms-alzheimers-dementia.asp):

1. Memory loss
2. Difficulty performing familiar tasks
3. Problems with language
4. Disorientation to time and place
5. Poor or decreased judgment
6. Problems with abstract thought
7. Misplacing things
8. Changes in mood or behavior
9. Changes in personality
10. Loss of initiative.

The role of the primary care physician in the diagnosis of dementia is to exclude a potentially treatable illness such as vitamin B_{12} deficiency, depression, or a thyroid disturbance; and to refer to a specialist for a definitive diagnosis. Screening tools like the Mini-Mental State Examination (MMSE)[31] can be used to detect and monitor response to treatment for early dementia with positive predictive value of 50% or less.[32] A brief 6-item, reliable screener with diagnostic properties comparable to the full MMSE is in the public domain and included in Table 8-6.[33]

Delirium. The 3-minute diagnostic assessment[34] and 4A's test[35] are examples of the highly sensitive and specific tools that are now available to assess

TABLE 8-5. DSM-5 Criteria for Dementia and Delirium	
DSM-5 CRITERIA FOR MAJOR NEUROCOGNITIVE DISORDER (DEMENTIA)	**DSM-5 CRITERIA FOR DELIRIUM**
A. Evidence of significant decline from a previous level of performance in 1 or more of the following cognitive domains: • Learning and memory • Language • Executive function • Complex attention • Perceptual-motor • Social cognition	A. Disturbance in attention (reduced ability to direct, focus, sustain, and shift attention) and awareness B. Develops over a short period of time (hours to days), represents a change from baseline, and tends to fluctuate during the course of the day
B. Cognitive deficits interfere in daily activities; assistance is required with complex instrumental activities of daily living	C. An additional disturbance in 1 or more of the following cognitive domains: a. Learning and memory b. Orientation c. Language d. Visuospatial ability e. Perception
C. Cognitive deficits do not occur exclusively in the context of delirium	D. The disturbances are not better explained by another preexisting, evolving, or established neurocognitive disorder
D. Cognitive deficits are not better explained by another mental disorder	E. Evidence that the disturbance is caused by a medical condition, substance intoxication or withdrawal, or medication side effect

DSM-5 = *Diagnostic and Statistical Manual of Mental Disorders*, 5th edition.

the risk of delirium and monitor response to treatment. To make the diagnosis of delirium, you must establish the patient's baseline mental status and the acuteness of any changes, usually by interviewing a knowledgeable informant. An acute change in mental status from baseline will distinguish delirium from mimicking conditions such as dementia, depression, and psychosis. A careful history and physical examination followed by a targeted evaluation for electrolyte or metabolic derangements, infection, and organ failure will often reveal the underlying cause(s). The reader is referred to standard medical textbooks for further information on delirium and dementia.[36]

Treatment

The biopsychosocial management of *neurocognitive disorders/dementia* is an integral part of primary care medicine. A multifactorial intervention comprising elements of the MHCM (regular exercise and healthy diet, cardiovascular risk factor modification, management of psychosocial stress, and treatment of major depression) may be superior to noninvasive brain stimulation and immunomodulators in the treatment and prevention of dementia.[37] Also, some data indicate that prevention can be enhanced by correcting socioeconomic deficiencies and by participation in intellectual activities.[38,39] Cholinesterase inhibitors are effective in slowing cognitive decline in clinically detected Alzheimer disease, but their effect on people whose dementia is detected by screening is uncertain.[32]

In addition to treating underlying causes, management of *delirium* focuses on mitigating risk factors such as immobility, functional decline, visual or hearing impairment, dehydration, and sleep deprivation. We advise you to reserve antipsychotic and other sedating medications for severe agitation that

TABLE 8-6. Brief Screener for Cognitive Impairment

COGNITIVE SCREENER

Now I am going to name 3 objects. After I have said them, I want you to repeat them. Remember what they are because I am going to ask you to name them again in a few minutes. Please repeat these words for me:

1. Apple-table-penny (You may repeat these words until patient is able to repeat them)
2. What is the year? _ _ _ _ (ONLY THE EXACT YEAR RECEIVES CREDIT)

   0 = INCORRECT

   1 = INCORRECT
3. What is the month? _____ (ONLY THE EXACT MONTH RECEIVES CREDIT)

   0 = INCORRECT

   1 = CORRECT
4. What is the day of the week? _____ (ONLY THE EXACT DAY OF WEEK RECEIVES CREDIT)

   0 = INCORRECT

   1 = CORRECT
5. What were the three objects I asked you to remember?

   (ORDER OF RECALL NOT IMPORTANT)

   _____ APPLE   0 = INCORRECT

   1 = CORRECT

   _____ TABLE   0 = INCORRECT

   1 = CORRECT

   _____ PENNY   0 = INCORRECT

   1 = CORRECT

TOTAL SCORE FROM ITEMS 2-5= ____/6

IF SCORE IS LESS THAN 4, CONSIDER COGNITIVE IMPAIRMENT

poses risks to the patient or others and when necessary to avoid interruption of essential medical therapies.[30]

Comorbid Conditions

Depression should always be excluded as it often masquerades as, or coexists with, dementia.[40] Delirium is often comorbid with dementia and other chronic medical and mental health disorders like depression and anxiety. When delirium is superimposed on preexisting dementia, there is an accelerated rate of cognitive decline, increased length of hospital stays, and higher rates of rehospitalization and death compared to patients with dementia but no delirium.[30]

EATING DISORDERS

Introduction

Eating disorders are among the more lethal mental health problems you will face in medical settings. Moreover, they can lead to both serious medical complications and even suicide. Even though most of these patients will require referral to a mental health professional and others for management, you will play a key role in initial diagnosis and timely referral as well as in coordination of care for often severe associated medical problems.

At least 30 million people suffer from an eating disorder in the United States.[41] Eating disorders are classified in DSM-5 as **anorexia nervosa**, **bulimia nervosa**, and **binge-eating disorder**,[5] summarized in Table 8-7.

Eating disorders are associated (comorbid) with almost all core DSM mood, anxiety, impulse control, and substance use disorders.[42]

Diagnosis and Screening

The essential *diagnostic distinction* among patients with the 3 disorders is that they usually are, respectively, underweight, normal weight, and overweight. All 3 disorders share a fundamental preoccupation with food and weight and, often, body image, and all are largely uncontrolled—not a matter of conscious choice. Complicating diagnoses is that anorexia nervosa and bulimia nervosa may convert back and forth at times. Comorbidity of depression and anxiety is prominent, and their treatment is a key part of management.

The Eating Disorder Screen for Primary Care (ESP) consists of the 4 questions you would ask of the patient suspected of having an eating disorder[43]; see Table 8-8. If it is positive (3 or 4 abnormal responses), further investigation and consultation is needed.

Anorexia Nervosa. Anorexia nervosa affects females about 10 times more often than males and has a 12-month prevalence of 0.4%. It typically begins in adolescence or young adulthood, often after a stressful event, and it seldom begins before puberty or after 40 years of age.[5] Its origin is multifactorial with cultural, environmental, and genetic influences.[5,44,45] Not only are suicide rates increased, but these patients

TABLE 8-7. The Eating Disorders and Subtypes From DSM-5

	CRITERIA	SYMPTOMS/SIGNS	MEDICAL COMPLICATIONS	MEDICAL TREATMENT
Anorexia nervosa • **Restricting** • **Binge eating[a] and purging**	1. BMI[b] < 18.5 2. Persistent energy intake restriction 3. Fear weight gain or becoming fat 4. Persistent behavior that interferes with weight gain 5. Self-perception of overweight or misshapen	1. Amenorrhea 2. Weakness 3. Bloating and abdominal pain 4. Cold sensitivity 5. Depression 6. Anxiety 7. Decreased libido 8. Hypotension, orthostatic 9. Childlike secondary sexual features	1. ECG: Bradycardia, low voltage, increase QTc and PR intervals, and ST-T wave changes 2. Decreased magnesium, sodium, and phosphorus 3. Hypoglycemia 4. Sick thyroid syndrome	1. Nutrition 2. Electrolyte/water balance—includes refeeding syndrome with severe phosphate depletion 3. Arrhythmias and heart failure 4. Osteoporosis and fractures 5. Risk of infection 6. Pancreatitis *Often need hospitalization, especially with BMI < 17.0*
Bulimia nervosa • **Purging** • **Nonpurging**	1. Normal weight 2. Recurrent binge eating 3. Inappropriate measures to prevent weight gain (purging; excessive exercise; laxatives; enemas; diuretics; fasting) 4. Self-perception unduly focused on body shape/weight	1. Irregular menses 2. Depression 3. Anxiety 4. Bloating and constipation 5. Sore throat 6. Dyspepsia 7. Eroded tooth enamel 8. Swollen parotid and submandibular glands 9. Calluses of knuckles	1. ECG: Bradycardia, low voltage, increase QTc, U waves 2. Decreased chloride and potassium with metabolic alkalosis; decreased magnesium and phosphate 3. Increased pancreatic enzymes 4. Mallory-Weiss syndrome	1. Nutrition 2. Electrolyte correction 3. Dehydration 4. Esophageal rupture and bleeding 5. Aspiration pneumonia 6. Rib fracture and pneumothorax 7. Post-binge pancreatitis
Binge-eating disorder	1. Overweight 2. Recurrent binge eating 3. There is no compensating behavior to lose weight	1. Bloating and discomfort 2. Dyspepsia 3. Depression 4. Anxiety 5. Overweight	1. Those expected with chronic overweight: Coronary artery disease, hypertension, type 2 diabetes, elevated LDL and triglycerides, NASH 2. Osteoarthritis 3. Obstructive sleep apnea 4. Cholecystitis 5. Gastric dilation and rupture	1. Treatment of standard medical conditions 2. Gastric rupture

DSM-5 = *Diagnostic and Statistical Manual of Mental Disorders*, 5th ed.; ECG = electrocardiogram; LDL = low-density lipoprotein; NASH = nonalcoholic steatohepatitis.

[a]Binge eating must occur at least once per week for 3 months and is defined as eating an amount of food larger than normal over 2 hours for which the patient experiences lack of control.

[b]BMI = body mass index (kg weight divided by height in meters[2]) where 18.5 is lower limit of normal.

TABLE 8-8. Eating Disorder Screen for Primary Care (ESP)

1. Are you satisfied with your eating patterns? (A "no" to this question was classified as an abnormal response).
2. Do you ever eat in secret? (A "yes" to this question was classified as an abnormal response).
3. Does your weight affect the way you feel about yourself? (A "yes" to this question was classified as an abnormal response).
4. Do you currently suffer with or have you ever suffered in the past with an eating disorder? (A "yes" to this question was classified as an abnormal response).

Scoring: Zero or one "abnormal" responses—no likelihood of an eating disorder

Three or more "abnormal" responses—high likelihood of an eating disorder

also can have extraordinarily severe medical problems attendant on weight loss and its treatment. As noted in Table 8-7, severe nutritional and metabolic changes can occur, as well as an increased predisposition to infection, osteoporosis, and fractures. The prognosis varies along a continuum from mild with no more than 1 episode to lifelong problems and multiple hospitalizations for medical and psychiatric problems.

Bulimia Nervosa. Bulimia nervosa again affects females in about a 10:1 ratio over males, and it has a 12-month prevalence of 1% to 1.5% and occurs primarily in older adolescents and young adults.[5] Its origin also is multifactorial with cultural, environmental, and genetic influences.[5,44,45] Onset often occurs with stress or after losing weight via diet. Suicide rates are higher, and as shown in Table 8-7, medical complications can be prominent, particularly the hypokalemic metabolic alkalosis that results from repeated self-induced vomiting and the chloride loss this practice produces. Expected hypokalemic changes on the electrocardiogram (ECG) are seen, and pancreatitis may complicate the course. While there is some tendency for bulimia nervosa to dissipate over time without treatment, treatment improves outcomes.

Binge-Eating Disorder. Binge-eating disorder is a lesser variant of the other 2 eating disorders although patients continue to exhibit lack of control of eating habits. It is about twice as common in females

as males where the respective 12-month prevalence raters are 1.6% and 0.8%.[5] While some patients may be normal weight, binge-eating disorder also differs from the psychopathology of obesity because most of the latter do not have uncontrollable bingeing. Also, obese patients without bingeing do not have the same lower quality of life, psychiatric comorbidity, functional impairment, or subjective distress as patients with binge-eating disorder.[5] The medical problems are those one would expect with chronic overeating, as seen in Table 8-5, for example, coronary artery disease and hypertension. A rare complication is gastric dilation and rupture from overeating.[46]

Treatment

The MHCM provides the overarching treatment approach for all 3 disorders. In addition to your medical care and your care of comorbid mental disorders, for example, depression and anxiety, a mental health professional with expertise in eating disorders usually is needed as part of the care team in moderate and severe cases. Also, a nutritionist often will be a key part of the team, particularly in anorexia nervosa where weight gain is needed but is not as simple as telling the patient to increase their intake of calories because patients frequently resist this suggestion. The MHCM emphasis on patient education and establishing a strong, nonjudgmental relationship is essential for all members of the care team. Patients may have many misunderstandings about their eating habits, their weight, and the disorder and require patient support while, at the same time, providing more helpful and healthy information. Also, goal setting is essential as a long-range guide for both the patient and the team, and commitment to the care plan often must be revisited, for example getting to 90% or more of their expected body weight. Most of the treatment plan will be under the guidance of the mental health professional, but you will often need to treat the comorbid depression and anxiety.

In patients with anorexia nervosa, medical problems can become prominent and life threatening, and patients often require hospitalization for medical management of malnutrition and its attendant cardiovascular and metabolic changes.[47,48] Patients particularly at risk and requiring hospitalization are those with comorbid medical problems, alcohol abuse, recent weight loss, and minimal caloric intake for the preceding 5 to 7 days. Severe arrhythmias, hypotension, and hypothermia may occur along with severe electrolyte and water imbalance.

Especially problematic can be the *refeeding syndrome*.[47,48] In malnourished patients already depleted of phosphate, resumption of calories containing carbohydrates further reduces the phosphorus (it is used in the increased carbohydrate metabolism) and can lead to arrhythmias and heart failure (usual cause of death), rhabdomyolysis, seizures, respiratory failure, and coma. This can occur with either enteral or parenteral calorie administration. To reduce the likelihood of the refeeding syndrome, you can take several measures. (1) Make a careful assessment of all the clinical and laboratory parameters, shown in Table 8-7, before beginning refeeding and correct the electrolyte abnormalities *before* refeeding begins, which can be completed in the first 18 to 24 hours; (2) treat and monitor them daily for the first week and 3 times weekly thereafter if the patient is stable; (3) begin initial refeeding at approximately 20 kcal/kg body weight over the first week, increasing it thereafter by 200 to 300 calories daily every 2 to 3 days. In severely malnourished patients with a body mass index (BMI) of 14 kg/m^2 or less, the caloric intake should be reduced further at the outset. Monitor for changes in blood pressure and pulse rate or the development of edema; because of the expected bradycardia, an increase in the pulse rate to "normal" can be the first sign of heart failure. In addition to nutritional needs, patients also require thiamine and B vitamins at the outset, usually initiated before refeeding and continued during feeding; later, calcium and vitamin D can be added. Hepatic enzymes may increase during refeeding and usually are not significant and can be reduced by decreasing caloric intake briefly.

Patients with bulimia nervosa are at much less risk although, at times, may require hospitalization for correction of hypochloremic, hypokalemic metabolic alkalosis, and any related fluid and electrolyte disturbances. Also, the uncommon cases of Mallory-Weiss bleeding and even more uncommon of esophageal rupture are emergencies to be kept in mind. Gastroesophageal reflux disease is more common and can be addressed on an outpatient basis. Many patients require dental consultation because of recurrent purging.

Patients with binge-eating disorder also are far less severe than anorexia nervosa and have no unique problems. Rather, standard management of the many problems that attend chronically overeating and obesity will be where you focus your treatment, except for rare instances of gastric rupture.

SUMMARY

You now have learned about the common core of mental health problems about which medical clinicians can manage effectively, and you have heard, in this chapter, about some other common problems in medical settings. In Chapters 9 and 10, we will consider the less common, more severe psychiatric disorders where your role will be early diagnosis and referral and co-managing medical problems with psychiatrists and other mental health professionals.

PATIENT RESOURCES

From the National Institute of Mental Health:

Free Booklets and Brochures

- **Eating Disorders: About More Than Food**—A brochure about the common eating disorders anorexia nervosa, bulimia nervosa, and binge-eating disorder, and various approaches to treatment. Order a free copy.

Multimedia

- Watch: Eating Disorders Myths Busted—A video series by NIMH: Cynthia Bulik, PhD, an NIMH grantee at the University of North Carolina, debunks 9 myths about eating disorders.
- NIMH Twitter Chat on Eating Disorders.
- NIMH Twitter Chat on Binge-Eating Disorder.

REFERENCES

1. Haavik J, Halmoy A, Lundervold AJ, Fasmer OB. Clinical assessment and diagnosis of adults with attention-deficit/hyperactivity disorder. *Expert Rev Neurother.* 2010; 10(10):1569-1580.
2. Okie S. ADHD in adults. *N Engl J Med.* 2006;354(25): 2637-2641.
3. Kessler RC, Adler L, Barkley R, et al. The prevalence and correlates of adult ADHD in the United States: results from the National Comorbidity Survey Replication. *Am J Psychiatry.* 2006;163(4):716-723.

4. Agnew-Blais JC, Polanczyk GV, Danese A, Wertz J, Moffitt TE, Arseneault L. Young adult mental health and functional outcomes among individuals with remitted, persistent and late-onset ADHD. *Br J Psychiatry.* 2018;213(3):526-534.

5. American Psychiatric Association. *Diagnostic and Statistical Manual of Mental Disorders.* 5th ed. Washington, DC: American Psychiatric Association; 2013.

6. Sibley MH, Rohde LA, Swanson JM, et al. Late-onset ADHD reconsidered with comprehensive repeated assessments between ages 10 and 25. *Am J Psychiatry.* 2018;175(2):140-149.

7. Ustun B, Adler LA, Rudin C, et al. The World Health Organization Adult Attention-Deficit/Hyperactivity Disorder Self-Report Screening Scale for DSM-5. *JAMA Psychiatry.* 2017;74:520-526.

8. Owen GT, Burton AW, Schade CM, Passik S. Urine drug testing: current recommendations and best practices. *Pain Physician.* 2012;15(3 suppl):ES119-ES133.

9. Kooij SJ, Bejerot S, Blackwell A, et al. European consensus statement on diagnosis and treatment of adult ADHD: the European Network Adult ADHD. *BMC Psychiatry.* 2010;10:67.

10. Rohde LA. Efficacy of stimulants beyond treatment of core symptoms of attention-deficit/hyperactivity disorder. *JAMA Psychiatry.* 2017;74:822-823.

11. Montano B. Diagnosis and treatment of ADHD in adults in primary care. *J Clin Psychiatry.* 2004;(65 suppl 3): 18-21.

12. Australian Government Department of Health 2004. http://www.health.gov.au/internet/publications/publishing .nsf/Content/drugtreat-pubs-modpsy-toc~drugtreat-pubs-modpsy-3~drugtreat-pubs-modpsy-3-7~drugtreat-pubs-modpsy-3-7-aws. Accessed July 4, 2018.

13. Lunney JR, Lynn J, Hogan C. Profiles of older medicare decedents. *J Am Geriatr Soc.* 2002;50(6):1108-1112.

14. Cohen-Mansfield J, Skornick-Bouchbinder M, Brill S. Trajectories of end of life: a systematic review. *J Gerontol B Psychol Sci Soc Sci.* 2018;73(4):564-572.

15. Steinhauser KE, Christakis NA, Clipp EC, McNeilly M, McIntyre L, Tulsky JA. Factors considered important at the end of life by patients, family, physicians, and other care providers. *JAMA.* 2000;284(19):2476-2482.

16. Chaudhry SI, Murphy TE, Gahbauer E, Sussman LS, Allore HG, Gill TM. Restricting symptoms in the last year of life: a prospective cohort study. *JAMA Intern Med.* 2013;173(16):1534-1540.

17. Yogananda MN, Muthu V, Prasad KT, Kohli A, Behera D, Singh N. Utility of the revised Edmonton Symptom Assessment System (ESAS-r) and the Patient-Reported Functional Status (PRFS) in lung cancer patients. *Support Care Cancer.* 2018;26(3):767-775.

18. Quill T, Holloway R, Shah M, Caprio T, Olden A, Storey J. *Primer of Palliative Care.* 5th ed. Glenview, IL: Academy of Hospice and Palliative Medicine; 2010.

19. Quill TE, Abernethy AP. Generalist plus specialist palliative care—creating a more sustainable model. *N Engl J Med.* 2013;368(13):1173-1175.

20. Casarett DJ, Inouye SK; American College of Physicians-American Society of Internal Medicine End-of-Life Care Consensus Penal. Diagnosis and management of delirium near the end of life. *Ann Intern Med.* 2001;135(1):32-40.

21. Kim SL, Tarn DM. Effect of primary care involvement on end-of-life care outcomes: a systematic review. *J Am Geriatr Soc.* 2016;64(10):1968-1974.

22. Tavares N, Jarrett N, Hunt K, Wilkinson T. Palliative and end-of-life care conversations in COPD: a systematic literature review. *ERJ Open Res.* 2017;3(2).

23. Mitchell GK, Senior HE, Johnson CE, et al. Systematic review of general practice end-of-life symptom control. *BMJ Support Palliat Care.* 2018;8(4):411-420.

24. Brighton LJ, Koffman J, Hawkins A, et al. A systematic review of end-of-life care communication skills training for generalist palliative care providers: research quality and reporting guidance. *J Pain Symptom Manage.* 2017;54(3):417-425.

25. Walczak A, Butow PN, Bu S, Clayton JM. A systematic review of evidence for end-of-life communication interventions: who do they target, how are they structured and do they work? *Patient Educ Couns.* 2016;99(1):3-16.

26. Cardona-Morrell M, Benfatti-Olivato G, Jansen J, Turner RM, Fajardo-Pulido D, Hillman K. A systematic review of effectiveness of decision aids to assist older patients at the end of life. *Patient Educ Couns.* 2017;100(3):425-435.

27. Quill TE, Ganzini L, Truog RD, Pope TM. Voluntarily stopping eating and drinking among patients with serious advanced illness—clinical, ethical, and legal aspects. *JAMA Intern Med.* 2018;178(1):123-127.

28. Galvin JE, Sadowsky CH, Nincds A. Practical guidelines for the recognition and diagnosis of dementia. *J Am Board Fam Med.* 2012;25(3):367-382.

29. Schmitz N, Deschenes SS, Burns RJ, et al. Cardiometabolic dysregulation and cognitive decline: potential role of depressive symptoms. *Br J Psychiatry.* 2018;212(2):96-102.

30. Oh ES, Fong TG, Hshieh TT, Inouye SK. Delirium in older persons: advances in diagnosis and treatment. *JAMA.* 2017;318(12):1161-1174.

31. Galasko D, Hansen LA, Katzman R, et al. Clinical-neuropathological correlations in Alzheimer's disease and related dementias. *Arch Neurol.* 1994;51(9):888-895.

32. Boustani M, Peterson B, Hanson L, Harris R, Lohr KN; U.S. Preventive Services Task Force. Screening for dementia in primary care: a summary of the evidence for the U.S. Preventive Services Task Force. *Ann Intern Med*. 2003;138(11):927-937.

33. Callahan CM, Unverzagt FW, Hui SL, Perkins AJ, Hendrie HC. Six-item screener to identify cognitive impairment among potential subjects for clinical research. *Med Care*. 2002;40(9):771-781.

34. Marcantonio ER, Ngo LH, O'Connor M, et al. 3D-CAM: derivation and validation of a 3-minute diagnostic interview for CAM-defined delirium: a cross-sectional diagnostic test study. *Ann Intern Med*. 2014;161(8):554-561.

35. Bellelli G, Morandi A, Davis DH, et al. Validation of the 4AT, a new instrument for rapid delirium screening: a study in 234 hospitalised older people. *Age Ageing*. 2014;43(4):496-502.

36. Jameson J, Fauci A, Kasper D, Hauser S, Longo DL, Loscalzo J, eds. *Harrison's Principles of Internal Medicine*. 20th ed. New York, NY: McGraw-Hill; 2018.

37. Rakesh G, Szabo ST, Alexopoulos GS, Zannas AS. Strategies for dementia prevention: latest evidence and implications. *Ther Adv Chronic Dis*. 2017;8(8-9):121-136.

38. Cadar D, Lassale C, Davies H, Llewellyn DJ, Batty GD, Steptoe A. Individual and area-based socioeconomic factors associated with dementia incidence in England: evidence from a 12-year follow-up in the English longitudinal study of ageing. *JAMA Psychiatry*. 2018;75(7):723-732.

39. Lee ATC, Richards M, Chan WC, Chiu HFK, Lee RSY, Lam LCW. Association of daily intellectual activities with lower risk of incident dementia among older Chinese adults. *JAMA Psychiatry*. 2018.

40. Robinson L, Tang E, Taylor JP. Dementia: timely diagnosis and early intervention. *BMJ*. 2015;350:h3029.

41. Maguen S, Hebenstreit C, Li Y, et al. Screen for disordered eating: improving the accuracy of eating disorder screening in primary care. *Gen Hosp Psychiatry*. 2018;50:20-25.

42. Hudson JI, Hiripi E, Pope HG, Jr., Kessler RC. The prevalence and correlates of eating disorders in the National Comorbidity Survey Replication. *Biol Psychiatry*. 2007;61(3):348-358.

43. Cotton MA, Ball C, Robinson P. Four simple questions can help screen for eating disorders. *J Gen Intern Med*. 2003;18(1):53-56.

44. National Institute of Mental Health 2016. https://www.nimh.nih.gov/health/topics/eating-disorders/index.shtml. Accessed July 1, 2018.

45. National Alliance on Mental Illness 2018. http://namimi.org/eating-disorders?gclid=CjwKCAjw9-HZBRAwEiwAGw0Qccy0xiuD6FCMoO8QNXzMUiyxKiCdQXYQnT85kRDvd86zlIQhVdvqSxoCRqAQAvD_BwE. Accessed July 1, 2018.

46. Dewangan M, Khare MK, Mishra S, Marhual JC. Binge eating leading to acute gastric dilatation, ischemic necrosis and rupture—a case report. *J Clin Diagn Res*. 2016;10(3):PD06-PD07.

47. Crook MA, Hally V, Panteli JV. The importance of the refeeding syndrome. *Nutrition*. 2001;17(7-8):632-637.

48. Mehanna HM, Moledina J, Travis J. Refeeding syndrome: what it is, and how to prevent and treat it. *BMJ*. 2008;336(7659):1495-1498.

9

Psychotic Disorders

INTRODUCTION

We consider psychotic disorders to reside primarily in the domain of psychiatry. But primary care and other medical physicians almost always see these patients at some early point during their illness journey and can play a significant role in their care. By recognizing that your patient may have a psychotic disorder—or be in the process of developing one—early referral is possible. The duration of untreated psychosis is directly related to time to recovery.[1] Hence, primary care physicians play a pivotal role in reducing the duration of untreated psychosis and modifying long-term outcome.[2,3] Also, you can play a key role in co-managing, with a psychiatrist, patients' often very prominent medical problems.

Unfortunately, there are many barriers to early recognition and treatment. First, "lack of insight," which is perhaps the most frequent symptom of psychotic disorders, often delays seeking care by the patient.[4] Second, self-stigma and societal stigma associated with the diagnosis of a psychiatric disorder, particularly a psychotic disorder, are prominent and difficult obstacles.[4] Third, the customary separation of mental illness from general medicine means that medical clinicians are often unfamiliar with psychotic disorders, not considered part of their domain. Finally, substance use disorder is observed in 50% of patients presenting with early psychosis. This greatly impedes the diagnosis of a psychotic disorder, symptoms too readily ascribed to the substance use.[5]

Psychotic symptoms are experienced by 3% of the general population and up to 20% of patients seeking primary care.[6,7] Further, up to a third of the general population will at some time during their lives experience psychotic symptoms.[8] Worldwide, schizophrenia occurs in about 1% of the population, and it is the fifth (for men) and sixth (for women) leading cause of work disability.[9]

Neurobiological Basis. Our understanding of the neurobiological basis of psychotic disorders emerged in the 1950s following the serendipitous discovery of chlorpromazine. It became the first effective antipsychotic and dramatically transformed the lives of patients from sequestration in remotely-located institutions to recovery.[10] It was discovered that antipsychotic agents work by blocking postsynaptic dopamine (D_2) receptors in the mesolimbic pathway.[10] The later discovery that amphetamines enhance the release of dopamine in this pathway and induce psychotic symptoms further corroborated this notion.[11] This led to the "dopamine hypothesis." The observation that psychotomimetic agents such as LSD and mescaline, which are serotonin 5-HT_{2A} agonists, also induce psychotic symptoms, led to the "serotonin hypothesis" and the subsequent discovery of antipsychotic drugs targeting serotonin 5-HT_{2A} receptors. Finally, the discovery that phencyclidine (PCP) induces the full spectrum of schizophrenic symptoms (positive, negative, and cognitive) led to the "glutamate N-methyl-D-aspartate (NMDA) receptor deficit hypothesis."[11]

Key Symptoms. The symptoms of schizophrenia, the quintessential psychotic disorder, are generally classified as positive, negative, and cognitive, summarized

TABLE 9-1. Symptoms of Schizophrenia

Positive Symptoms (of psychosis)
1. Hallucinations
   a. Altered perception in any senses (visual, tactile, olfactory, auditory)
   b. May be part of spiritual belief system; eg, hearing God or Jesus speaking to them
   c. Need to consider other causes
      i. Organic mental syndromes, such as delirium tremens, uremia, hepatic encephalopathy, head injury
      ii. Temporal lobe epilepsy
      iii. Migraine aura
2. Delusions
   a. Persisting belief at odds with reality
      i. Delusions of grandeur
      ii. Delusions of parasitosis
      iii. Delusions of persecution—paranoia
   b. Often part of fixed belief system around environmental, spiritual, social, or cultural needs
   c. Often bizarre and not possible; eg, time travel, friend of a celebrity
3. Disorganized behaviors and/or speech
   a. Socially inappropriate actions
      i. Dress—unkempt, dirty, ill-fitting, unbuttoned, weather or context inappropriate, states of undress, multiple layers, bizarre make-up
      ii. Swearing extensively, speaking offensively
      iii. Toileting in public
      iv. Unusual fads, nonconformist behaviors
4. Thought disorder (illogical thinking)
   a. Tangential thinking
   b. Flight of ideas
   c. Word salad
   d. Loose associations
   e. Peculiar neologisms
   f. Unintelligible ideas

Negative Symptoms (of resulting dysfunction)
1. Poverty of ideas
2. Flat affect
3. Apathy and withdrawal
4. Lack of motivation

Cognitive Symptoms
1. Judgment and executive function
2. Working memory
3. Attention
4. Concentration
5. Intellectual function
6. Social awareness

in Table 9-1. The *positive symptoms* are those of the psychosis itself: hallucinations, delusions, illogical thinking, and disorganized behaviors and speech. The *negative symptoms* are deficits of normal function: poverty of ideas, flat affect, withdrawal/apathy, impoverished speech, and lack of motivation. *Cognitive symptoms* include deficits of attention, concentration, intellect, working memory, social cognition, and executive function. Unfortunately, negative symptoms and neurocognitive and social cognitive deficits often precede the emergence of positive psychotic symptoms by many years, obscuring the underlying diagnosis. Furthermore, the cognitive deficit symptoms may be misattributed to a depressive disorder or to attention deficit disorder and inadvertently managed with psychostimulants.[12] In addition to positive, negative, and cognitive symptoms, untreated schizophrenia is associated with a gradual decline in social, interpersonal, and occupational function.

Psychotic Spectrum Disorders. In Table 9-2, the *primary psychotic disorders* represent conditions in which psychotic symptoms are predominant and not explained by another disorder. They include schizophrenia, schizoaffective disorder, brief psychotic

TABLE 9-2. Psychotic Spectrum Disorders

Primary Psychotic Disorders
Schizophrenia, schizoaffective disorder, brief psychotic disorder, schizophreniform disorder, and delusional disorders

Secondary Psychotic Disorders
1. Another psychiatric disorder: Major depression, bipolar disorder, posttraumatic stress disorder (PTSD), borderline personality disorder, dissociative disorders
2. Neurologic disorder:
   a. Acute: Meningitis, encephalitis, collagen disease vasculitis, other vasculitides
   b. Chronic: Dementia, Parkinson disease, Wilson disease, Huntington chorea, stroke, multiple sclerosis, and traumatic brain injury
3. Physical disorder: Intermittent porphyria, Tay Sach's disease, thiamine deficiency, electrolyte imbalance (hyponatremia, hypercalcemia), renal failure, hepatic failure
4. Prescription medications: Corticosteroids, psychostimulants, anticholinergic agents
5. Substance use disorder: Opioid intoxication, alcohol withdrawal

TABLE 9-3. Differential Diagnosis of Medical Conditions That Can Present With Psychosis

MEDICAL CONDITION	EXAMPLE
Neoplasms	Mental status changes are common in primary and metastatic brain tumors.
Neurovascular events	Hemi-neglect and seizures can resemble delusions.
Seizures	Temporal lobe seizures can be associated with olfactory and religious delusions.
Neurodegenerative disorders	Dementia, Huntington's disease, and Creutzfeldt-Jakob disease are all associated with psychosis.
White matter diseases	Metachromatic leukodystrophy, X-linked adrenoleukodystrophy, Pelizaeus-Merzbacher disease, cerebrotendinous xanthomatosis, adult-onset Niemann-Pick type C, and multiple sclerosis may be associated with symptoms of psychosis.
Systemic lupus erythematosus	Psychosis occurs in 5%-15% of patients.
Delirium	Electrolyte disturbances and poor oxygenation associated with many illnesses may cause psychosis. Steroids, opiates, benzodiazepines, and any polypharmacy frequently cause delirium.
Endocrine disorders	Hypo- and hyperthyroidism, Addison's and Cushing's diseases, and hyper- and hypoparathyroidism may cause psychosis.
Intoxications	Amphetamines, cocaine, phencyclidine (PCP, angel dust), methylenedioxypyrovalerone (bath salts), hallucinogens (eg, lysergic acid diethylamide or LSD, mescaline, psilocybin), dextromethorphan at high doses, and cannabis are among the drugs that can trigger psychotic symptoms.
HIV, AIDS	HIV-associated psychosis can occur directly from the viral infection and typically presents with a sudden onset (no prodrome), delusions (87% of patients), hallucinations (61% of patients), and mood symptoms (81% of patients). HIV-associated dementia can involve delusions.
Other infections	Patients with syphilis, tuberculosis, or other central nervous system infections may develop psychotic symptoms.
Limbic encephalitis	Limbic encephalitis is subacute and involves short-term memory loss, psychosis, behavior changes, and seizures involving the temporomedial lobes and amygdalae.
Mitochondrial disorders	Mitochondrial disorders usually involve multiple organ systems, so a past medical history of multiple medical problems affecting several organs is often suggestive.

disorder, schizophreniform disorder, and delusional disorders. *Secondary psychotic disorders* are conditions in which psychotic symptoms are caused by another psychiatric disorder, by a neurological or physical disorder, or by a drug or substance-induced disorder.

Differential Diagnosis. Let's now look at how to make a specific diagnosis.

- *Nonpsychiatric disorders*: Acute or subacute, *isolated psychotic symptoms* are usually due to

medical/neurologic causes or to a medication/substance cause, as summarized in Table 9-3; that is, all the secondary psychotic disorders except the "other psychiatric disorders." Hallucinations may occur in the context of *delirium*, along with disturbances in attention and other cognitive problems, when the psychosis is due to a medical condition, substance abuse or withdrawal, exposure to a toxin, or a combination of causes. If psychosis is present only in the context of delirium and is demonstrated by evidence (from the history, physical examination, or laboratory findings) to be the direct physiologic consequence of a general medical condition, then the diagnosis is *psychotic disorder due to another medical condition*. When hallucinations or delusions develop in the context of intoxication with or withdrawal from a drug, medication, or toxin, and do not occur exclusively during the course of a delirium, then the diagnosis is *substance/medication-induced psychotic disorder*. Hallucinations that occur during the transition from wakefulness to sleep or the transition from sleep to waking (called, respectively, hypnagogic and hypnopompic hallucinations) are observed in narcolepsy and do not signify a psychiatric disorder.[13] Auditory and visual hallucinations that occur in bereavement are considered as normal human experiences. These are often comforting in nature and are described as benign hallucinations.

Generally, visual hallucinations suggest delirium, while auditory hallucinations suggest a primary psychotic disorder. Tactile hallucinations are commonly observed in drug intoxication, olfactory and gustatory hallucinations in temporal lobe epilepsy. Persecutory delusions are often observed in patients with Alzheimer and Lewy body dementia and Parkinson's disease.

- *All psychiatric disorders*: Subacute to chronic cognitive, behavioral, or emotional symptoms are the usual presentation of true psychiatric disorders—the primary psychotic disorders and other psychotic disorders due to another psychiatric disorder (such as depression or bipolar disorder). These conditions typically present with the progressive worsening of symptoms in a subacute or chronic fashion. Clinicians then differentiate primary from secondary psychiatric disorders as follows:

  - Secondary psychotic disorders

    - Major depressive disorder—See Chapter 4 for the severe, psychotic type of depression where depressive symptoms precede the onset of psychosis, the latter remitting with treatment of the depression. Auditory hallucinations and delusions occur in about 14% of patients with major depressive disorder. These are typically mood-congruent and often disparaging and commanding self-harm. In contrast to the bizarre and paranoid delusions observed in schizophrenia, the delusions observed in depression carry themes of guilt, sin, poverty, serious somatic illness, and nihilism.

    - Bipolar disorder—See Chapter 4 for bipolar I disorder, wherein psychotic symptoms often occur during the peak of a manic episode. Grandiose delusions (eg, affluence, power, physical strength, divinity) are commonly associated with mania.

    - Posttraumatic stress disorder (PTSD)—See Chapter 5 where severe PTSD flashbacks and reexperiencing of the traumatic event may cause auditory and visual hallucinations.

    - Personality disorder—With severe personality disorders, brief psychotic periods may appear, reviewed in Chapter 10. For example, patients with borderline personality disorder infrequently experience auditory hallucinations that resemble the ones observed in patients with major depression or PTSD.

    - Dissociative disorders—These disorders are rare and may appear to be experienced as psychotic. The diagnoses will require psychiatric input.

- Primary psychotic disorders: When other etiologies have been ruled out and the symptoms are attributed to a primary psychotic disorder, careful attention is paid to the timing, the nature of the symptoms, and associated features to arrive at a diagnosis.

  - Brief psychotic disorder—This is a condition resembling schizophrenia but lasts *less than a month* (and at least 1 day).

  - Schizophreniform disorder—This condition resembles schizophrenia but lasts *less than 6 months* (and at least 1 month). It almost invariably progresses to schizophrenia.

  - Schizophrenia—Lasts *more than 6 months*. See discussion below.

  - Schizoaffective disorder—This combination of schizophrenia and a mood disorder (unipolar or bipolar) lasts *greater than 6 months* but also must have a 2-week period where psychotic symptoms are present when the mood disorder is quiescent.

  - Delusional disorders—These are psychotic disorders characterized by usually isolated delusions, that is, without hallucinations, negative or cognitive symptoms, and deterioration of social function. They last *longer than 1 month.*

We now expand on the primary psychotic disorders and then address their treatment, emphasizing what the medical clinician can do.

SCHIZOPHRENIA

Introduction. The all-cause standardized mortality for schizophrenia is 12 times higher than in the general population.[14,15] About a third of patients with schizophrenia attempt suicide. One in every 10 dies of suicide.[14] Nevertheless, medical problems, not suicides, are the major reason deaths exceed expectations. Metabolic, cardiovascular, cerebrovascular, pulmonary, and substance use disorders are more prevalent than in the general population.[14] Although much is written about metabolic consequences of antipsychotic drugs,[16] it is increasingly apparent that schizophrenia is independently associated with adverse health outcomes. Because of this, schizophrenia has been described as a "systemic disorder." Adverse health outcomes are multifactorial and may relate to lifestyle (sedentary living, cigarette smoking, overeating), substance misuse, and the neuroimmune and neuroendocrine sequelae of psychosis. For instance, medication-naïve patients with schizophrenia display elevated levels of inflammatory markers such as homocysteine, C-reactive protein, interleukin-6, and tumor necrosis factor.[16] The Recovery after Initial Schizophrenia Episode (RAISE) study revealed that metabolic disorders are present at disease onset and that medication-naïve patients had elevated levels of serum cortisol, total cholesterol, triglycerides, and excessive visceral adiposity compared to nonaffected age-matched individuals.[17] The Clinical Antipsychotic Trials of Antipsychotic Effectiveness (CATIE) study revealed that obesity, hypertension, and dyslipidemia are twice as common among patients with schizophrenia as compared to those in the general population.[18] Hence, whereas the care of patients with schizophrenia generally resides in the mental health sector, primary care physicians are consulted to manage the common physical disorders.[7] The high frequency of comorbid substance use increases the risk of medical illnesses such as hepatic and neurologic disorders.[8]

Compounding all these risk factors is the stark reality that patients with schizophrenia are less likely to receive routine health maintenance, annual physical examinations, and recommended medical screening procedures.[19] Transportation difficulties, embarrassment, and adverse health care experiences are all barriers to screening. Fear of pain and discomfort additionally interfere even though schizophrenia is associated with increased pain tolerance. Less likely to experience pain, they are less likely to seek medical care.[20] The lack of insight commonly observed in patients with psychotic disorders applies to physical diseases as well. This means that patients with primary psychotic disorders are just as likely to not seek treatment for physical symptoms as for psychological symptoms.[19]

Diagnosis. Schizophrenia is characterized by the hallmark positive, negative, and cognitive symptoms noted earlier and in Table 9-1. See Table 9-4 for the *Diagnostic and Statistical Manual of Mental Disorders,* 5th Edition (DSM-5) criteria for a diagnosis.[21] Symptoms generally emerge during late adolescence or early adulthood. The age of onset is early to mid-20s in men and mid- to late-20s in women.[21] The symptoms tend to occur in 3 progressive phases, which we now outline to help you make an early diagnosis in the prodromal phase.

- *Prodromal phase (mood and cognitive symptoms):* Two-thirds of patients who go on to develop schizophrenia experience prodromal symptoms. These are observed for 2 to 5 years before the emergence of psychosis. Depressed mood, sleep disturbances, social withdrawal, lack of motivation, impaired attention and concentration, and attenuated psychosis are prominent.

- *Psychotic phase (positive symptoms):* During a psychotic episode patients display predominantly positive symptoms: delusions, hallucinations, and/or disorganized thoughts, speech, and behavior. Erratic, risk-taking behavior and self-neglect can lead to psychiatric attention.

- *Residual phase (negative symptoms):* Following the first episode of psychosis, the illness course is characterized by recurrence and gradual deterioration of social, occupational, and interpersonal function. This is accompanied by loss of gray matter volume in the cerebral cortex.[22,23] Positive symptoms generally

TABLE 9-4. DSM-5 Criteria for Schizophrenia (F20.9)

A. Two (or more) of the following, each present for a significant portion of time during a 1-month period (or less if successfully treated). At least 1 of these must be (1), (2), or (3):
   1. Delusions.
   2. Hallucinations.
   3. Disorganized speech (eg, frequent derailment or incoherence).
   4. Grossly disorganized or catatonic behavior.
   5. Negative symptoms (ie, diminished emotional expression or avolition).
B. For a significant portion of the time since the onset of the disturbance, level of functioning in one or more major areas, such as work, interpersonal relations, or self-care, is markedly below the level achieved prior to the onset (or when the onset is in childhood or adolescence, there is failure to achieve expected level of interpersonal, academic, or occupational functioning).
C. Continuous signs of the disturbance persist for at least 6 months. This 6-month period must include at least 1 month of symptoms (or less if successfully treated) that meet criterion A (ie, active-phase symptoms) and may include periods of prodromal or residual symptoms. During these prodromal or residual periods, the signs of the disturbance may be manifested by only negative symptoms or by 2 or more symptoms listed in criterion A present in an attenuated form (eg, odd beliefs, unusual perceptual experiences).
D. Schizoaffective disorder and depressive or bipolar disorder with psychotic features have been ruled out because either (1) no major depressive or manic episodes have occurred concurrently with the active-phase symptoms, or (2) if mood episodes have occurred during active-phase symptoms, they have been present for a minority of the total duration of the active and residual periods of the illness.
E. The disturbance is not attributable to the physiologic effects of a substance (eg, a drug of abuse, a medication) or another medical condition.
F. If there is a history of autism spectrum disorder or a communication disorder of childhood onset, the additional diagnosis of schizophrenia is made only if prominent delusions or hallucinations, in addition to the other required symptoms of schizophrenia, are also present for at least 1 month (or less if successfully treated).

DSM-5, *Diagnostic and Statistical Manual of Mental Disorders,* 5th edition. Reprinted with permission from the *Diagnostic and Statistical Manual of Mental Disorders,* Fifth Edition, (Copyright ©2013). American Psychiatric Association. All Rights Reserved.

respond to treatment, while negative symptoms respond less well. The burden of negative symptoms is cumulative, growing steadily with each successive psychotic episode. It is widely believed that prevention of relapse can diminish the negative symptom burden, preserve functional capacity, and perhaps arrest the progressive loss of gray matter volume.[23]

Hence, early recognition of prodromal symptoms in primary care and prevention of relapse in the mental health sector provide opportunities to fundamentally alter the illness trajectory.

The assessment of a patient presenting with a psychotic disorder requires gathering a comprehensive medical and social history, emphasizing the availability of support personnel and services. Patients who are experiencing an acute psychotic episode are frequently unable to provide a detailed and coherent story. It is often necessary to seek information from collateral sources: family members, care providers, and medical records. The initial evaluation should include a standard medical history and physical examination, a mental status evaluation, physical examination, and screening laboratory tests: CBC, UA, comprehensive panel, TSH, urine drug screen, and a brain CT scan. The purpose of the initial assessment is to establish a psychiatric diagnosis and identify possible alternative causative or concurrent medical conditions.

Screening. The Prodromal Questionnaire-16 (PQ-16) in Table 9-5 is a validated self-rated screening tool for psychotic symptoms that can be used in a primary care setting.[24] Nine items reflect perceptual abnormalities/hallucinations, 5 items concern unusual thought content/delusional thinking/paranoia, and 2 items measure negative symptoms. A score of 6 or more is suggestive of a psychotic disorder.

Treatment. We will now briefly review treatment so you have some idea of what your psychiatry consultant will be doing and why. We do not recommend that you treat patients, nor do you need to know the usual drug

TABLE 9-5. The Prodromal Questionnaire-16 (PQ-16)						
			IF TRUE: HOW MUCH DISTRESS DID YOU EXPERIENCE?			
	TRUE	FALSE	NO (0)	MILD (1)	MODERATE (2)	SEVERE (3)
1. I feel uninterested in the things I used to enjoy.	❏	❏	❏	❏	❏	❏
2. I often seem to live through events exactly as they happened before (déjà vu).	❏	❏	❏	❏	❏	❏
3. I sometimes smell or taste things that other people can't smell or taste.	❏	❏	❏	❏	❏	❏
4. I often hear unusual sounds like banging, clicking, hissing, clapping, or ringing in my ears.	❏	❏	❏	❏	❏	❏
5. I have been confused at times whether something I experienced was real or imaginary.	❏	❏	❏	❏	❏	❏
6. When I look at a person, or look at myself in a mirror, I have seen the face change right before my eyes.	❏	❏	❏	❏	❏	❏
7. I get extremely anxious when meeting people for the first time.	❏	❏	❏	❏	❏	❏
8. I have seen things that other people apparently can't see.	❏	❏	❏	❏	❏	❏
9. My thoughts are sometimes so strong that I can almost hear them.	❏	❏	❏	❏	❏	❏
10. I sometimes see special meanings in advertisements, shop windows, or in the way things are arranged around me.	❏	❏	❏	❏	❏	❏
11. Sometimes I have felt that I'm not in control of my own ideas or thoughts	❏	❏	❏	❏	❏	❏
12. Sometimes I feel suddenly distracted by distant sounds that I am not normally aware of.	❏	❏	❏	❏	❏	❏
13. I have heard things other people can't hear like voices of people whispering or talking.	❏	❏	❏	❏	❏	❏
14. I often feel that others have it in for me.	❏	❏	❏	❏	❏	❏
15. I have had the sense that some person or force is around me, even though I could not see anyone.	❏	❏	❏	❏	❏	❏
16. I feel that parts of my body have changed in some way, or that parts of my body are working differently than before.	❏	❏	❏	❏	❏	❏

Scoring: A score of 6 or more is suggestive of a psychotic disorder.

doses. Rather, become familiar with the drug side effects and their medical consequences so that you can co-manage these patients' medical problems with the psychiatrist. We will not address medical treatment because you will already be familiar with that and can consult standard resources when necessary.[13]

Pharmacotherapy of Psychotic Disorders. Antipsychotics represent a cornerstone in the pharmacotherapy of patients with psychotic disorders.[5] The discovery in 1952 of the so-called typical or first-generation antipsychotics (FGA), such as chlorpromazine, revolutionized the treatment of psychotic disorders. The atypical or second-generation antipsychotics (AAP), which were introduced in the 1980s, represent a further evolution that continues to this day.[10]

- Typical antipsychotics are selective dopamine D_2 receptor antagonists. These medications selectively target positive symptoms, by diminishing dopamine transmission in the mesolimbic dopamine pathway.[5]

- AAP are more varied. Some are serotonin ($5HT_2$) and dopamine (D_2) receptor antagonists,[10] again decreasing dopamine transmission in the mesolimbic pathways and alleviating positive symptoms; additionally, at the same time they enhance dopamine transmission in the mesocortical pathway alleviating negative, cognitive, and impulsive symptoms. Ideally, they have a neutral effect on dopamine transmission in the nigrostriatal and tuberoinfundibular pathways, minimizing extrapyramidal (eg, acute dystonias, pseudoparkinsonism, tardive dyskinesia) and endocrine adverse effects (eg, hyperprolactinemia, gynecomastia, galactorrhea). Some newer AAPs, such as aripiprazole, combine partial dopamine D_2 receptor agonism with serotonin $5-HT_2$ receptor antagonism to regulate rather than block dopamine receptors, diminishing dopamine activity in hyperactive circuits, and enhancing it in hypoactive circuits. The AAPs thus offer a broader spectrum of action, are associated with fewer adverse effects, are better tolerated, and are more widely prescribed than older typical antipsychotics.

Acute agitated psychotic states may sometimes require the urgent administration of parenteral antipsychotics. Among typical antipsychotics, haloperidol is most commonly used. Olanzapine and ziprasidone

are atypical antipsychotics available in parenteral preparations. Whereas the efficacy of these compounds is similar, haloperidol is somewhat more likely to induce acute dystonias than olanzapine and ziprasidone. Intramuscular short- and long-acting antipsychotics are often augmented with the simultaneous administration of a parenteral benzodiazepine (eg, lorazepam).

Psychosocial Interventions for Psychotic Disorders. Unfortunately, even in the best of circumstances, approximately 50% of patients with primary psychotic disorders experience residual symptoms and functional deficits. This remains true despite adherence to recommended pharmacotherapy. Hence, intensive "wrap-around" services are required to prevent functional disability. Integrative approaches that thoughtfully combine (1) family support and psychoeducation, (2) supported education and employment, (3) individual resiliency training, (4) social skills training, (5) positive psychology, (6) mindfulness, (7) acceptance commitment therapy, (8) cognitive behavior therapy, (9) behavioral activation, (10) cognitive enhancement training, (11) case management, and (12) motivational interviewing, are essential components of the extended care of patients. These manualized approaches have traditionally been reserved only for the most severely disabled patients.[25-27]

However, the RAISE study, which front-loaded intensive multimodal interventions, challenged this practice.[28,29] This study demonstrated that the downward spiral of primary psychotic disorders can be modified with early, multimodal, and intensive interventions. This approach is analogous to deploying "disease modifying" interventions early in patients diagnosed with rheumatoid arthritis. With greater than 50% of early phase psychosis patients receiving appropriate care,[30] the data strongly indicate that early intervention is effective and should become standard of care.[30,31] The greatest problem with early intervention, however, has been patients disengaging due to a multiplicity of causes.[32]

Cognitive behavioral interventions such as relaxation training, behavioral activation, cognitive reappraisal and restructuring, and mindfulness meditation are effectively deployed in patients with severe psychotic disorders, just as in patients with anxiety and depressive disorders.[25-27] Delusions are traditionally defined as fixed beliefs that are not amenable to change in spite of conflicting evidence. The cognitive therapist, however, views delusions as misperceptions that are amenable to change with targeted interventions: normalizing, exploring antecedents, and examining the evidence. Much like in patients with depression, negative symptoms of schizophrenia (eg, apathy, anhedonia) are associated with diminished expectancies of pleasure and success in social activities. Behavioral activation and graded task assignments modify these aberrant negative expectancies and enhance social function. Patients with severe and persistent psychotic disorders can be engaged in therapy. They are capable of acquiring enduring self-help behavioral skills. However, the integration and delivery of guided self-help interventions in this subpopulation requires specialty expertise and familiarity with motivational interviewing skills.[33,34]

The Side Effects of Antipsychotic Medications. Side effects, summarized in Table 9-6, are important to the primary care physician during medical management

of the schizophrenic or other psychiatric patient taking antipsychotics. They will enter into your differential diagnosis as you consider alternative explanations for a medical problem, and they may be important causes of an evolving and medically relevant problem such as the metabolic syndrome.

Gastrointestinal Side Effects

Antipsychotic medications with potent anticholinergic properties, such as clozapine and olanzapine, can produce adverse effects such as dryness of mouth and constipation. Xerostomia (dry mouth), which is not dose dependent, can lead to dental caries if not controlled. Treatment includes using saliva stimulants or saliva substitutes. Sugarless gums or candies that contain aspartame, mannitol, sorbitol, or xylitol stimulate saliva production. Oral moisturizers include glycerate polymer (Biotene) and the hydroxyethyl cellulose solution (Oralube). Constipation can rarely progress to life-threatening obstipation, bowel obstruction, and

TABLE 9-6. Antipsychotics and Side-Effect Profile

	TARGET DOSE (mg/d)	METABOLIC EFFECT[a]	EPS	PRL	SEDATION	ANTICHOLINERGIC	HYPOTENSION
Quetiapine XR *Seroquel XR*	300-800	++	+/−	−	+++	+	+++
Risperidone[b] *Risperdal*	4-6	++	++	+++	++	−	++
Aripiprazole *Abilify*	10-30	+	+	−	+	−	+
Ziprasidone[c] *Geodon*	160	+	+	+	++	−	+
Olanzapine *Zyprexa*	10-20	+++	+	+	++	++	+/−
Clozapine[d] *Clozaril*	300-450	+++	+	+	++	++	++

EPS = extrapyramidal syndrome; PRL = prolactin.
[a]Obtain fasting blood sugar at baseline, 12 weeks, and yearly.
[b]May have marked prolactin increase; if clinical suspicion, obtain levels.
[c]May prolong QTc (corrected QT interval on baseline ECG); if rises above > 500 milliseconds, discontinue medication.
[d]Severe myeloid suppression and neutropenia potential: absolute neutrophil count weekly for first 6 months, biweekly for next 6 months, monthly thereafter (see text). Seizures are frequent at doses exceeding 600 mg/day.

megacolon. Aripiprazole is uniquely associated with nausea and hiccups.

Atypical antipsychotics can produce a transient elevation of hepatic transaminases where alanine aminotransferase (ALT) exceeds aspartate aminotransferase (AST). Serial monitoring of transaminases is initially required until levels normalize. Antipsychotic-induced weight gain can result in protracted elevated transaminase levels, heralding the onset of nonalcoholic steatohepatitis (NASH). If switching to an antipsychotic with a more benign metabolic profile does not resolve the condition, an intense weight-loss effort should be undertaken. The causative AAPs can generally be continued cautiously, but should be withheld if liver enzymes exceed 3 times the upper limits of normal. Cholestatic jaundice is associated with typical antipsychotics such as chlorpromazine but not with the AAPs. Excessive drooling (sialorrhea), which occurs in a third to half of patients on clozapine and can also be observed with risperidone and olanzapine, is not dose dependent. The anticholinergic agent oral glycopyrrolate, which does not cross the blood-brain barrier, and is not associated with central cognitive effects, is the drug of first choice. However, oxybutynin, topical ipratropium bromide spray and the selective M_4 receptor antagonist pirenzepine can also be used.

Cardiovascular Side Effects

Antipsychotics with potent α_1-adrenergic blockade (eg, risperidone and clozapine) can induce significant postural hypotension and compensatory reflex tachycardia. These agents need to be titrated cautiously, with close monitoring of blood pressure and heart rate. When conservative measures such as increasing fluid volume and compression stockings are insufficient, midodrine or fludrocortisone can be used. Some of the older, seldom used typical antipsychotics (thioridazine, chlorpromazine, and pimozide), can prolong the QTc, and may be associated with a risk of torsades de pointes.[35] Although AAPs, like antidepressants,[36] can be prescribed without a baseline electrocardiogram (ECG) or ECG monitoring in patients without a history suggesting heart disease, a baseline ECG is recommended if any of the following are present: the patient is already taking a drug known to prolong the QTc (especially methadone), known heart disease or significant ECG abnormality, bradycardia,

electrolyte disturbance, a personal history of syncope, a family history of sudden death under age 40 years, or congenital prolonged QTc syndrome. If the QTc on the baseline ECG is greater than 500 milliseconds, an alternative drug should be selected. When using an AAP, an ECG is indicated if the patient presents with symptoms such as lightheadedness or syncope, and the AAP should be discontinued if the QTc exceeds 500 milliseconds.[35,37] The risk in large community studies is quite low, but there has been a small association with unexplained sudden death, likely related to cardiac arrhythmias such as torsades de pointes.[37]

Thrombophlebitis is a possible adverse effect of antipsychotics, and pedal edema can often be induced by antipsychotics because of peripheral vasodilatation. It is recommended that the condition be managed conservatively with elevation of the legs, compression stockings, and diuretics. However, if the condition persists then the offending agent should be discontinued.

Metabolic and Endocrine Side Effects

Increased appetite and weight gain are common side effects of AAPs. Clozapine and olanzapine are the leading offenders. Quetiapine and risperidone occupy the middle range. Ziprasidone and aripiprazole are safest. However, weight gain can be observed with all AAPs, often accompanied by increased appetite. The combination of life-style modification (diet and exercise) and weight loss medications are recommended. Metformin and topiramate have demonstrated modest benefit in patients receiving antipsychotics. Lorcaserin, a $5-HT_{2C}$ agonist weight loss compound, the combination of bupropion and naltrexone, and the combination of topiramate and phentermine are also useful for weight loss. The therapeutic benefits of pharmacologic weight loss medications are modest and transient; the benefits are often lost when the agents are discontinued. Some AAPs are associated with increased serum levels of LDL and triglycerides and low levels of HDL.

Glycemic Dysregulation and Diabetes

AAPs are associated with the risk of impaired glucose metabolism and diabetes. The risk is greatest with clozapine and olanzapine, which inhibit glucose-induced insulin release from the pancreatic beta cells.[38] Antipsychotic-induced diabetes has been observed even in the absence of drug-related weight gain.

The American Diabetic Association and American Psychiatric Association recommend monitoring of fasting plasma glucose levels at baseline, after 12 weeks, and annually thereafter. Co-administration of metformin does not appear to diminish the risk of developing diabetes[39] but may reduce weight gain.

Hyperprolactinemia, Galactorrhea, and Gynecomastia

Because dopamine suppresses the production of prolactin from the anterior pituitary, dopamine antagonists are associated with hyperprolactinemia. Clinical manifestations include macromastia and galactorrhea in women, gynecomastia in men, and diminished libido in both. Long-term risks include osteoporosis and infertility. While we do not recommend routinely measuring serum prolactin levels for patients on antipsychotic medications, it is advisable to do so when patients experience clinical signs or symptoms that suggest hyperprolactinemia. You can manage this condition by either switching to a prolactin-sparing agent or augmentation with a dopamine agonist such as bromocriptine or amantadine. Recently, adjunctive low-dose aripiprazole, a partial dopamine agonist, has proved effective in managing antipsychotic-induced hyperprolactinemia.

SIADH

Syndrome of inappropriate antidiuretic hormone secretion (SIADH) may occur after days to months of exposure to an antipsychotic. Neuropsychiatric signs may develop when serum sodium levels fall below 120 mEq/L. Elimination of the causal agent and fluid restriction are first-line interventions. Rapid correction of hyponatremia (aggressive infusion of hypertonic saline) can lead to central pontine myelinolysis, and severe hyponatremia must be corrected gradually, in a medical setting.[13]

Neurologic Side Effects

Cognitive side effects (sedation, memory impairment, confusion) are more common in the elderly. Extrapyramidal syndromes may be acute and/or long-term as well as reversible or irreversible. These are generally observed during initiation of an antipsychotic, especially with rapid up-titration of the dose. *Acute dystonias* are brief involuntary spasms of the muscles of the face, neck, jaw, and trunk. They may include trismus, blepharospasm, oculogyric crisis, laryngospasm (with stridor), or truncal dystonia (opisthotonos). They are more common in men and in younger individuals. They are sometimes associated with the use of antipsychotics in patients with cocaine withdrawal. Benztropine or diphenhydramine are recommended and effective. Parenteral preparations produce rapid relief of symptoms, and are preferred to oral formulations.

Akathisia, an intolerable restlessness and difficulty remaining still, typically affects the lower extremities with the feeling of the need to pace or move the feet. Objective signs include fidgetiness, pacing, and anxiety. Unmanaged akathisia can become so bothersome that it can lead to suicide. *Pseudoparkinsonism* is manifest as a cluster of symptoms that may be indistinguishable from idiopathic Parkinson's disease. Patients often display a characteristic coarse, low-frequency resting tremor of the hands or lips, which is less apparent with action. Impaired postural reflexes can lead to accidental falls, difficulty ambulating, suppression of the gag reflex, leading to aspiration, and drooling of saliva.

Tardive dyskinesias (*TD*) may emerge following many years of exposure to antipsychotics. These side effects are characterized as repetitive involuntary stereotypic or choreathetotic movements, occurring in 10% to 20% of patients who receive FGA and in less than 1% of patients who receive second-generation antipsychotics. While these movements most commonly affect the muscles of facial expression and the bucco-linguo-masticatory triad, peripheral limbs, fingers, and toes can also be affected. Truncal rocking and writhing movements are also observed.

Neuroleptic malignant syndrome is a life-threatening complication associated with the initiation and rapid up-titration of parenteral, high-dose antipsychotics. Two-thirds of cases occur in the initial week of therapy. Untreated, mortality approaches 20%. The clinical manifestations include 3 symptom clusters and abnormal laboratory findings. Neuromuscular (catatonia, tremor), autonomic (tachycardia, hyperpyrexia, diaphoresis), and cognitive (delirium) symptoms prevail. Leukocytosis, elevated serum creatine phosphokinase, and myoglobinuria may occur. Management includes withdrawal of the offending antipsychotic, supportive care for hyperthermia, hydration, benzodiazepines, dopamine agonists such as bromocriptine, and intravenous muscle relaxants (eg, dantrolene).

Seizures may occur with all antipsychotics as a result of lowering the seizure threshold, but none as much as clozapine. Seizures are observed in 5% of patients maintained on doses of clozapine that exceed 600 mg/d. They are more likely with rapid dose escalation, when the drug is prescribed in combination with other agents that can lower the seizure threshold, such as bupropion, and in patients with a past history of seizures.

Genitourinary Side Effects

Urinary hesitancy and retention can be induced by antipsychotics with substantial anticholinergic properties, such as clozapine, olanzapine, and quetiapine. Risk factors include benign prostate hypertrophy and concomitant use of α-adrenergic agents (eg, the serotonin and norepinephrine reuptake inhibitor [SNRI] duloxetine). The parasympathomimetic agent bethanechol is used to manage urinary hesitancy.

Enuresis and urinary stress incontinence has been observed as an infrequent adverse effect associated with clozapine, risperidone, and olanzapine. Oxybutynin and intranasal desmopressin may provide relief.

Sexual Dysfunction

The rate of sexual dysfunction reported in FDA registration trials of antipsychotics in schizophrenia is extremely low (< 1%). However, in the CATIE study, sexual dysfunction occurred in 27% of patients assigned to risperidone and olanzapine, 20% on quetiapine, and 19% on ziprasidone.

Diminished libido is recognized as a direct consequence of antipsychotic-induced hyperprolactinemia. However, in the CATIE study the rates of sexual dysfunction were unrelated to changes in serum prolactin. Even agents associated with reductions in prolactin levels had an incidence of sexual dysfunction approaching 20%. A meta-analysis of antipsychotic-induced sexual dysfunction identified the following in descending order: clozapine > haloperidol > risperidone > olanzapine > aripiprazole > ziprasidone > quetiapine.[40] Aripiprazole and ziprasidone are least likely to impair sexual desire.

Erectile dysfunction related to arousal and orgasmic dysfunction, among antipsychotics studied, was least with aripiprazole and quetiapine. *Ejaculatory dysfunction*, either ejaculatory failure or retrograde ejaculation, described mainly with FGA, are related

to adrenergic α$_2$-blockade, and can be managed with imipramine, yohimbine, or cyproheptadine.

Hematologic Side Effects

Severe neutropenia due to clozapine-induced myeloid suppression is most likely to occur during the first 6 months of treatment. It is recommended that patients started on clozapine have their absolute neutrophil count (ANC) monitored weekly for the first 6 months, biweekly for the next 6 months, and monthly thereafter. Mild neutropenia (ANC < 1000/mm) requires that clozapine is stopped, and monitoring increased to 2 times a week. Severe neutropenia (agranulocytosis), a potentially lethal adverse effect, with ANC less than 500/mm requires permanent discontinuation of clozapine, daily ANC monitoring, and consultation with a hematologist. The clozapine REMS website provides comprehensive information on this subject (www.clozapinerems.com). *We recommend that the use of clozapine be determined only by your psychiatry consultant.*

Ocular Side Effects

Blurring of vision is a common adverse effect. It is caused by anticholinergic effects that impair muscles of accommodation in the eye, generally affecting near rather than distant vision. On eye examination, patients may reveal pupillary dilatation and, rarely, in susceptible older individuals, antipsychotics can induce *an acute exacerbation of angle closure glaucoma. Cataracts* also have been described as a possible consequence of long-term use of the older typical antipsychotics. There is minimal risk from the AAPs. *Retinitis pigmentosa,* melanin deposits in the retina, is uniquely associated with long-term exposure to thioridazine but not with other antipsychotics.

Other Medication Considerations

- *Pregnancy and lactation*: Reproductive age women should be informed of the risks and benefits of antipsychotics in pregnancy and lactation. When confronted with the need for antipsychotics during pregnancy, the website supported by the Massachusetts General Hospital Reproductive Health (www.womensmentalhealth.org) provides up-to-date information on this constantly evolving landscape. Antipsychotics are not associated with teratogenicity, but the newborn may display withdrawal effects, excessive sedation, tremor, increased or decreased muscle tone, and difficulty feeding.[41]

- *Cigarette smoking*: Antipsychotic medications primarily metabolized through the hepatic P-450 1A2 metabolic pathway (such as clozapine and olanzapine) are susceptible to the influence of the enzyme inducing effect of the hydrocarbons of cigarette smoke on serum levels. When patients abruptly stop smoking (such as following admission to a hospital), the serum levels can rise, triggering profound sedation and seizures with clozapine. Conversely, following discharge from the hospital and resumption of smoking, serum levels may decline precipitating symptom relapse.

- *The frail elderly*: All antipsychotics carry a black box warning of the risk of death when used in elderly individuals with dementia. The choice of an antipsychotic in older patients should be made after balancing the risks of tardive dyskinesia, orthostatic hypotension, sedation, and accidental falls. Regardless of medication chosen, the least effective dose should be used.

- *Antipsychotic discontinuation syndrome*: Withdrawal symptoms can be expected when an antipsychotic is stopped abruptly. Nausea, vomiting, diarrhea, diaphoresis, muscle aches and pains, insomnia, and anxiety may be related to cholinergic rebound. Exacerbation of psychosis is most commonly associated with abrupt withdrawal of clozapine. It is recommended that switching from one antipsychotic to another should be accomplished by gradual cross-titration over 2 to 3 weeks.

OTHER PRIMARY PSYCHOTIC DISORDERS

Schizoaffective disorder is characterized by co-occurrence of psychotic and mood symptoms. Psychotic symptoms include the positive, negative, and disorganization symptoms associated with schizophrenia. Mood symptoms include those observed in a major depressive episode or a manic episode. Typically, when psychotic symptoms occur in patients with mood disorders they are short-lived, occur during the peak of an episode and then gradually fade away as mood symptoms remit. Conversely, in schizoaffective disorder psychotic symptoms are persistent and predominant, occurring even following the resolution of mood symptoms. Major mood episodes are present for at least half the duration of the illness. The condition occurs in 1% of the population and is more commonly observed in women than men.

Schizophreniform disorder is characterized by 2 or more core symptoms of schizophrenia (delusions, hallucinations, disorganized speech, and negative symptoms) for a period of time that is longer than one but less than 6 months. Unlike schizophrenia, a decline in social or occupational function is not observed. A third of patients with an initial diagnosis of schizophreniform disorder experience a complete recovery, without recurrences. The remaining two-thirds progress relentlessly to develop schizophrenia.

Brief psychotic disorder is characterized by delusions, hallucinations, or disorganized speech lasting for more than 1 day but resolving within 1 month. Characteristically, people experiencing a brief psychotic disorder will change from a nonpsychotic state to a psychotic state suddenly (eg, within 2 weeks) without a prodrome. A full return to the premorbid level of functioning is required by DSM-5 to make this diagnosis. Ruling out psychoses due to medications or abused substances is essential before making the diagnosis.

Delusional disorder is characterized by 1 or more delusions, without prominent hallucinations, disorganized behavior or speech, and with a duration of symptoms of 1 month or longer. Social, occupational, and interpersonal functioning is not impaired. There are 5 defined subtypes.

1. Persecutory subtype, characterized by circumscribed paranoid delusions—the most common.
2. Grandiose subtype, characterized by delusions of power, wealth, strength, or divinity.
3. Jealous subtype, characterized by a theme of an unfaithful partner.
4. Somatic subtype, characterized by delusions involving bodily functions or sensations. Common variants include the delusion that one emits a foul odor, that one is infested with parasites, or that parts of the body are not functioning or are misshapen. An interesting subset is the shared delusional disorder where another person shares the belief, for example, that they as well as the patient are infested with bugs or parasites.

5. Erotomanic subtype (Clerambault syndrome), characterized by the belief that another person (typically of higher social status) is in love with the individual. Erotomanic delusions can also be observed in schizophrenia or bipolar disorder.

CONCLUSION

Primary care physicians can play a pivotal role throughout the life journey of patients with psychotic disorders. Patients with prodromal schizophrenia or early psychosis are more likely to present at a primary care than a mental health setting, with complaints of depression, attention or concentration deficits, apathy, or avolition. Recognizing prodromal symptoms, acquiring information from ancillary sources, and making an early referral to psychiatry can change disease outcome. The presence of (1) primary psychotic disorders such as schizophrenia, (2) suicidal ideation or behavior, and (3) acute agitated psychotic states warrants referral to mental health professionals. Further along in the illness journey, physicians in every specialty are called upon to manage the complex medical sequelae of severe and persistent mental disorders, and to alleviate the adverse effects that accompany antipsychotic medications. This provides an opportunity to enhance quality of life and prevent premature mortality.

Additional Resources

CBT Radio Podcast. Cognitive-Behavioral Therapy for Psychosis. May 17, 2010.

Hagen R, Turkington D, Berge T, Grawe RW. *CBT for Psychosis–A Symptom-Based Approach*. London: Routledge; 2011.

Hogarty GE. *Personal Therapy for Schizophrenia & Related Disorders—A Guide to Individualized Treatment*. New York, NY: The Guilford Press; 2002.

Penn DL, Meyer PS, Gottlieb JD, et al. *Individual Resiliency Training (IRT)*. NAVIGATE, 2014. www.navigateconsultants.org.

Wright JH, Turkington D, Kingdon DG, Ramirez-Basco M. *Cognitive-Behavior Therapy for Severe Mental Illness—An Illustrated Guide*. Washington, DC: APPI; 2009.

Wright NP. *Treating Psychosis: A Clinician's Guide to Integrating Acceptance & Commitment Therapy, Compassion-Focused Therapy & Mindfulness Approaches within the Cognitive Behavioral Therapy Tradition*. Oakland: New Harbinger; 2014. www.treatingpsychosis.com

www.earlypsychosis.ca.

www.navigateconsultants.org.
www.ontrackny.org.

Patient Self-Help Resources

CBT-i Coach Android/iPAD app for Insomnia.

Cognitive Enhancement Training website www.brainhq.com.

Depression CBT Self-Help Guide Android app (relaxation, guided imagery, mindfulness and cognitive restructuring tools).

eCBT Mood iPAD app (cognitive restructuring).

E-COUCH www.ecouch.anu.edu.au (tools for self-management of anxiety)

Fit Brains & BrainHQ Android/IPAD apps for Cognitive Enhancement Training

Freeman D, Freeman J, Garety P. *Overcoming Paranoid and Suspicious Thoughts—A Self-Help Guide Using Cognitive Behavioral Techniques*. New York, NY: Basic Books; 2008. www.paranoidthoughts.com. Accessed on January 17, 2019.

Gloucestershire Hearing Voices and Recovery Groups: www.hearingvoices.org.uk.

Greenberger D, Padesky CA. *Mind over Mood–Change How You Feel by Changing the Way You Think*. 2nd ed. New York, NY: Guilford Press; 2016.

Hayes SC, Smith S. *Get out of Your Mind and Into Your Life—The New Acceptance and Commitment Therapy*. New York, NY: MJF Books; 2005.

http://www.nytimes.com/2007/03/25/magazine/25voices.t.html?_r=0.

Mindshift Android/iPAD app (relaxation, guided imagery, mindfulness).

Torrey EF. *Surviving Schizophrenia—A Family Manual*. 6th ed. New York, NY: Harper Perennial; 2013.

Turkington D, Kingdon D, Rathod S, et al. *Back to Life, Back to Normality: Cognitive Therapy, Recovery and Psychosis*. New York, NY: Cambridge University Press; 2009.

Van Dijk S. *Calming the Emotional Storm—Using Dialectical Behavior Therapy Skills to Manage Your Emotions & Balance Your Life*. Oakland, CA: New Harbinger Publications; 2012.

Watkins J. *Hearing Voices—A Common Human Experience*. South Yarra, Australia: Michelle Anderson Publishing; 2008.

REFERENCES

1. Perkins DO, Gu H, Boteva K, Lieberman JA. Relationship between duration of untreated psychosis and outcome in first-episode schizophrenia: a critical review and meta-analysis. *Am J Psychiatry*. 2005;162(10):1785-1804.

2. Deakin J, Lennox B. Psychotic symptoms in young people warrant urgent referral. *Practitioner*. 2013; 257(1759):25-28, 3.

3. Anderson KK, Norman R, MacDougall AG, et al. Disparities in access to early psychosis intervention services: comparison of service users and nonusers in health administrative data. *Can J Psychiatry*. 2018;63(6): 395-403.

4. El-Adl M, Burke J, Little K. First-episode psychosis: primary care experience and implications for service development. *Psychiatric Bulletin*. 2009;33:165-168.

5. Starzer MSK, Nordentoft M, Hjorthoj C. Rates and predictors of conversion to schizophrenia or bipolar disorder following substance-induced psychosis. *Am J Psychiatry*. 2018;175(4):343-350.

6. Olfson M, Lewis-Fernandez R, Weissman MM, et al. Psychotic symptoms in an urban general medicine practice. *Am J Psychiatry*. 2002;159(8):1412-1419.

7. Griswold KS, Del Regno PA, Berger RC. Recognition and differential diagnosis of psychosis in primary care. *Am Fam Physician*. 2015;91(12):856-863.

8. Saunders K, Brain S, Ebmeier KP. Diagnosing and managing psychosis in primary care. *Practitioner*. 2011;255(1740): 2-3, 17-20.

9. GBD 2015 Disease and Injury Incidence and Prevalence Collaborators. Global, regional, and national incidence, prevalence, and years lived with disability for 310 diseases and injuries, 1990-2015: a systematic analysis for the Global Burden of Disease Study 2015. *Lancet*. 2016;388(10053):1545-1602.

10. Nasrallah H, Tandon R. Classic antipsychotic medications. In: Schatzberg A, Nemeroff CB, eds. *The American Psychiatric Association Publishing Textbook of Psychopharmacology*. 5th ed. Arlington, VA: American Psychiatric Association Publishing; 2017.

11. Stahl S. *Stahl's Essential Psychopharmacology: Neuroscientific Basis and Practical Applications*. 4th ed. New York, NY: Cambridge University Press; 2013.

12. Levy E, Traicu A, Iyer S, Malla A, Joober R. Psychotic disorders comorbid with attention-deficit hyperactivity disorder: an important knowledge gap. *Can J Psychiatry*. 2015;60(3 suppl 2):S48-S52.

13. Jameson J, Fauci A, Kasper D, Hauser S, Longo DL, Loscalzo J, eds. *Harrison's Principles of Internal Medicine*. 20th ed. New York, NY: McGraw-Hill; 2018.

14. Brown S, Inskip H, Barraclough B. Causes of the excess mortality of schizophrenia. *Br J Psychiatry*. 2000;177:212-217.

15. Shiers D, Lester H. Early intervention for first episode psychosis. *BMJ*. 2004;328(7454):1451-1452.

16. Borovcanin MM, Jovanovic I, Radosavljevic G, et al. Interleukin-6 in schizophrenia—is there a therapeutic relevance? *Front Psychiatry*. 2017;8:221.

17. Correll CU, Robinson DG, Schooler NR, et al. Cardiometabolic risk in patients with first-episode schizophrenia spectrum disorders: baseline results from the RAISE-ETP study. *JAMA Psychiatry*. 2014;71(12):1350-1363.

18. Meyer JM, Davis VG, Goff DC, et al. Change in metabolic syndrome parameters with antipsychotic treatment in the CATIE Schizophrenia Trial: prospective data from phase 1. *Schizophr Res*. 2008;101(1-3):273-286.

19. Aggarwal A, Pandurangi A, Smith W. Disparities in breast and cervical cancer screening in women with mental illness: a systematic literature review. *Am J Prev Med*. 2013;44(4):392-398.

20. Stubbs B, Thompson T, Acaster S, Vancampfort D, Gaughran F, Correll CU. Decreased pain sensitivity among people with schizophrenia: a meta-analysis of experimental pain induction studies. *Pain*. 2015;156(11):2121-2131.

21. American Psychiatric Association. *Diagnostic and Statistical Manual of Mental Disorders*. 5th ed. Washington, DC: American Psychiatric Association; 2013.

22. Mitelman SA, Shihabuddin L, Brickman AM, Hazlett EA, Buchsbaum MS. Volume of the cingulate and outcome in schizophrenia. *Schizophr Res*. 2005;72(2-3):91-108.

23. Vita A, De Peri L, Deste G, Sacchetti E. Progressive loss of cortical gray matter in schizophrenia: a meta-analysis and meta-regression of longitudinal MRI studies. *Transl Psychiatry*. 2012;2:e190.

24. Ising HK, Veling W, Loewy RL, et al. The validity of the 16-item version of the Prodromal Questionnaire (PQ-16) to screen for ultra high risk of developing psychosis in the general help-seeking population. *Schizophr Bull*. 2012;38(6):1288-1296.

25. Wright J, Turkington D, Kingdon D, Ramirez-Basco M. *Cognitive-Behavior Therapy for Severe Mental Illness—An Illustrated Guide*. Washington, DC: American Psychiatric Association Publishing; 2009.

26. Wright N, Turkington D, Kelly O, Davies D, Jacobs A, Hopton J. *Treating Psychosis: A Clinician's Guide to Integrating Acceptance and Commitment Therapy, Compassion-Focused Therapy and Mindfulness Approaches Within the Cognitive Behavioral Therapy Tradition*. Oakland, CA: New Harbinger; 2014.

27. Hagen R, Turkington D, Berge T, Grawe R. *CBT for Psychosis—A Symptom-Based Approach*. London, UK: Routledge; 2011.

28. Insel TR. RAISE-ing our expectations for first-episode psychosis. *Am J Psychiatry*. 2016;173(4):311-312.

29. Azrin S, Goldstein A, Heinssen R. Early intervention for psychosis: the recovery after an initial schizophrenia episode project. *Psychiatric Annals*. 2015;45:548-553.

30. Macnaughton E. Expanding the reach of early psychosis intervention. *Can J Psychiatry*. 2018;63(6):354-355.

31. Correll CU, Galling B, Pawar A, et al. Comparison of early intervention services vs treatment as usual for early-phase psychosis: a systematic review, meta-analysis, and meta-regression. *JAMA Psychiatry*. 2018;75(6): 555-565.

32. Solmi F, Mohammadi A, Perez JA, Hameed Y, Jones PB, Kirkbride JB. Predictors of disengagement from early intervention in psychosis services. *Br J Psychiatry*. 2018;213(2):477-483.

33. Levounis P, Arnaout B, Marienfeld C. *Motivational Interviewing for Clinical Practice*. Arlington, VA: American Psychiatric Association Publishing; 2017.

34. Miller W, Rollnick S. *Motivational Interviewing—Helping People Change*. 3rd ed. New York, NY: The Guilford Press; 2013.

35. Wenzel-Seifert K, Wittmann M, Haen E. QTc prolongation by psychotropic drugs and the risk of torsade de pointes. *Dtsch Arztebl Int*. 2011;108(41):687-693.

36. Beach SR, Kostis WJ, Celano CM, et al. Meta-analysis of selective serotonin reuptake inhibitor-associated QTc prolongation. *J Clin Psychiatry*. 2014;75(5):e441-449.

37. Beach SR, Celano CM, Sugrue AM, et al. QT Prolongation, torsades de pointes, and psychotropic medications: a 5-year update. *Psychosomatics*. 2017;59:105-122.

38. Chintoh AF, Mann SW, Lam L, et al. Insulin resistance and secretion in vivo: effects of different antipsychotics in an animal model. *Schizophr Res*. 2009; 108(1-3):127-133.

39. Ehret M, Goethe J, Lanosa M, Coleman CI. The effect of metformin on anthropometrics and insulin resistance in patients receiving atypical antipsychotic agents: a meta-analysis. *J Clin Psychiatry*. 2010; 71(10):1286-1292.

40. Serretti A, Chiesa A. A meta-analysis of sexual dysfunction in psychiatric patients taking antipsychotics. *Int Clin Psychopharmacol*. 2011;26(3):130-140.

41. Cohen LS, Viguera AC, McInerney KA, et al. Reproductive safety of second-generation antipsychotics: current data from the Massachusetts General Hospital National Pregnancy Registry for Atypical Antipsychotics. *Am J Psychiatry*. 2016;173(3):263-270.

10

Personality Disorders

INTRODUCTION

Personality is a complex concept—and an important one: it reflects human beings' basic psychological infrastructure.[1,2] This means that it plays a critical role in determining how people live their lives and negotiate the myriad challenges that life presents. In medicine, personality has direct effects on the propensity to seek health care, the ease and accuracy of providing a medical history, adherence to treatment, and the adequacy of health-related social support networks. It further predicts self-care and lifestyle issues, for example choice of employment (or profession), eating and drinking habits, exercise, and risk-taking behaviors, including substance use and sexual habits.[3]

In Chapter 5 on anxiety disorders we discussed the difference between obsessive compulsive disorder (OCD) and obsessive compulsive personality disorder, the major difference being patients with OCD are anxious and distressed by their thoughts and behaviors while those with the personality disorder are not.

Before discussing these and other personality disorders, however, let's first expand on another point from Chapter 5: that many obsessive and compulsive personality traits reflect neither OCD nor obsessive compulsive personality disorder. Like all personality traits, most are quite normal—defined as functioning to help people adapt most effectively to life, which is especially important in choosing a life pathway or career.[4] We described the **adaptive** features of *obsessive* and *compulsive traits* with the example of their being necessary for becoming a successful surgeon, while other personality traits also are valuable in becoming

a successful physician—or any other person—such as the importance of dependency traits for a successful marriage or of histrionic traits for making one attractive.

Adaptive *dependency personality traits*, for example, are one of these essential traits for all people and associated to "attachments" so vital to making and maintaining human relationships. Medical students and residents are dependent on faculty to provide them with the education and training required to become successful physicians and to function with increasing independence in their patient care. In contemporary medical practice we are all dependent on multilayered systems involved in the care of our patients. These systems involve other health care professionals we are dependent on from the various levels of nursing personnel, to laboratory technicians, to pharmacists. We are also dependent on each other for consultation and coverage. Primary care practitioners are dependent on a wide range of fellow professionals and paraprofessionals from the pathologist who provides biopsy reports to their "front-office" personnel and secretaries who schedule appointments and maintain efficient patient flow.

Adaptive *personality traits of suspiciousness* are also very important because clinicians are detectives who investigate all forms of injury and illness. Suspiciousness informs our judgments from the workups for each individual patient to being more attentive and wary of the knowledge and skill levels of a senior medical student compared to those of a senior or chief resident. It is also a good practice to be more wary of the histories provided to us by those we suspect of substance abuse than other forms of illness. We even use terms reflecting this quality, such as "high level of suspicion" and "a suspicious lesion." In respect to our attention to responsibilities to patients and each other, it would indeed be foolish to ignore a suspicious odor of alcohol on the breath of a trainee or colleague on duty.

The operative word in each of the examples is "adaptive." Each example above requires the mature appreciation that there are circumstances when obsessiveness, compulsiveness, dependency, and/or suspiciousness are useful, even necessary, for our best functioning as physicians and in life.

When the traits become exaggerated, they can become harmful and interfere with effective learning and psychosocial functioning. That is, they have become **maladaptive**, which defines the *personality disorders* we'll address in this chapter. Rather than help the person live an effective, happy life, as in the earlier examples, they interfere with having one. For example, from the above situations, dependency and suspiciousness (paranoia) can become sufficiently exaggerated that they dominate all aspects of a patient's life. This almost always interferes with healthy functioning, often severely.[4,5] In fact, pathological exaggeration of any personality trait defines the various personality disorders we'll discuss.

Healthy adaptive functioning requires an expanded repertoire of psychological strategies and behaviors that are appropriate in a wide range of interpersonal, social, and occupational settings. It is helpful to think of patients with a personality disorder as being limited or constrained in their manner or style of dealing with others in social and work situations and in managing their lives. Instead, they respond in the same, exaggerated way to most situations. Regardless of the interpersonal, social, or occupational circumstance, this rigidity in how one acts in the complex situations life presents permeates every facet of their life so extensively that they cannot respond with appropriate adaptive congruence and flexibility. They appear to respond in much the same way to almost every situation. This is especially true for their health-related behaviors.

THE PERSONALITY DISORDERS

Personality disorders are common in the general population, affecting up to 15% of the U.S. population.[6]

Personality disorder behaviors may diminish with advancing age, but it is important to remember these disorders are lifelong.[7,8] Patients with personality disorders are high utilizers of both mental health and primary care services primarily due to their difficulty in fully cooperating with their care. This inability to fully cooperate with a negotiated care plan increases overall morbidity.[9] Further complicating their care, personality disorders are highly comorbid with other mental disorders, especially anxiety and depression, and worsen their prognoses.[10-12] As described in earlier chapters, due to the shortage of psychiatrists, primary care clinicians often become "front-line" managers of these patients.

In this chapter, we provide descriptions of each personality disorder according to *The Diagnostic and Statistical Manual of Mental Disorders*, 5th ed. (DSM-5) criteria[6] and provide brief examples of the manner in which these patients present problems in health care settings. We also provide guidance on early recognition, general management, and referral to mental health professionals.[4]

DSM-5 defines personality disorders as an enduring pattern of inner experience and behavior that deviates markedly from the expectations of the individual's culture, is pervasive and inflexible, has an onset in adolescence or early adulthood, is stable over time, and leads to distress or impairment in functioning.[6] Whereas patients with adaptive personality traits establish a good patient-clinician relationship, patients with personality disorders are a source of frustration to the clinician and the expanded clinic staff. These patients are typically described as "difficult" and their responses to treatment are often disappointing.[12,13]

DSM-5 first presents personality disorders in a "categorical" manner with features common to each of the disorders. Many clinician-researchers argue, however, that personality features are sufficiently complex and fluid that they find the categorical approach too limiting. DSM-5 therefore also offers an alternative "dimensional" model based on the level of impairment: some, moderate, severe, and extreme impairment. The categorical and dimensional models are complementary. Both provide clinicians expanded methodologies to assess and clarify areas of dysfunction in those patients they suspect of having a personality disorder or of possessing dysfunctional traits that may impair patients' abilities to cooperate with their care.

The next step in reaching a diagnosis is to identify general descriptive features of personality dysfunction. DSM-5 further divides the personality disorders into 3 "clusters" emphasizing descriptively how these patients may present. *Cluster A* patients exhibit odd and/or eccentric behavior; *Cluster B* patients exhibit erratic, emotional, or dramatic behavior; and *Cluster C* patients exhibit anxious and fearful behavior. These clustered features are likely to be accentuated when patients are under the stress of physical illness and they assist the clinician in narrowing down a more specific diagnosis. Table 10-1 lists the categorical personality disorders according to the cluster where they occur. Thus, first identify the cluster representing the patient's symptoms to narrow down the differential diagnosis. Then, use the criteria we provide below to identify which of the 3 or 4 specific personality disorders is present.

Diagnosis. Patients who have personality disorders are common in all medical practices and specific diagnosis can be difficult because many times diagnostic features overlap. Further, clinicians rarely see patients at their best because illnesses are stressful and reactions to stress alter ordinary emotions and behavior; that is, they make the basic personality structure, be it an adaptive trait or a disabling disorder, more apparent and manifest. What clinicians observe during medical visits may be completely normal behavioral stress responses even if it suggests a personality disorder. Differentiating normal stress responses from disordered responses requires careful observation, reflection, time, and patience. Primary care clinicians see patients repeatedly and are in an ideal position to determine ingrained and maladaptive behavioral styles in their patients. If the patient has a personality disorder, it will be at least partially observable when they are not under some medical stress, such as seeing them when an illness has resolved or outside your practice.

Patients who develop reputations as being "difficult" require more careful evaluation and are more likely to have personality disorders.[14] Hence, your office staff and others contacting the patient can be helpful. Screening instruments are also helpful when a personality disorder is suspected. The simplest of these is the Standardized Assessment of Personality-Abbreviated Scale (SAP-AS) found in Table 10-2, an 8-item yes/no questionnaire.[15] The alpha coefficient for the total score is 0.68 and Lin's concordance coefficient for the total score is 0.89. A score of 3 or more on this screen identified 94% of psychiatric patients with DSM-IV personality disorder; sensitivity 0.94 and specificity 0.85.

TABLE 10-1. Personality Disorders

Cluster A: Odd and/or eccentric behavior
1. Paranoid—distrustful and suspicious others out to harm them
2. Schizoid—detached, difficult to establish a relationship, nonemotional
3. Schizotypal—difficulty with close relationships, eccentric behavior, cognitive and/or perceptual distortion; part of schizophrenia spectrum of disorders

Cluster B: Erratic, emotional, or dramatic behavior
1. Antisocial—pervasive disregard and violation of rights of others, conduct disorder before age 15
2. Borderline—impulsivity; instability of relationships, self-image, and emotions
3. Histrionic—excessive emotionality and attention-seeking
4. Narcissistic—grandiosity (fantasy as well as behavior), need for admiration, lack of empathy

Cluster C: Anxious and fearful behavior
1. Avoidant—social inhibition; hypersensitivity to criticism; feels inadequate
2. Dependent—need to be cared for; submissive and clinging; fear separation
3. Obsessive-compulsive—preoccupied with orderliness, perfectionism, and being in control of emotions and others

---

TABLE 10-2. Standardized Assessment of Personality-Abbreviated Scale

1. In general, do you have difficulty making and keeping friends?
2. Would you normally describe yourself as a loner?
3. In general, do you trust other people?
4. Do you normally lose your temper easily?
5. Are you normally an impulsive sort of person?
6. Are you normally a worrier?
7. In general, do you depend on others a lot?
8. In general, are you a perfectionist?

Scoring: Score "yes" if the patient feels the statement applies to them most of the time or in most situations.

A total of 3 "yes" responses indicate a personality disorder is likely.

We now address the specific (categorical) personality disorders with examples of typical patient behaviors, the feelings and reactions of clinicians and staff, and general strategies to promote optimal outcomes.

Paranoid Personality Disorder. Patients suffering from paranoid personality disorder generally surprise, confuse, and unnerve both clinicians and staff because they look for, expect, and perceive threat and malevolence from everyone and anywhere. Patients with this disorder seem to be perpetually "on guard" and may become hostile and argumentative in their interactions. The questions they ask and the manner in which they ask them imply skepticism and hyper-suspiciousness. Many times these patients conform to the concept of "the self-fulfilling prophecy" in that their interactional style evokes guarded or hostile responses from other people, serving only then to confirm their overdetermined expectations.

- *Clinical example:* In training and in practice we developed a systematic survey of local pharmacies for their prices for various medications. We shared the information with patients, especially those experiencing financial hardship or without health care coverage. Most patients are pleasantly surprised that we offer this advice and are very appreciative of the courtesy. A patient who had, during his visit, exhibited features of paranoid personality disorder, responded very differently. "You think I don't know what's going on here. You and the pharmacist at that drug store have a "kick-back" arrangement don't you?"

- *Clinician emotional reactions:* The comment was both surprising and off-putting, evoking a feeling of irritation that required instant containment. Other common responses to patients with paranoid personality disorder include fear (often of being sued) as well as anger and frustration. To respond in a manner that is, in any way, argumentative is likely to perpetuate the problem, rather than lead to a solution.

- *Clinician therapeutic response:* In a friendly tone: "I never really considered that possibility but I suppose in some rare cases that might be true. We would consider it a favor if you might do your own survey and, at your recheck appointment, let us know if you were able to find this prescription at a better price."

Schizoid Personality Disorder. These patients have a history of leading constrained and, at times, nearly solitary lives. They often indicate being satisfied with this lifestyle and do not miss or even desire interactions with others. During schooling, they are often identified by teachers and fellow students as "loners" as they have few, if any, friendships and do not participate in extracurricular activities. They typically seek employment where they work alone or in jobs requiring minimal interaction with fellow employees. They find interactions with others unpleasant and generally drift toward a life of increasing isolation and, many times, never date or marry. Because of the more intimate features of sharing their medical history and the physical examination, they tend to delay seeking care so that they may present at their initial visit with advanced illness.

- *Clinical example:* A 53-year-old, overweight, single man was brought to the clinic by his elder brother who was tired of hearing about the patient's headaches and "spells of feeling dazed, dizzy, and weak." He waited in his brother's car prior to his examination because the waiting area "was too full." He was reluctant to provide history, declined a patient gown, and insisted on being examined through his clothing. He was found to have hypertension and evidence of end-organ involvement. He admitted not liking to see physicians and wanted to end the visit as quickly as possible. "Just give me a prescription and I'll get out of your hair."

- *Clinician emotional reactions:* In contrast to the paranoid patient, this man's overall behavior elicits a more empathic response. Due to the self-imposed constraint and isolation in these patients' lives, it is common for clinicians to "feel sorry" for them. Clinicians then generally feel an increased responsibility to provide care but find the patients' resistance and nonresponse to expressions of empathy frustrating.

- *Clinician therapeutic response:* "Your brother was right to bring you in today because your blood pressure is high now and most likely has been for some time. This can be treated and will require follow-up visits. We will make these visits as short and efficient as possible." Provide as thorough an examination as the patient will allow and give brief verbal feedback and instructions in a neutral tone of voice.

Provide ample written information the patient may review later. Follow-up appointments need to be reinforced, but gently. Efforts should be made to reschedule the patient at the beginning of the day or other times when the waiting area is quiet. Follow-up visits should be shorter than with other patients and with interactions being clear, straightforward, and efficient. Positive feedback should be clear and measured when these patients cooperate with their care and adhere to their treatment plans.

Schizotypal Personality Disorder. These patients may dress and behave in odd and idiosyncratic fashions and express unusual beliefs, which may even sound delusional. Indeed, this personality disorder is a risk factor for schizophrenia, especially when cannabis, opioids, or amphetamines are used.[12,16] Their beliefs about their illness and subsequent treatment may also sound unusual. They often describe their symptoms in vague, metaphoric, or circumstantial manners. Their emotional responses generally are muted but they also may appear anxious, likely because they are uncomfortable in social situations. Their social anxiety is especially high in novel settings so the circumstance of a first clinic visit can be very stressful. Their anxiety does not usually diminish with subsequent visits and increasing familiarity with clinic staff. They may, like patients with schizoid personality, want the clinic visit to be short.

- *Clinical example:* A 45-year-old woman arrives for a first clinic visit. Scheduling staff share that she requested a clinician who is nonjudgmental, has at least 1 tattoo, and is either an Aquarius or a Pisces. She presents wearing purple eye shadow, lipstick, and nail polish and is wearing a purple paisley dress. Her bright orange athletic shoes present a stark contrast. She has both professionally and nonprofessionally applied purple tattoos on her forearms, hands, neck, and chest. Her chief complaint is: "my periods go on forever and I have never enjoyed blood sport." She sang throughout her pelvic examination and showed no emotion when her treatment plan was discussed.

- *Clinician emotional reactions:* The eccentric dress and behavior of the patient may evoke a feeling of mere curiosity but also feelings of guardedness and/or amusement. Clinicians and staff may also be unnerved by unusual questions or the patient's appearance and awkward social interactions.

- *Clinician therapeutic response:* Stay focused on the clinical tasks and maintain a neutral posture during history taking and examination. Discuss with staff that they must refrain from staring and staff should expeditiously move the patient into an examination room if he or she is receiving stares or chuckles from others in the waiting area. Instructions should be provided in a clear, straightforward manner and follow-up appointments made prior to departure to prevent the patient from feeling unwelcome or rejected.

Antisocial Personality Disorder. The antisocial personality disorder is more common among men than women and often heralded by a history of a conduct disorder as a teen, often with legal problems. The most common feature of these patients is a general disregard and lack of empathy for others, including repeated violation of their rights, which may become apparent by their behavior even in the waiting area. They usually are sensitive to authority and may behave quite differently to clinicians than support staff, showing clinicians more respect. They are capable of being interpersonally charming, especially if they desire something. This feature may change suddenly to irritability and progressive threatening behavior or comments if what they desire is withheld. Their histories may reveal problems with substance use, multiple prior marriages or relationships, frequent job changes, and legal difficulties. They may make requests for controlled medications and have prepared stories about all prior non-controlled medication treatments not working for them. They may also be the patients to run high balances for prior unpaid visits as patterns of irresponsibility are common.

- *Clinical example:* A 28-year-old man presents to the clinic with the complaint of back pain. He reports that surgery has been suggested but he does not have insurance coverage as he is "between jobs." He reports he was a patient at a pain clinic but "they expected cash up-front and I couldn't afford it anymore." Examination reveals little in the way of objective findings. He is reluctant to go for X-rays. "I told you, I can't afford it." He then requests opioid medications and is familiar with brand names. When it is explained these are not indicated he requests: "Valium to cut down on my muscle spasms." When this also denied after explanation he responds: "at least give me some Neurontin, that's not controlled and lots of people take it for pain." He is clearly irritated by the conservative treatment plan suggested and seems ambivalent about a follow-up appointment.

■ *Clinician emotional reactions:* The most common emotional response is a sense of uneasiness, caution, irritation, and even fear, especially when the superficial charm is followed by an inappropriate request, as for a nonindicated controlled substance. You may also experience the feelings of being manipulated, "scammed," intimidated, or threatened.

■ *Clinician therapeutic response:* In this case, the goal is to contain any emotional overreaction to the above feelings. Treatment plans must be explained in clear, firm, and straightforward ways with explanations of why certain inappropriate requests are not consistent with good medical care. Personal and staff safety should always be first priority if threats become overt. These patients are most likely to raise their voices or even yell at the clinician or staff. This behavior should be managed with immediate and firm intervention. "Questions or complaints about your care are welcome in our clinic but you must express them politely and in a normal tone of voice. If you cannot do this you will have to seek care elsewhere." Call the police if they become disorderly.

Histrionic Personality Disorder. The most descriptive term for patients with this disorder is "drama." They tend to present themselves in a manner that will attract attention. This includes dressing in flashy and/or revealing clothing and they behave in ways that are flirtatious and seductive. They crave being the center of attention in every setting, even if it makes them look bad, and the medical clinic is no exception. Their manner of interacting many times seems shallow, superficial, and lacking in authenticity. Their interaction with the clinician may be flattering and over-ingratiating. After a few visits they may become "hyper-familiar," including calling the clinician by first name. They are influenced by authority and can be very suggestible which, although posing risk, may be useful in promoting cooperation with their care and positive placebo responses to treatment. They may hold strong but not well-founded opinions about treatment that may interfere with their care. They

do not do well with detailed explanations and often appear to not comprehend.

■ *Clinical example:* An attractive 30-year-old, twice divorced, unemployed, woman presents with the chief complaints of anxiety, depression, muscle aches, and fatigue. "I think I have fibro." She shares a long, complicated history of developmental hardship and multiple relationships. She is attractively but seductively dressed with the front of her blouse unbuttoned to expose her breasts. She is also wearing "bling" jewelry and has multiple ear piercings. She states she requested a male clinician because "I don't get along well with other women." She frequently reaches out and touches the clinician on the forearm during history taking and comments positively about his appearance. Her symptoms are nonspecific and her anxiety and depression are consistent with present turmoil in her life. Her musculoskeletal tenderness does not conform to a syndrome or specific diagnosis. She seems disappointed when no medications are prescribed but cooperates with lab orders and a follow-up appointment. She asks to be assigned to the clinician's patient panel because: "I like you and you seem to understand my situation."

■ *Clinician emotional reactions:* Clinicians vulnerable to flattery or seductive behaviors may be influenced and "taken with" the patient's appearance, demeanor, compliments, and positive attention.

■ *Clinician therapeutic response:* Maintain a caring posture but do not respond to the patient's use of flattery. The patient may encourage the clinician to reciprocate their familiarity but avoid it. Addressing these patients more formally using "Mr.," "Ms.," and their last name assists to maintain clear boundaries. Avoid end-of-day or after-hours appointments.

Narcissistic Personality Disorder. The hallmark of this disorder is self-importance that is sometimes evident in the beginning of the visit by the presumptuous manner in which they deal with staff. They emphasize that they are special, often presenting in a pretentious and boastful manner. They embellish their accomplishments and may even "fish for compliments." They are concerned with hierarchy, authority, and status and may insist upon an appointment with the senior-most clinician. They display entitlement. Their presentation is interpreted frequently by staff as haughty, arrogant, condescending, and snobbish. They may arrive at the clinic without an appointment and expect to be "worked into" the schedule. If their expectations of praise from others are not reciprocated, they may be dismissive and critical of staff or prior clinicians' care. They commonly "work in" to their history irrelevant information that implies high status. Antisocial features frequently overlap with narcissism and these patients may also respond to frustration by raising their voice or yelling, especially at support staff. Clinician responses should be identical to that described with antisocial personality disorder if this behavior is displayed.

- *Clinical example:* A 44-year-old man arrives 15 minutes late for his appointment at the clinic for a recheck of his hypertension. He does not apologize for his tardiness and is abrupt with staff and irritated when asked to wait. He frequently paces and checks his watch and cell phone. When seen, he complains about the wait, other patients in the waiting area, and that "you don't have any magazines for smart people." He reports he is under stress at work and that others always look to him to solve problems. He describes himself as "one of the big dogs at the plant." He emphasizes that he is in a hurry because there is yet one more crisis at work and others are depending on him to manage it. His hypertension is not under control and he implies that he must not be on the correct medication and "my physiology is different than other peoples." At the end of the visit, he does not stop to pay but tells the clerk, "just bill my account" and hurriedly leaves.

- *Clinician emotional reactions:* Clinicians may not be put-off because patients with this disorder often treat them more respectfully. Clinicians may even be surprised at the negative assessments of these patients by the support staff. Clinicians may also experience a range of reactions from amusement to irritation at the patients' embellishments, entitlement, and over-important presentations.

- *Clinician therapeutic response:* Caution is necessary not to retaliate in a way that the patient interprets as a "put down" because underneath the presumptuousness, they are emotionally fragile and sensitive to slights. If the clinician is running behind and appointments are indeed late, a polite apology is in order. The clinician may suggest that future

appointments be made as the first patient of day and that timely arrival is expected.

Avoidant Personality Disorder. The major features of these patients are their long-standing feelings of low self-esteem and inadequacy. Their behavioral responses may be identical to that of the patient with schizoid personality disorder. The major differential feature is that the avoidant patient is desirous of relationships with others but their fear of criticism, disapproval, or rejection, prevents them from engaging. Generally, they have histories of harsh developmental treatment and/or growing up with constant parental criticism. They may have been objects of bullying or teasing during their schooling. They are shy and fearful in social situations and are extremely sensitive to any comment or behavior that might be interpreted as criticism. They usually drift toward employment where they may work alone or with as few others as possible. Here, like the paranoid patient, their behavior may become a "self-fulfilling prophecy." They genuinely feel inferior to others and their fearful and overly cautious behavior in social interactions and situations may elicit the very criticism or ridicule they fear most. They strive to make themselves "invisible" when they must be in a public setting, for example public transportation, waiting areas, and shopping.

- *Clinical example:* A 36-year-old woman presents to the clinic for nonspecific GI complaints. The receptionist notes that she always sits in the waiting area as far away from others as possible with her "face buried in a magazine." During her examination she makes many self-deprecating remarks relating mostly to her weight and appearance. Her GI complaints coincide with the change in her work as a night cleaner at a hotel. In the past, she alone was assigned a set number of rooms that were her responsibility. New management mandated that rooms must be cleaned by a team to be safe and time efficient. Her assigned team member was a younger woman whom she felt was easily more attractive and intelligent than herself. Her teammate seemed to desire having conversations "about everything" as they performed their work. She felt obligated to try to converse but "knew" the new coworker assessed her as "ugly, dull, and stupid." She also stated that she "knew" the new coworker resented having to work with her.

■ *Clinician emotional reactions:* The typical response from clinicians is puzzlement because the harshness of the patient's self-criticism is typically inconsistent with their own assessment. In medical settings, these patients invoke genuine sympathy and empathy from others who recognize their near constant emotional pain.

■ *Clinician therapeutic response:* The empathic feelings of clinicians toward these patients are genuine but their behavior yields more positive results than verbal compliments. Because their low self-esteem is so evident and painful, many clinicians try to bolster them with early and "over-the-top compliments" which are easily interpreted as inauthentic.

Dependent Personality Disorder. These patients feel inadequate in most circumstances and this includes health care settings. They experience the need to be taken care of by others, and are fearful or anxious about becoming independent. They have great difficulty making decisions for themselves in most circumstances. They are often overly submissive, obsequious, and are manipulative in their efforts to get others to do things for them. Their emotional need for support can lead to becoming involved in and maintaining unbalanced and even abusive relationships with others. If employed, they avoid work that requires making decisions because they are worried about "getting it wrong." Their interpersonal and social relationships are usually limited to those on whom they are dependent. Developmental histories commonly include symptoms of separation anxiety disorder or chronic childhood illness. A positive feature of patients with dependency issues is that they are typically more receptive to mental health referral.

■ *Clinical example:* A 64-year-old woman is brought to clinic by her husband for routine follow-up for type 2 diabetes. The couple does not have children and the patient herself has never been employed. Staff describes the behavior of the husband as "doting and parental," which is consistent with the behavior observed by the clinician. The patient seems to need frequent reassurance from her husband and he interjects her historical responses with added detail. She has continued to gain weight, despite adequate dietary education "because my husband is such a good cook." She is devastated when told her care now requires a schedule of insulin. "I couldn't possibly stick myself with a needle." The husband quickly reassures her not to worry as he will administer her insulin for her.

■ *Clinician emotional reactions:* These patients evoke a variety of feelings from clinicians ranging from genuine sympathy to disdain. Risks involve the clinician allowing her/his feelings to affect care by becoming either overinvolved in wanting to help or to becoming emotionally distant when extra caring efforts are met with only more demands.

■ *Clinician therapeutic response:* Both patient and husband require reassurance. The importance of competent and conscientious self-care cannot be overemphasized. Emphasis is then placed upon effective step-by-step training in her new management strategy. She requires supervision in the clinic setting to manage the entire process of injecting herself. The husband will require encouragement, support, and specific instruction to refrain from taking responsibility for her if possible.

Obsessive Compulsive Personality Disorder. Patients with this disorder exhibit overdetermined needs for self-control. They prefer their lives to be orderly and predictable and are much concerned about cleanliness. Consistent with their need for orderliness, they value details, precision, rules, and organization. Unlike the patients with OCD (discussed earlier and in Chapter 5) who are bothered by their symptoms, patients with the personality disorder embrace their perfectionism and consider it an asset. They have high standards for themselves and others and are typically rigid in their moral beliefs. They are formal in their interactions and generally dress conservatively and impeccably with great attention to detail. They persevere in their beliefs and behaviors at the expense of efficiency and leisure. They are deferential to those above them in social or work hierarchies and expect loyalty and obedience by those below them. In work settings they may have difficulty completing tasks due to their perfectionism. They are emotionally unexpressive and avoid emotional topics. They recognize clinicians as authority figures and generally follow instructions. They are sensitive to the efficient functioning of the clinic and expect a smooth, trouble-free visit, including being seen promptly at their scheduled appointment time. They are perceived by staff as stiff, formal, and joyless.

■ *Clinical example:* A 28-year-old man employed as a computer programmer presents to the clinic with symptoms consistent with bacterial sinusitis. He expresses irritation to staff and the clinician about being made to wait past the appointment time. He is professionally dressed, formal, and polite in his interactions, and listens carefully to treatment instructions. He states he must return to work quickly and seems reassured he will not require a follow-up appointment unless he does not respond to treatment. He phones the following day with a list of questions for the clinician and inquires if the antibiotic prescription instructions which are 3 times daily should be every 8 hours or evenly distributed during his waking hours. He also asks if it should be taken with a specific amount of water or juice. He has read the precautionary literature provided by the pharmacy and has a number of questions about adverse effects. Finally he reports that attempts at irrigating his sinuses with saline are too messy and disgusting but he will persevere as instructed.

■ *Clinician emotional reactions:* Clinicians generally do not mind patients with this personality disorder as they tend to be deferential and follow instructions closely. Clinicians may feel challenged or impatient by these patients' needs for precise and comprehensive explanations when they have extended questions about their care—or if they are dominating talkers in a busy office.

■ *Clinician therapeutic response:* These patients may require a more formal demeanor by the clinician than other patients. The formality is reassuring to these patients and careful, systematic explanations of the treatment plan are appreciated. They also respond positively to suggestions that they research their diagnoses and treatment recommendations. It may also be helpful to suggest that they schedule appointments at the beginning of the day to prevent their feelings of impatience or irritation by the delays common in busy medical practice.

Borderline Personality Disorder. Although listed in Cluster B, we present this disorder last because it is the most complex, demanding, and frustrating of all the personality disorders. As well, because it has been the most extensively studied, we have better information for medical management. The "borderline" term for the disorder reflects historical clinical observations

that these patients occupy a middle ground between the older concepts of neurosis and psychosis. In general, these patients have difficulty functioning in an adaptive manner to life's demands (thus neurosis) and, especially in times of severe stress, can show compromise in their ability to test reality (thus psychosis). The diagnostic names for the disorder have periodically changed over time but the present terminology in DSM-5 in now firm.[17] As with any chronic illness with exacerbations and remissions, the earlier the diagnosis is made and appropriate management started, the better the long-term clinical outcome.[18]

The hallmark feature seen in these patients is instability in their overall manner of functioning. It generally takes a number of primary care visits to make the diagnosis if this is not already known from psychiatry.[19] This tendency toward instability is especially seen in their fluctuating moods and they often also meet criteria for bipolar disorder.[20,21] Substance abuse is also common, many times being their attempts to self-medicate their unstable moods.[22]

These patients present, especially in more stressful times, with wide-ranging mood instability both high and low. They have long-standing histories of volatility in many of their social relationships and they are extraordinarily sensitive to rejection and perceived abandonment. They waver broadly in their self-image and have a pattern of impulsivity. They also find it difficult to be alone and are bothered by feelings of emotional emptiness. They are the patients most likely to engage in cutting, burning, or other forms of self-injury. They are also the patients most likely to make suicidal threats and gestures and remain at chronic self-destructive risk. During times of poor reality testing, they may require treatment with antipsychotic agents. Patients with borderline personality disorders are especially high utilizers of psychiatric care services at all levels.[23] Periodic psychiatric hospitalization may be required, especially during times of heightened self-destructive behavior. If available, day hospitalization is preferable to acute in-patient hospitalization. Hospitalization should be limited to these critical times and brief due to patients becoming either too comfortable with the level of increased support or becoming disruptive to the in-patient milieu.

These patients present a significant challenge to the primary care clinicians, especially if they also have concomitant medical illness. They vary widely in their abilities to cooperate with care and may show wide variability in their presentations from visit to visit. They are also challenging to the clinic staff due to the phenomenon of "splitting" where the patient pits some staff against others. Clinicians will often discover that clinic staff has wide-ranging opinions about these patients for this reason. For example, if you find that certain office staff can't stand the patient while others quite like them, look for a borderline personality. Clinicians must be sensitive to this feature of the disorder as the patients may sow discord between colleagues as well by their tendency to overvalue some and devalue others. A corollary feature of this clinical phenomenon of splitting is a tendency toward binary thinking, dividing others as "all good" or "all bad."

Screening. Due to the variability and confusing nature of symptoms over time, a screening instrument is helpful to clarify the diagnosis of borderline personality disorder. The McLean Screening Instrument for Borderline Personality Disorder (MSI-BPD) is very helpful in addition to a clinician's longitudinal experience of a patient's emotions and behavior.[24] It consists of the 10 yes–no questions outlined in Table 10-3. Using a cutoff score of 7 yes answers results in a sensitivity of 0.90 and a specificity of 0.93 in patients 25 years or younger and a sensitivity of 0.81, and a specificity of 0.85 in patients older than 25 years. Review of the questions' content highlights the clinical issues of mood instability and the commonality of the coexistence of mood disorder.

- *Clinical example:* A 26-year-old single woman presents to the clinic for a follow-up visit for diabetes which has been stable for the past 6 months. She reports enjoying this period of stability but is looking forward to her new job and is in a new relationship. She comments that she is lucky to have the best boyfriend as well as the "best doctor ever." She describes a good relationship with her psychiatrist and case manager at the community mental health center and feels her psychotropic medication doses and combinations are "just right." Examination of her arms and legs reveal well healed linear scars from prior episodes of cutting. Further examination reveals both healing superficial cuts and punctate burn marks over her abdomen. She explains they are left over from the recent break-up with a former boyfriend. She expressed regret over her

TABLE 10-3. McLean Screening Instrument for Borderline Personality Disorder (MSI-BPD)

1. Have any of your closest relationships been troubled by a lot of arguments or repeated breakups?
2. Have you deliberately hurt yourself physically (eg, punched yourself, cut yourself, burned yourself)? Have you made a suicide attempt?
3. Have you had at least 2 other problems with impulsivity (eg, eating binges, and spending sprees, drinking too much and verbal outbursts)?
4. Have you been extremely moody?
5. Have you felt angry a lot of the time? Have you often acted in an angry or sarcastic manner?
6. Have you often been mistrustful of other people?
7. Have you frequently felt unreal or as if things around you were unreal?
8. Have you felt empty for a long time?
9. Have you often felt that you had no idea of who you are or that you have no identity?
10. Have you made desperate efforts to avoid feeling abandoned or being abandoned, such as repeatedly calling someone to reassure yourself that he or she still cared, begged them not to leave you, and clung to them physically?

Scoring: 7 or more yes answers highly suggest a diagnosis of borderline personality disorder.

self-damaging behavior. "I was not trying to kill myself," she explained and then indicated hurting herself helped her deal with negative events because it provided an "emotional release." This experience reflects a phenomenon called "non-suicidal self-injury." It is common and may predict subsequent suicidal gestures or attempts; DSM-5 indicates the need for further study.[25]

- *Clinician emotional reaction:* In this instance, the clinician may feel a sense of anxiety and foreboding due to the recent and apparently abrupt changes in her romantic relationship as well as the stresses involved with pending new employment. Clinicians' emotions may vary widely due to the variable presentation of these patients. Feelings may range from genuine sympathy to resentment to fear. Risks for physicians include over-indulgence and "need to rescue," to frustration, dread, and wishes that the patient seek care elsewhere. Such often unrecognized feelings can lead to compromise in clinical objectivity.

■ *Clinician therapeutic response:* Genuine reinforcement of her present success at diabetic self-care and stress management strategies like exercise and sufficient restful sleep are useful. Expression of caution in respect to recent changes in relationship and employment status is in order also. Caring statements encouraging her to share these potential stressors with her psychiatrist and case manager are appropriate. A firm appointment for her regular diabetes follow-up care should be scheduled to promote further stability, prevent feelings of rejection, and monitor and reinforce any adaptive ways of coping she describes in the interim.

CONCLUSION

Patients with personality disorders are pervasive in primary care practice. Following the described recommendations for the screening, diagnosis, and primary care management of these patients, improved overall clinical outcomes and, equally importantly, the primary care clinicians' professional satisfaction and well-being often follow.

While we recommend throughout this book that you actively treat depression, anxiety, and prescription substance misuse, we warn that comorbid personality disorders make this task more difficult since these patients tend to be more refractory. Their association with poor relationships and nonadherence makes their prognosis less optimistic.[12] Using guidelines already given, make referrals to mental health professionals. See Chapter 11 for the details of referral. The caveat is that patients with comorbid personality disorders are likely to be less responsive and require earlier referral than typical patients with an analogous diagnosis.

Primary care clinicians should develop a cooperative partnership with local mental health professionals to become part of the expanded and integrated team approach. Long-term psychotherapy, cognitive-behavioral therapy, counseling, and other forms of treatment may be helpful; the evidence for this best established for borderline personality disorder.[12]

Here are some general guidelines for working with all personality disorders.

1. The following are management goals in the primary care setting for patients with a personality disorder.
   a. Emotional support, emphasis on long-term care, and strengthening the therapeutic relationship
   b. Increased availability during periods of crisis
   c. Attention to the treatment of comorbid psychiatric disorders, especially anxiety and depression
   d. Reinforcing motivation to adhere to the treatment plan
   e. Strategies for stress and harm reduction
   f. Referral and advice regarding practical supports including emergency services, housing, social welfare agencies, financial and educational assistance, and child/elder care

2. As reinforced in each case above and discussed in Chapter 11, clinicians must monitor the feelings (emotional reactions) they experience during visits with these patients. Special caution is indicated when clinicians perceive feeling differently about patients than is usual for themselves, especially negativity and declining empathy; alternatively, undue attraction to the patient and a desire to help them or otherwise interact with them beyond what is usual are also warning signs.

3. These patients can be difficult and trying. If possible, schedule these patients at times when clinicians are at their best, most rested, and most patient themselves. With some, you may need to schedule more time. Also, do not schedule a number of them on the same day. Further, do not schedule patients with histrionic or borderline personality disorder at the end of the day or after hours.

4. Pay attention to and directly solicit the feelings and feedback from clinic staff. Communication is critical and team meetings should include special coverage of the needs and vicissitudes of each difficult patient and the role of each member of the care team. See Chapter 11 for guidelines for team care. Open staff communications are essential to prevent or manage the phenomena of the "splitting" characteristic of patients with borderline personality disorders. Staff may need to be trained not to refer to these patients as their psychiatric disorder or to refer to them in pejorative terms, for example "borderline," "flake," "drama queen," or "Oscar the grouch." Help your staff understand that patients have identities beyond their disorders.

5. After clinician-patient relationships are established, a discussion about referral for mental health care is in order, if this contact is not already established. Explain how newer techniques, such as dialectical behavior therapy, have been demonstrated to

stabilize mood and improve overall levels of function.[26] Expect patients with personality disorders to react with puzzlement and or reluctance. Gentle reminders of how their behaviors have interfered with their ability to enjoy life are helpful. When patients are under stresses, try to help them relate their stress to their emotional and behavioral styles as a way to obtain acceptance to referral. Open communication and cooperation between primary care and mental health care is essential.

6. Be available to colleagues and clinic staff who are experiencing difficulty managing their feelings about their patients with personality disorder. Better yet, create a Balint Group to meet on a regular basis to discuss difficult cases.[27-29]

7. For most patients with personality disorders, it is wise to avoid one's usual more outgoing, friendly, and interactive approach. Rather, be more formally professional, stick to the problem at hand, and be efficient. Once a relationship is established, the clinician can experiment with being more interactive.

We now transition to the final chapter to provide some suggestions to further improve mental health care.

REFERENCES

1. Shapiro D. *Neurotic Styles*. New York, NY: Basic Books; 1965.
2. Reich W. *Character Analysis*. New York, NY: Pocket Books; 1976.
3. Amador C, Xia C, Nagy R, et al. Regional variation in health is predominantly driven by lifestyle rather than genetics. *Nat Commun*. 2017;8(1):801.
4. Fortin VI AH, Dwamena F, Frankel R, Lepisto B, Smith R. *Smith's Patient-Centered Interviewing— An Evidence-Based Method*. 4th ed. New York, NY: McGraw-Hill, Lange Series; 2018.
5. Metzger JA. Adaptive defense mechanisms: function and transcendence. *J Clin Psychol*. 2014;70(5):478-488.
6. American Psychiatric Association. *Diagnostic and Statistical Manual of Mental Disorders*. 5th ed. Washington, DC: American Psychiatric Association; 2013.
7. Mattar S, Khan F. Personality disorders in older adults: diagnosis and management. *Prog Neurol Psychiatry*. 2017;21:22-27.
8. Videler A, VanderFeltx-Cornelis C, Rosi G. Psychotherapeutic treatment levels for personality disorders in older adults. *Clin Gerontol*. 2015;38:325-341.
9. Kealy D, Steinberg PI, Ogrodniczuk JS. "Difficult" patient? Or does he have a personality disorder? *J Fam Pract*. 2014;63(12):697-703.
10. Angstman KB, Seshadri A, Marcelin A, Gonzalez CA, Garrison GM, Allen JS. Personality disorders in primary care: impact on depression outcomes within collaborative care. *J Prim Care Community Health*. 2017;8(4):233-238.
11. Bentall RP. Understanding the association between personality and severe mental illness. *JAMA Psychiatry*. 2017;74(7):671-672.
12. Kendell RE. The distinction between personality disorder and mental illness. *Brit J Psychiatry*. 2002;180:110-115.
13. Laird-Fick H, Freilich L, Han C, Smith R. Deconstructing difficult encounters. *J Clin Outcomes Manag*. 2012;19:557-562.
14. Davison S. Principles of managing patients with personality disorder. *Adv Psychiatr Treatment*. 2002;8:1-9.
15. Moran P, Leese M, Lee T, Walters P, Thornicroft G, Mann A. Standardised Assessment of Personality— Abbreviated Scale (SAPAS): preliminary validation of a brief screen for personality disorder. *Br J Psychiatry*. 2003;183:228-232.
16. Hjorthoj C, Albert N, Nordentoft M. Association of substance use disorders with conversion from schizotypal disorder to schizophrenia. *JAMA Psychiatry*. 2018;75(7):733-739.
17. Kernberg OF, Michels R. Borderline personality disorder. *Am J Psychiatry*. 2009;166(5):505-508.
18. Zimmerman M. Improving the recognition of borderline personality disorder. *Current Psychiatry*. 2017;184:1789-1794.
19. Biskin RS, Paris J. Diagnosing borderline personality disorder. *CMAJ*. 2012;184(16):1789-1794.
20. Paris J, Black DW. Borderline personality disorder and bipolar disorder: what is the difference and why does it matter? *J Nerv Ment Dis*. 2015;203(1):3-7.
21. Bayes AJ, Parker GB. Clinical vs. DSM diagnosis of bipolar disorder, borderline personality disorder and their co-occurrence. *Acta Psychiatr Scand*. 2017;135(3):259-265.
22. Carpenter RW, Wood PK, Trull TJ. Comorbidity of borderline personality disorder and lifetime substance use disorders in a nationally representative sample. *J Pers Disord*. 2016;30(3):336-350.
23. Comtois KA, Carmel A. Borderline personality disorder and high utilization of inpatient psychiatric hospitalization: concordance between research and clinical diagnosis. *J Behav Health Serv Res*. 2016;43(2):272-280.
24. Zanarini MC, Vujanovic AA, Parachini EA, Boulanger JL, Frankenburg FR, Hennen J. A screening measure for BPD: the McLean Screening Instrument for Borderline Personality Disorder (MSI-BPD). *J Pers Disord*. 2003;17(6):568-573.

25. Kerr PL, Muehlenkamp JJ, Turner JM. Nonsuicidal self-injury: a review of current research for family medicine and primary care physicians. *J Am Board Fam Med.* 2010;23(2):240-259.

26. Gunderson JG. Mechanisms of change in treatments of personality disorders: commentary on the special section. *J Pers Disord.* 2018;32(Supplement):129-133.

27. Balint M. Method and technique in the teaching of medical psychology. II. Training general practitioners in psychotherapy. *Brit J Med Psychol.* 1954;27:37-41.

28. Scheingold L. Balint work in England: lessons for American family medicine. *J Fam Prac.* 1988;26:315-320.

29. Salander P, Sandstrom M. A Balint-inspired reflective forum in oncology for medical residents: main themes during seven years. *Patient Educ Couns.* 2014;97(1):47-51.

11

Enhancing Your Own Care

In this chapter, we consider 3 issues that can improve your conduct of mental health care: working as a team, referral, and personal awareness. The first 2 issues consider how best to get help from others by enlarging your care team, while the latter addresses what you can do to enhance your own success in conducting effective mental health care.

WORKING AS A TEAM

In this section, we explore ways in which primary care health providers can incorporate other team members to maximize mental health care in primary care settings. As we discuss the benefits of collaborative care models (CCMs), we'll focus on how you can extend this care beyond the boundaries of a single practice and what an individual practice can do, based on principles developed in patient-centered medical homes.

Working As a Team Within the Primary Care Office

Some practices have formal CCMs. CCMs include mental health specialists (usually a psychiatrist) embedded within or external to the practice. Although there are many models of CCM,[1] in the generic one, the psychiatrist, usually off-site, supervises mental health care by consulting with the second component of a CCM, an onsite (full-time or part-time) care manger, hopefully with some mental health care training. Guided by the psychiatrist on a weekly or biweekly basis, typically by telephone, the care manager provides day-to-day mental health care in consultation with the primary care

provider who largely functions to write prescriptions advised by the psychiatrist.[2,3] Studies have found that these models improve outcomes for depression as well as chronic medical conditions like diabetes mellitus.[3-8] Unfortunately, reflecting the dearth of psychiatrists, there has been little widescale penetration into US care when viewed from a population perspective. If you are among those fortunate to have a CCM team available, make use of them not only for your patients, but also as an educational resource.

Nevertheless, because most practitioners to not have access to a CCM team, we need to think about ways that you can construct and mobilize your own core teams based on the chronic care model that guides collaborative care.[9] This means enlisting your partners and staff in your own offices to fulfill at least some of the functions of CCM team members. After all, these are the people interacting with your patients at check-in, by phone, during visits, and when you are out of town. The skills and roles will vary among different practices, from highly developed patient-centered medical homes to traditional primary care offices.

Identifying core team members can help in several ways with the ongoing care of your patients with mental health disorders. These benefits include:

- Identifying high-risk patients
- Identifying problematic and/or positive behaviors
- Reinforcing care plans
- Coordinating care outside of office visits
- Facilitating contact with community resources

Doing so requires shared vision and strong leadership backed by open communication, clearly defined roles, and common processes.[10,11] For example, if you are caring for a group of patients with chronic pain, your goals might be to: (1) decrease utilization of the emergency department; (2) decrease diagnostic testing; and (3) decrease specialist referrals. To replace this, your strategy would be to: (1) promote continuity by regularly scheduled, frequent office visits with the provider and/or other skilled office staff; (2) emphasize coping skills and symptom management at these visits; and (3) ensure that calls outside of office hours do not result in emergency department visits. To be successful, you will need the support of your scheduling staff, nurse, a social worker (if available), and partners who share call. Patients with chronic pain (or other medically unexplained symptom problems like irritable bowel syndrome and chronic fatigue or other mental health problems) will need to be clearly identified and general management protocols agreed upon—and the roles of different team members identified. For example, the scheduling staff would ensure open slots in your schedule so that a chronic pain patient can be seen on a regular basis, and they would work with you (and the patient) to avoid nonscheduled visits. A skilled nurse or medical assistant might engage in a 5-minute phone check-in each week with the patient, at the same time helping out with any necessary community resources and doing simple problem-solving. You are thus establishing not just a strong clinician-patient relationship but also a therapeutic relationship for the patient with your office staff. Your on-call physician colleague is also included and would know not to fill opioid or benzodiazepine prescriptions, except with your advance approval, when they were covering your patients in your absence. As part of forming your office team, you will need to meet regularly with office staff, encourage them in what can be a new but exciting role, and do some training such as teaching them to use NURS in their patient interactions. They can also be helpful in identifying problem patients who will benefit from a systematic team approach, and they should be encouraged to be proactive and engaged contributors to the team. You will find that this team effort greatly lessens your own burden and enhances office esprit. Staff like to be involved and feel like they have an important role in patient care.

To guide you, the functions and actions described in Table 11-1 come from studies of CCMs.[3,5-8,10,11]

Organizations have implemented the changes as sets, either all at once or incrementally. Activities range from simple interventions such as distributing screening instruments to patients as part of the check-in process, to more labor-intensive endeavors such as creating patient registries. Every team member can—and should—have a role to play, perhaps an area where they are primarily responsible, depending on their skills and interest.

All teams need clearly defined roles and expectations to be successful. One way to support this objective in a primary care office is to create small "pods" that include some combination of physician, physician assistant or nurse practitioner, nurse, medical assistant, and front office staff. Pod members should be working in the same space to enhance real-time communication.[10,11] Additional strategies like daily huddles and white boards at staff stations help. Pods can come together in weekly staff meetings to share best practices and problem-solve.

Huddles are structured activities to support the vision and goals of team-based care. Pod members meet briefly, say, at the beginning of a clinic session, to review the patients scheduled, the care to be provided, and any outstanding concerns.[10,11] Huddles also can be used to review patient registries and determine next steps. For example, the nurse and practice physicians might review a registry of patients with major depressive disorder and determine who needs lab tests ordered or an assessment for remission of symptoms on a Patient Health Questionnaire-9 (PHQ-9).

Collaborating Outside the Core Office Team

CCM is a wonderful opportunity to provide mental health care within primary care practices if it's available. Most of us, however, rely on collaborating with consultants external to our practices. This is especially important for complex patients and for specialized services, like counseling or psychotherapy. When should we refer? Who is the "right" professional to add to the patient's team? And how do we communicate effectively and coordinate care?

Table 11-2 summarizes the many indications for referral but they generally fall into 3 categories:

- Emergency care, such as suicidal ideation or psychosis;

- Failure to respond to first- and second-line therapies for conditions otherwise within your scope of practice;

TABLE 11-1. Key Functions and Actions to Provide Team-Based Care for Patients

FUNCTIONS	ACTIONS	EXAMPLES
Identifying high-risk patients	**Screening** for: • Depression (eg, Patient Health Questionnaire-9[a]) • Anxiety (eg, Generalized Anxiety Disorders 7-item) • Bipolar disorder (eg, The Mood Disorder Questionnaire) • Drug and alcohol misuse (eg, CAGE, CAGE-AID) • Risk of substance misuse (eg, Opioid Risk Tool) • Social determinants of health **Creating registries** of patients with chronic diseases	• **Front office staff** distributes screening forms at check-in.[a] • **Medical assistant** administers screening forms as part of intake for visit.[a] • **Nurse or social worker** screens patients with depression for comorbidities. • **Nurse** creates and maintains registries.
Identifying problematic and/or positive behaviors	**Reconciling medications** **Monitoring controlled substance prescriptions** **Observing patient behaviors**	• **Medical assistant or Nurse** completes medication reconciliation and updates medical record.[a] • **Nurse** maintains registry of patients on controlled substances and runs reports from prescription monitoring system. • **Nurse** maintains registry of patients being treated for depressive disorders and monitors for remission.[a] • **Team members** participate in huddles to discuss patient care. • **Team members** report concerns based on interactions at check-in, during telephone conversations, and other interactions
Reinforcing care plans	**Maintaining consistent interactions and expectations** **Following policies or protocols on medication prescribing and refills**	• **Front office staff** schedule patient with primary care provider to facilitate continuity. • **Nurse (as care manager), physician, and patient** meet together during visits. • **Team members** give patients a team business card to reinforce roles and available resources. • **Nurse or social worker** reinforces treatment plans with patients outside of formal visits. • **Physician and physician extender** use evidence-based protocols for patient management (ie, psychotropic medication prescribing, follow up for chronic pain, minimizing serial testing for medically unexplained symptoms).

(Continued)

TABLE 11-1. Key Functions and Actions to Provide Team-Based Care for Patients (*Continued*)

FUNCTIONS	ACTIONS	EXAMPLES
Coordinating care	**Educating patients** **Administering medications in the office** **Monitoring adherence and effectiveness of therapy** **Scheduling appointments** with primary team, diagnostic services, or consultants **Communicating with consultants** **Providing or identifying resources** (eg, for medications, transportation, housing, exercise) **Performing handovers** for complicated patients	• **Physician extender, Nurse, or social worker** teaches patient about self-care practices. • **Nurse or social worker** calls to ensure patient is taking medication. • **Nurse or social worker** conduct in-person visits. • **Social worker** provides contacts for counselors. • **Social worker** provides brief counseling directly. • **Team members** participate in huddles to discuss goals for specific visits or chronic disease management. • **Medical Assistants** use pre-visit planning sheets or templates to prepare for visits or obtain data during visits. • **Physicians or other team members** perform structured handovers for patients in case of contact outside business hours or during absences. • **Nurse** manages patient portal to facilitate between-visit care and to engage patients in self-management. • **Team members** work from buckets or electronic "to do" lists.

ªPerformance indicators for patient-centered medical home certification.

TABLE 11-2. Indications for Referral

1. Suicidal or homicidal ideation
2. Psychosis, whether due to schizophrenia, bipolar I disorder, or other causes
3. Other indications for inpatient management, such as substance abuse
4. Failure of your primary care treatment, eg, for depression or anxiety
5. Worsening of dysfunctional behaviors, irrespective of other indications
6. Resistance of the patient to becoming engaged in your treatment
7. The patient requests a referral
8. Multiple and/or severe stressors
9. When your treatment has been successful in identifying a need for and a patient's desire for counseling

■ To receive care that is outside your scope of practice, such as counseling for mood disorders, pharmacological treatment of complex mental health disorders (eg, bipolar disorder, schizophrenia, substance abuse), electroconvulsive therapy, or diagnostic testing (eg, neuropsychiatric testing).

Table 11-3 summarizes the roles of other health professionals in caring for patients with mental disorders. Some of these professionals may prescribe medications (ie, psychiatrists), while others provide nonpharmacological management (ie, psychologists, licensed medical social workers, other counselors) or diagnostic testing (ie, neuropsychologists). It is important to understand what services the provider offers and be clear about the type of assistance you are seeking. For example, you might be able to schedule a

TABLE 11-3. Health Professionals for Care of Mental Health Disorders

HEALTH PROFESSIONALS	ROLES	CONSIDERATIONS

Psychiatrists	• Treatment of resistant mood disorders (ie, failed first- and second-line therapies) with medications, electroconvulsive therapy, or other advanced modalities
	• Management of psychotropic medications, particularly in patients with:
	  • Bipolar disorder
	  • Depressive disorder with psychotic features
	  • Mood disorders refractory to first- and second-line therapy
	  • Comorbid personality disorders or complex psychiatric conditions
	• Mental health emergencies, in inpatient settings (ie, suicidal or homicidal ideation)
		• Subspecialties: Child and adolescent psychiatry, geropsychiatry, addiction medicine
		• Adult patients and their families typically need to self-refer
		• Children may be referred by primary care providers

Neuropsychiatrists	• Specialized testing to assess cognitive abilities and evaluate for attention deficit hyperactivity disorder	• Requires a referral • Not all services may be covered by insurance
Addiction medicine specialists	• Management of patients with substance misuse • Methadone and buprenorphine therapy	• May be trained as psychiatrists or medical physicians
Other health providers for treatment of pain or somatic complaints	• Medical management of chronic pain • Oversight of nonpharmacologic measures for pain or somatic dysfunction • Invasive procedures for treatment of pain	• Referral may be required • Wide range of skills and services to consider: pain medicine, physical medicine and rehabilitation, physical and occupational therapy, osteopathic manipulative medicine
Psychologists	• Counseling therapy for mood disorders, personality disorders, some patients with medically unexplained symptoms • May have a particular area of focus—cognitive behavioral therapy, panic disorder, or chronic pain	• Adult patients and their families typically need to self-refer • Children may be referred by primary care providers
Licensed medical social workers	• Depending on training, may provide counseling or may aid patients and families in negotiating health systems and identifying resources	• Adult patients and their families typically need to self-refer • Children may be referred by primary care providers • Resource coordination function may be available as part of home health care services, or a local commission on aging

patient with bipolar disorder with a psychologist, but that person will not assume management of mood stabilizing medications. On the other hand, most psychiatrists no longer perform psychotherapy or counseling if that is your patient's need.

Close communication between psychiatrists, therapists, care managers, primary care clinicians, and patients is a core component of CCM. Privacy laws in the United States create a barrier to communication between mental health and primary care providers. Psychiatrists and therapists, for example, cannot routinely send consultant notes to primary care providers. Patients can sign *releases of information* to allow communication to coordinate care, though, and this need should always be addressed. Authorization can include copies of medical records and direct oral communication, and extend to care managers, social workers, or other team members within the primary care setting—perhaps having it part of a contract. Involving these team members can be invaluable for facilitating communication—and therefore care.

Form Your Care Team

With planning, you can leverage resources within your offices and communities to provide patient-centered, team-based care. Physician extenders, nurses, medical assistants, social workers, and front office staff can work together to provide care within the office and outside of office visits. Shared vision and leadership coupled with clearly defined roles and communication are critical to successfully implementing team-based care.

Some patients need care beyond what you can provide in your office—either because of the acuteness and/or complexity of their illnesses or the scope of your practice. You can work with a range of other professionals to join you in co-managing patients so that they receive the care they need. Your team members—notably care managers and social workers—can facilitate communication with these providers and patients. Team care is fun, alleviates some of the burden of caring for difficult patients, and is good for office esprit.

REFERRAL

We have frequently pointed out the need for referral with the various conditions we have discussed in earlier chapters. The indications for referral mentioned earlier are summarized in Table 11-2. We now address the critical process of the referral itself and what is needed to make it successful.[12]

One of the most overlooked parts of making a successful referral is the patient! Once you have identified a need, this must be shared with the patient. From the outset, one message is essential: that you will not abandon them. Patients' prior experiences in the medical system often associate a physician's recommendation for referral as meaning you are giving up on them or simply wanting to get rid of them, especially in patients with chronic pain or other unexplained symptom syndromes. As well, there remains even today significant stigma about seeing a psychiatrist or a counselor. Accordingly, it is important not to imply they are a "psych case" but, rather, that they need help beyond your level of expertise—and that you will continue with their care in a co-managing role. It frequently helps to "normalize" their mental health problem by saying that anyone with such distress would be depressed, upset, or anxious; for example, "...if I had that problem in my own life, I'd feel depressed, who wouldn't..." Further, it may take several visits over several weeks to months for a patient to agree to a referral. During this time, be patient and understanding unless there is an emergency; see below for involuntary commitment of patients. Using plentiful amounts of NURS (Naming, Respecting, Understanding, Supporting), convey your empathy about their reluctance and assure them that you will continue to work with them. Nor will it help to try to force them. It does often help, however, to bring in significant others in their life, and this should always be tried. Generally, patients will agree in due time. If not and there is no emergency, you simply follow them the best you can. In this situation you may want to get a signed contract that they have refused referral.

Later, following a successful referral, be sure to obtain progress information from the consultant. Then share this progress with the patient so they know you are continuing to be actively involved—and interested—in their care. During your follow-up visits, it is key to inquire how the referral is going from the patient's standpoint. Are they satisfied and making progress; also, do they like the consultant or not? If the latter, you should be in touch with the consultant to ascertain the problem. At times, you may need to facilitate a replacement consultant.

In nonemergency situations, it is essential to talk with the consultant beforehand. They will need to know what you have done—how the patient has responded and the details of medications, for example—and what you'd like to see happen, for example, help with medications in someone whose depression has not cleared, electroconvulsive therapy in an older person with refractory depression, counseling, testing a patient's cognitive capacity, grief management, or behavioral management of panic disorder.

Because many patients present with physical symptoms and comorbid medical problems, the consultant needs to know this and the medications employed, especially a psychiatrist who will be making medication adjustments and concerned about drug interactions. Further, consultants need to know that you already have excluded underlying organic disease explanations in patients with chronic pain so that consultants do not inadvertently recommend to the patient that they need additional workup. Rather, ask the consultant to first discuss with you any ideas they have about additional investigation.

In emergency situations, if patients refuse care by a psychiatrist and/or to go to the emergency department, your task is simple but can be taxing: you have to get them to the emergency room where they can be involuntarily committed for up to 72 hours.[13] While you can also commit them from your office, we recommend that the psychiatry personnel in the emergency room do it in conjunction with the admitting psychiatrist. This saves you time and mental health professionals will be much more familiar with the local legal requirements and ramifications of involuntary commitment. Your task is to get them to the emergency room.

Never let them drive themselves or allow a relative to take them to the emergency department. Instead, have an ambulance take them. If this somehow does not work (because, for example, adequate personnel are unavailable or for a difficult patient)—or if the patient escapes your care—call the police and they will take the patient to the emergency room. You also, of course, contact the emergency room to provide information about the patient's condition and imminent arrival and then follow-up to be sure they arrived and are under adequate care.

PERSONAL AWARENESS

So far, this book has focused on the patient. Now it's time to focus on you. Indeed, you will be the most important determinant of your success in conducting mental health care. We know from considerable research that the clinician-patient relationship you establish with the patient is one of the most important determinants of good outcomes. In fact, it's been demonstrated to be the common denominator in many successful psychotherapy and medical interventions.[14-19] That is, the relationship contributes as much to the outcome as do the medications or therapy. So, this relationship is worth a heavy investment.

The relationship deserves special mention in mental health care because you have not been well trained in this aspect of medicine, particularly in dealing with the most difficult of all patients—those with chronic pain, especially when seeking opioids and/or benzodiazepines. This is a well-known setup for the physician to exhibit negative reactions to the patient wherein a harmful relationship develops.[12,20-22] Harmful responses vary along a spectrum from passively prescribing the medications patients desire as the easiest way to get rid of them quickly to seeing them last in a busy clinic to not giving return appointments to arguing with them angrily to actively firing them from your practice; the limited and infrequent conditions for the latter are outlined in Chapter 3 (Section 3)—basically, if they are not participating in the therapeutic program. While often understandable, negative physician reactions to the patient are nonetheless a huge deterrent to effective care. In the following, we address how you can best deal with what are often subconscious and therefore mostly reflexive reactions on your part. What do you do? It's simple: make yourself aware of your feelings and their impact on your behaviors with the patient.[20,23]

To identify difficulties with your personal reactions to patients, it helps to begin by becoming more familiar with all emotions you have, whether positive or negative, whether inside or outside medicine. First, begin to identify any emotions you experience in all aspects of your life. There are any number of interesting and fun ways to do this, but it takes time and will not simply happen just because you want it to.

Here are some activities to foster your emotional awareness—do them regularly:

1. Read stories of patients' courage in the face of severe pain and/or suffering.
2. Read emotion-laden biographies and fiction.
3. Watch movies with considerable emotion, for example, the movie Wit with Emma Thompson.
4. Engage with emotionally expressive people.
5. Engage in emotionally relevant (to you) music and art.

In all these activities, first identify your emotion and then see what actual behavior it led to—what you did in response to the emotion. For example, if a story you read made you feel sad, what behavior on your part followed—read more, stop reading, tell someone about it, think about it later in the day? Here's another example, perhaps you became angry about a sleight from someone you cared about. What behavior followed that—ignoring that person the next day, talking to them about it, drinking a beer to get it off your mind? It is useful to seek positive as well as negative emotions, for example, that you felt good about a patient's compliment and spent more time with them.

There are some very productive activities you can employ to foster emotional awareness, and we recommend you employ all of them.

1. Talk about your positive as well as negative reactions to others and invite them to do so as well—this is also a great chance to use your NURS skills and see how they encourage the other person to share their emotions.
2. Various meditation exercises can help you focus on your emotions.[24-26] For example, meditate on interactions, both rewarding and difficult, with peers, patients, clinical circumstances, or in your personal life. Always note what the emotion was and how you responded to it. Table 11-4 describes a simple meditation exercise many have found useful and practice daily.
3. Keep a journal of your emotional experiences and the behaviors that followed; see Table 11-5.[27,28] One does this daily at a reasonably quiet time for no more than 10 minutes initially, being open to longer times as you begin to have more to write. Write about what's on your mind, what's most important to you—right now—and the emotions that go with it and the resulting behaviors.

TABLE 11-4. Breathing Meditation

1. In a quiet room where you will not be disturbed, sit on a chair or cross-legged on a pillow on the floor. Try to sit straight but be comfortable.
2. Close your eyes and pay attention to your breathing, focusing on each breath, saying to yourself, "In" with each inhalation and "Out" as you exhale. Breathe as you normally would, likely taking breaths of various depths. Beginning with a deep breath or two often helps get the process going, but don't hyperventilate.
3. Start counting your breaths, as "In…Out-1" → "In-Out-2" → (continue; you may want to start over or count backwards once you hit 100)
4. Continue focusing on your breathing, trying to "breathe from the stomach"—this means push your abdomen out to inhale and let it come back as you exhale; try not to move your chest when you breathe. As you count stay focused on the movement of your abdomen, in and out.
5. As you do this, your mind will likely wander to other thoughts, such as a task you need to do. This is perfectly ok. Once you realize it, though, simply drop the thought and return your focus to the breathing, the abdomen moving in and out, continuing to count.
6. If you have problems falling asleep, keep your eyes open and proceed the same way. Keep a constant focus of your eyes on, say, your shoelaces or a door knob.

When you first meditate, stop after 10 minutes or so. When you stop, slowly open your eyes, stretch your muscles, and get your bearings. Then gradually resume your regular day. You will feel quite relaxed and peaceful. As you become more accustomed to meditating, you can extend the meditations to 15 or 20 minutes, even meditating 2 times a day. Also, during a busy day, you can get a similar effect at, say, a meeting, by focusing on the breath for just a couple breaths, beginning with a deep breath or two.

There is a variation of this technique you can try, called progressive muscular relaxation. After you've begun the breathing meditation, change your focus to your muscles. You are going to tense a specific muscle area of your body for 10 seconds (to feel what tension is like) and then relax it, staying focused on just that small area of your body, to feel what a completely relaxed muscle group feels like. You then move to the next adjacent area. Most people begin by tensing and relaxing one foot, then the calf, the thigh, the buttocks (do the right side first and then the left), the abdomen, the chest, the back, the neck, the shoulders, the arms (right then left), and the face. When you finish this sequence, return to the breathing for a few minutes before you stop.

TABLE 11-5. Journaling Guidelines

When writing a journal, do not simply record what you did during the day. Rather, focus on your emotional reactions to daily events—and how you responded to them. Find out how your thoughts and emotions meshed or did not mesh. Look for patterns over time in your emotional reactions. Many people find the same pattern with patients, friends, and families. Indeed, when working with your emotions by journaling you should look for these connections. Here are some guidelines for your writing.

1. What were the most memorable things that happened to you today? Positive? Negative? What were your emotions and what behavior did the emotion produce?
2. What were the 3 most important things you learned about yourself today? How will you apply this new knowledge?
3. Did you experience any particularly strong emotions or feelings today (positive or negative)? Describe.
4. Describe how one of your emotions led to a behavior that you previously had not been aware of.
5. In what ways would you most like to change your own behavior if you could—have you changed any behaviors in your past? How did that come about?
6. Are there other issues you've become aware of that you would like to change? List them.

4. Following any patient interaction, ask yourself what your emotional reaction was to them and how it affected your own actions—hurried, spent more time than usual, looked at electronic health record more/less than usual, interested/bored, attracted/repulsed?
5. If you are in a group (practice, residency), a tremendous opportunity exists to work on improved emotional awareness—and to develop close collegial relationships. Members meet regularly in so-called Balint Groups—of as few as 2-3 members and as many as 8-10—to discuss their emotions and thoughts about difficult patients. Meeting from weekly to monthly, group members can, over time, help one another to better recognize emotional blind spots and resulting behaviors with patients. Please refer to the literature if you are interested in developing such a group.[29-33]

What do you do when you recognize an emotion that leads to a counterproductive behavior on your part? You simply say to yourself, "I'm feeling (angry, bored, sad, or afraid) and in the past I would have reacted by (forgetting to make a follow-up appointment, working on the electronic chart while the patient talked, changing the topic, or referring the patient). Now that I recognize my (negative reaction), it's up to me to decide if I want to continue to act the same way." Repeatedly acknowledging something one wants to change in their thoughts, feelings, and behaviors often leads to improvement. You are raising it to your full consciousness and making a rational decision what to do. Also, don't forget to NURS yourself. This is not easy and patients are not easy and progress will take time, and it takes courage to look hard at oneself.

You can make striking changes, though, as you get to know yourself better and stretch personally. This work fosters your innate capacity for adult growth and uncovers unexpected strengths and capabilities that can lead to more effective relationships with patients—and others.[34] Most physicians find that they like this process because one of the most exciting outcomes from this work is to gain insight not just into your interactions with patients but also with many others. You will know that personal awareness is worthwhile when your patients—and spouse—make positive comments about the changes they see in you. A comment such as "This was good conversation, I felt you really listening to me" could come from a patient—or a spouse! Improving your emotional intelligence benefits not just the doctor-patient relationship, but all your relationships whether professional or personal.

REFERENCES

1. AHRQ. Provider- and practice-level competencies for integrated behavioral health in primary care—a literature review. Kinman C, Gilchrist E, Payne-Murphy J, Miller BF, eds. Rockville, MD: AHRQ; 2015.
2. Woltmann E, Grogan-Kaylor A, Perron B, Georges H, Kilbourne AM, Bauer MS. Comparative effectiveness of collaborative chronic care models for mental health conditions across primary, specialty, and behavioral health care settings: systematic review and meta-analysis. *Am J Psychiatry*. 2012;169(8):790-804.
3. Goodrich DE, Kilbourne AM, Nord KM, Bauer MS. Mental health collaborative care and its role in primary care settings. *Curr Psychiatry Rep*. 2013;15(8):383.
4. Huffman JC, Niazi SK, Rundell JR, Sharpe M, Katon WJ. Essential articles on collaborative care models for the treatment of psychiatric disorders in medical settings: a publication by the Academy of Psychosomatic Medicine

Research and Evidence-Based Practice Committee. *Psychosomatics.* 2014;55(2):109-122.

5. Butler M, Kane RL, McAlpine D, et al. Does integrated care improve treatment for depression? A systematic review. *J Ambul Care Manage.* 2011;34(2):113-125.

6. McGregor M, Lin EH, Katon WJ. TEAMcare: an integrated multicondition collaborative care program for chronic illnesses and depression. *J Ambul Care Manage.* 2011;34(2):152-162.

7. Richards DA, Hill JJ, Gask L, et al. Clinical effectiveness of collaborative care for depression in UK primary care (CADET): cluster randomised controlled trial. *BMJ.* 2013;347:f4913.

8. Williams M, Angstman K, Johnson I, Katzelnick D. Implementation of a care management model for depression at two primary care clinics. *J Ambul Care Manage.* 2011;34(2):163-173.

9. Wagner EH, Austin BT, Von Korff M. Organizing care for patients with chronic ilness. *Millbank Q.* 1996;74:511-44.

10. Cromp D, Hsu C, Coleman K, et al. Barriers and facilitators to team-based care in the context of primary care transformation. *J Ambul Care Manage.* 2015;38(2):125-133.

11. Kates N, McPherson-Doe C, George L. Integrating mental health services within primary care settings: the Hamilton Family Health Team. *J Ambul Care Manage.* 2011;34(2):174-182.

12. Smith RC. Somatization disorder: defining its role in clinical medicine. *J Gen Intern Med.* 1991;6:168-175.

13. Mental Health America 2018. http://www.mental-healthamerica.net/positions/involuntary-treatment. Accessed May 22, 2018.

14. Quigley DD, Elliott MN, Farley DO, Burkhart Q, Skootsky SA, Hays RD. Specialties differ in which aspects of doctor communication predict overall physician ratings. *J Gen Intern Med.* 2014;29(3):447-454.

15. Kelley JM, Kraft-Todd G, Schapira L, Kossowsky J, Riess H. The influence of the patient-clinician relationship on healthcare outcomes: a systematic review and meta-analysis of randomized controlled trials. *PLoS One.* 2014;9(4):e94207.

16. Correll CU, Carbon M. Efficacy of pharmacologic and psychotherapeutic interventions in psychiatry: to talk or to prescribe: is that the question? *JAMA Psychiatry.* 2014;71(6):624-626.

17. Huhn M, Tardy M, Spineli LM, et al. Efficacy of pharmacotherapy and psychotherapy for adult psychiatric disorders: a systematic overview of meta-analyses. *JAMA Psychiatry.* 2014;71(6):706-715.

18. Greenberg R. The Return of Psychosocial Relevance in a Biochemical Age. The National Register; 2014.

19. Kendell RE. The distinction between personality disorder and mental illness. *Brit J Psychiatry.* 2002;180:110-115.

20. Smith RC, Dwamena FC, Fortin AH VI. Teaching personal awareness. *J Gen Intern Med.* 2005;20:201-207.

21. Marshall AA, Smith RC. Physicians' emotional reactions to patients: recognizing and managing countertransference. *Am J Gastroenterol.* 1995;90:4-8.

22. Smith RC, Zimny G. Physicians' emotional reactions to patients. *Psychosomatics.* 1988;29:392-397.

23. Fortin AH VI, Dwamena F, Frankel R, Lepisto B, Smith R. *Smith's Patient-Centered Interviewing—An Evidence-Based Method.* 4th ed. New York, NY: McGraw-Hill, Lange Series; 2018.

24. Benson H. *The Relaxation Response.* New York, NY: William Morrow and Company; 1975.

25. Epstein RM. Mindful practice. *JAMA.* 1999;282:833-839.

26. Kabat-Zinn J. *Wherever You Go, There You Are: Mindfulness Meditation in Everyday Life.* New York, NY: Hyperion; 1994.

27. Smyth JM. Written emotional expression: effect sizes, outcome types, and moderating variables. *J Consult Clin Psychol.* 1998;66:174-184.

28. Smyth JM, Stone AA, Hurewitz A, Kaell A. Effects of writing about stressful experiences on symptom reduction in patients with asthma or rheumatoid arthritis—a randomized trial. *JAMA.* 1999;281:1304-1309.

29. Balint M. Method and technique in the teaching of medical psychology. II. Training general practitioners in psychotherapy. *Brit J Med Psychol* 1954;27:37-41.

30. Balint M. The Doctor, His Patient, and The Illness. Revised. New York: International Universities Press, Inc.; 1957.

31. Courtenay MJF. A plain doctor's guide to Balint-work. *Journal Balint Society* 1992;20:20-21.

32. Salander P, Sandstrom M. A Balint-inspired reflective forum in oncology for medical residents: Main themes during seven years. *Patient Educ Couns* 2014;97:47-51.

33. Scheingold L. Balint work in England: lessons for American family medicine. *J Fam Prac* 1988;26:315-320.

34. Vaillant GE. *Adaptation to Life.* Boston, MA: Little, Brown and Company; 1977.

Index

Note: Page numbers followed by *f* and *t* indicate figures and tables, respectively.

A

AAP. *See* atypical antipsychotic
A-B-C model. *See* alarm-
    beliefs-coping model
Abilify. *See* aripiprazole
absolute neutrophil count (ANC),
    144
acamprosate, 95*t*, 106
acquired immunodeficiency
    syndrome (AIDS), 135*t*
acute coronary syndrome, 29
acute pain, 92–93
acute stress disorder (ASD), 73
Adderall. *See* dextroamphetamine
Addison's disease, 135*t*
ADHD. *See* attention-deficit/
    hyperactivity disorder
adjustment disorder, 30*t*, 43
adulteration, of urine, 87–88, 87*t*
AIDS. *See* acquired
    immunodeficiency
    syndrome
akathisia, 143
alanine aminotransferase (ALT),
    142
alarm-beliefs-coping model
    (A-B-C model), 60, 69
albuterol, 2*t*
alcohol
    AUDIT in, 103, 104*t*–106*t*
    CAGE questionnaire, 103, 103*t*
    counseling, 23
    misuse of, 101–107, 103*t*–106*t*
    NASH and, 142

Alcohol Use Disorders
    Identification Test (AUDIT),
    103, 104*t*–106*t*
Alcoholics Anonymous, 106
allergy testing, 22
Alliance of States with
    Prescription Monitoring
    Programs, 86
alprazolam, 68, 76, 98, 100,
    100*t*–101*t*
ALT. *See* alanine aminotransferase
Alzheimer dementia, 125–126, 136
American Diabetic Association,
    143
American Psychiatric Association,
    143
amphetamine, 122*t*
amygdala, 59
ANC. *See* absolute neutrophil
    count
anhedonia, 114*t*
anorexia nervosa, 127–129, 128*t*
Antabuse. *See* disulfiram
antidepressants. *See also*
    prescription misuse
    anxiety disorders and, 63–69,
    65*t*–68*t*
    in MHCM, 18, 19*t*, 21–22,
    24–25
    switching of, 40*t*, 41, 68, 68*t*
    TCA, 2, 3*t*, 36, 68, 78
antipsychotic discontinuation
    syndrome, 145
antipsychotic medication

CATIE study, 137, 144
    FGA, 140
    psychotic disorders and,
    141–145, 141*t*
    sexual dysfunction and, 144
    side effects of, 141–143, 141*t*
antisocial personality disorder,
    151*t*, 153–154
anxiety disorders, 3*t*, 8*t*
    ASD and, 73
    background on, 59
    common treatments of, 59–62,
    60*t*
    conclusions on, 78–79
    diagnosis of, 59–62, 60*t*
    GAD and, 62–69, 63*t*–68*t*
    GAD-7 in, 10
    introduction to, 59
    major depressive disorder,
    39
    OCD and, 77–78
    overlap of, 78, 79*t*
    panic disorder and, 69–72,
    70*t*–72*t*
    patient understanding of, 21
    PTSD and, 72–76, 74*t*–76*t*
    SNRI in, 64, 66*t*–68*t*, 67–68,
    71
    social phobia, 76–77
    specific phobias, 77
    SSRI in, 64, 65*t*, 67–68, 67*t*–68*t*,
    71
    switching antidepressants in,
    68, 68*t*